WJ
700
BER

MEDICAL RADIOLOGY
Diagnostic Imaging

Editors:
A. L. Baert, Leuven
M. Knauth, Göttingen
K. Sartor, Heidelberg

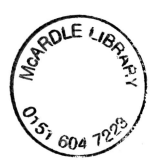

M. Bertolotto (Ed.)

Color Doppler US of the Penis

With Contributions by

C. Acampora · L. Barozzi · A. J. Bella · E. Belgrano · M. Belgrano · S. Benvenuto
W. O. Brant · S. Bucci · M. Coss · M. A. Cova · M. De Matteis · L. E. Derchi
V. Destéfano · M. Djouguela Fute · N. Gandolfo · F. Lacelli · G. Liguori · A. Lissiani
T. F. Lue · P. Martingano · F. Pozzi Mucelli · C. E. Neumaier · G. Ocello · P. Pavlica
N. Perrone · R. Pizzolato · M. Pow-Sang · C. Privitera · D. Sanabor · G. Savoca
L. Scofienza · G. Serafini · A. Spadacci · C. Trombetta · M. Ukmar · M. Valentino
R. Zappetti

Foreword by

A. L. Baert

With 153 Figures in 270 Separate Illustrations, 101 in Color and 4 Tables

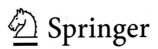

Michele Bertolotto, MD
Department Radiology
University of Trieste
Ospedale di Cattinara
Strada di Fiume 447
Trieste, 34124
Italy

Medical Radiology · Diagnostic Imaging and Radiation Oncology
Series Editors:
A. L. Baert · L. W. Brady · H.-P. Heilmann · M. Knauth · M. Molls · C. Nieder · K. Sartor

Continuation of Handbuch der medizinischen Radiologie
Encyclopedia of Medical Radiology

Library of Congress Control Number: 2007932228

ISBN 978-3-540-36676-8 Springer Berlin Heidelberg New York

This work is subject to copyright. All rights are reserved, whether the whole or part of the material is concerned, specifically the rights of translation, reprinting, reuse of illustrations, recitations, broadcasting, reproduction on microfilm or in any other way, and storage in data banks. Duplication of this publication or parts thereof is permitted only under the provisions of the German Copyright Law of September 9, 1965, in its current version, and permission for use must always be obtained from Springer-Verlag. Violations are liable for prosecution under the German Copyright Law.

Springer is part of Springer Science+Business Media

http//www.springer.com
© Springer-Verlag Berlin Heidelberg 2008
Printed in Germany

The use of general descriptive names, trademarks, etc. in this publication does not imply, even in the absence of a specific statement, that such names are exempt from the relevant protective laws and regulations and therefore free for general use.

Product liability: The publishers cannot guarantee the accuracy of any information about dosage and application contained in this book. In every case the user must check such information by consulting the relevant literature.

Medical Editor: Dr. Ute Heilmann, Heidelberg
Desk Editor: Ursula N. Davis, Heidelberg
Production Editor: Kurt Teichmann, Mauer
Cover-Design and Typesetting: Verlagsservice Teichmann, Mauer

Printed on acid-free paper – 21/3180xq – 5 4 3 2 1 0

To my father (July 13, 1940 – July 1, 2005)

To my wife
Rosaria
and beloved daughters
Noemi and *Sara*

Michele Bertolotto

Foreword

Ultrasound of the penis is a highly performing non-invasive imaging modality, which allows depicting superbly the normal anatomy of penile structures but also the macroscopic pathological changes occurring in various disease entities such as Peyronie's disease and priapism. Ultrasound plays also an important role in the optimal management of traumatic, post surgical and tumoral conditions of the penis and urethra.

In addition, the functional changes in penile blood flow as seen in erectile dysfunction can be studied appropriately with color Doppler ultrasound methods.

This superbly illustrated volume comprehensively covers our latest knowledge and insights on the technical possibilities of penile ultrasound and on its clinical role in relation to other non-invasive imaging modalities, particularly MRI.

I congratulate the editor, M. Bertolotto, and the contributing authors, all internationally recognised experts in the field, for this outstanding, well researched and superbly illustrated book.

I am convinced that this unique volume on a highly actual clinical topic will be of great interest for radiologists in training and for certified radiologists, but also for urologists and specialists in andrology.

I sincerely hope that it will meet the same success as the many other volumes previously published in the series: Medical Radiology – Diagnostic Imaging.

Leuven   ALBERT L. BAERT

Preface

Color Doppler ultrasound is increasingly used in clinical practice by both radiologists and clinicians. The advantages of new machines are particularly evident when imaging superficial structures since submillimetric anatomical details can be investigated and flow in very small vessels can be evaluated in real time without radiation.
Penile sonography, in particular, has gained many benefits from the introduction of new technologies. Improved spatial resolution enables evaluation of virtually all penile pathologies with an accuracy which, with few exceptions, cannot be reached by other, more expensive, imaging modalities.

During the 1990s, color Doppler ultrasound became the major tool for classification of organic causes of impotence. At present, the introduction into clinical practice of effective oral medications has greatly reduced the importance of this examination. However, other important applications of this technique are now emerging. In particular, the possibility to image the tunica albuginea with great anatomical detail opens new preoperative perspectives in evaluating patients with Peyronie's disease, trauma, priapism, and fibrosis.

Only a limited number of sonologists routinely perform penile ultrasound. Moreover, radiologists often have a superficial knowledge of what urologists really need from penile imaging studies, while clinicians often have insufficient knowledge of the diagnostic capabilities offered by latest generation equipment. This is unfortunate, because many patients with penile pathologies that could be successfully investigated and diagnosed with ultrasound usually undergo other, often more invasive, imaging tests or go directly to unnecessary surgery.

It only takes a little bit of effort to understand ultrasound penile anatomy and its changes in pathological conditions, and to appreciate what gray-scale and Doppler evaluation can show.

This book provides a comprehensive reference and practical guide on the technology and application of ultrasound to penile pathologies. For each topic a clinical introduction is provided, followed by a description of the current role of ultrasound and Doppler technique, and by discussion of further diagnostic information offered by other imaging modalities. It is addressed not only to radiologists and urologists primarily involved in urogenital imaging, but also to graduate students, and to all clinicians requiring a reference book for managing penile problems during their everyday clinical work.

The volume is the expression of the efforts of distinguished experts throughout the world. The contributing authors bring a wealth of international experience in penile clinics and imaging. I'm greatly indebted to them for their enthusiastic commitment and support.

Also, I would like to thank most sincerely the Medical Radiology series editor, Professor Albert Baert, for giving me the opportunity to publish this book.
I sincerely hope that the present book fulfills the expectations of our colleagues in their common clinical practice.

Trieste   MICHELE BERTOLOTTO

Contents

1. Instrumentation, Technical Requirements
   Lorenzo E. Derchi 1

2. Penile Anatomy
   Anthony J. Bella, William O. Brant, and Tom F. Lue 11

3. Physiology of Penile Erection and Pathophysiology of Erectile Dysfunction
   Anthony J. Bella, William O. Brant, and Tom F. Lue 15

4. Clinical Evaluation of Erectile Dysfunction in the Era of PDE-5 Inhibitors:
   The Residual Role of Penile Color Doppler US
   Emanuele Belgrano, Stefano Bucci, Giovanni Liguori, and
   Carlo Trombetta. 21

5. US Anatomy of the Penis: Common Findings and Anatomical Variations
   Michele Bertolotto, Andrea Lissiani, Riccardo Pizzolato and
   Micheline Djouguela Fute 25

6. US Evaluation of Erectile Dysfunction
   Pietro Pavlica, Massimo Valentino, and Libero Barozzi 39

7. Peyronie's Disease: Etiology and Treatment
   William O. Brant, Anthony J. Bella, and Tom F. Lue 55

8. US Evaluation of Patients with Peyronie's Disease
   Michele Bertolotto, Matteo Coss, and Carlo E. Neumaier 61

9. Pathophysiology and Treatment of Priapism
   Giovanni Liguori, Stefano Bucci, Sara Benvenuto,
   Carlo Trombetta, and Emanuele Belgrano 71

10. Imaging Priapism: The Diagnostic Role of Color Doppler US
    Michele Bertolotto, Fabio Pozzi Mucelli, Giovanni Liguori,
    and Daniela Sanabor 79

11. Penile Injuries: Mechanism, Presentation and Management
    Gianfranco Savoca 89

12. US Evaluation of Patients with Penile Traumas
    Michele Bertolotto, Carmelo Privitera, and Ciro Acampora 95

13. Penile Tumors: Classification, Clinics and Current Therapeutic Approach
    Mariela Pow-Sang and Victor Destefano 107

14 Penile Tumors: US Features
   Giovanni Serafini, Michele Bertolotto, Luca Scofienza,
   Francesca Lacelli, and Nicoletta Gandolfo 115

15 Surgical Treatment of Penile Disease: Current Indications
   Giovanni Liguori, Giuseppe Ocello, Stefano Bucci, Carlo Trombetta,
   and Emanuele Belgrano 125

16 US of the Postoperative Penis
   Michele Bertolotto, Paola Martingano, Andrea Spadacci,
   and Maria Assunta Cova 133

17 Penile Inflammation
   Giovanni Serafini, Michele Bertolotto, Francesca Lacelli,
   Luca Scofienza, and Nadia Perrone 147

18 Penile Scar and Fibrosis
   Michele Bertolotto, Paola Martingano, and Maja Ukmar 153

19 US Imaging of the Male Urethra
   Libero Barozzi, Pietro Pavlica, Massimo Valentino, and
   Massimo De Matteis 163

20 Miscellaneous Benign Diseases
   Michele Bertolotto, Pietro Pavlica, and Manuel Belgrano 175

21 Contrast-Enhanced US of the Penis
   Michele Bertolotto, Stefano Bucci, and Roberta Zappetti 183

   Subject Index 193

   List of Contributors 197

Instrumentation and Technical Requirements

Lorenzo E. Derchi

CONTENTS

1.1 Advances in Ultrasound Technology 1
1.2 Broadband Transducers 1
1.3 Coded Transmission 2
1.4 Multiple-Frequency and Wideband Imaging 4
1.5 Focusing 4
1.6 Transducer Selection and Handling 4
1.7 New Imaging Modalities 5
1.7.1 Advances in Doppler Imaging 5
1.7.2 Spatial Compounding 5
1.7.3 Frequency Compounding 6
1.8 Image Equalization Algorithms 6
1.9 Adaptive Filtering 7
1.10 Extended Field of View 7
1.11 Three-Dimensional (3D) Rendering 8
1.12 Three-Dimensional (3D) Imaging 8
1.13 Contrast-Specific Modes 9
References 9

L. E. Derchi
Professor and Chairman, Department of Radiology, DICMI University of Genova, Ospedale S. Martino, Largo Rosanna Benzi 8, Genova, 16132, Italy

1.1 Advances in Ultrasound Technology

The latest generation of beam-forming technologies and use of new broadband high-frequency probes have improved significantly the quality of ultrasound imaging, particularly in the examination of superficial structures. Penile sonography, in particular, has gained many benefits from the introduction of these new technologies. Improved spatial resolution allows evaluating normal and pathological structures generally of less than 1 mm with excellent detail, and increased color Doppler sensitivity for low flows allows full evaluation of the penile vasculature. Using higher frequency transducers with increased bandwidth and tissue penetration, in particular, has significantly increased the possibility of evaluating the tunica albuginea and its pathological changes in detail.

This chapter will review the main advances in ultrasound technology and address the clinical impact they have had or are likely to have in the future in imaging penile disease.

1.2 Broadband Transducers

The transducer is an essential element of ultrasound equipment, responsible for the generation of an ultrasound beam and the detection of returning echoes. It greatly influences spatial resolution, penetration and signal-to-noise ratio. In recent years, research in transducer technology has been focused on the development of piezoelectric elements with lower acoustic impedances and greater electromechanical coupling coefficients, as well as on improving the characteristics of absorbing backing layers and quarter-wave impedance matching layers (Claudon et al. 2002).

Currently, transducer arrays are formed by ceramic polymer composite elements. A variety of technical solutions have been applied to improve their mechanical characteristics. In particular, piano-concave elements can be used to provide a uniform elevation plane radiation pattern both in the near and in the far field (JEDRZEJEWICZ 1999). Similar results have been obtained producing multi-layered piezoelectric elements (WHITTINGHAM 1999b) or shaping the elements in other suitable ways. These refinements led to the use of very short pulses, increased bandwidth and better intrinsic collimation of the ultrasound beam (Fig. 1.1).

Capacitive micromachined ultrasonic transducers (CMUT) are now in an advanced state of development. Well-functioning prototypes have been produced, and commercially available probes based on this innovative technology will be soon commercially available. CMUTs have the potential to outperform conventional piezoelectric transducers in terms of bandwidth, sensitivity and electro-mechanical coupling efficiency (ORALKAN et al. 2002). The possibility to integrate both the CMUT transducer and the controlling electronics on a single silicon chip, reducing noise, interconnecting complexity and cost, appears very promising.

1.3
Coded Transmission

The issue of maximizing penetration depth retaining or enhancing spatial resolution constitutes one of the major challenges in ultrasound imaging. One of the original objectives in designing broadband transducers was to improve axial resolution without changing the emission frequency; in fact, the shorter the transmission pulses used in a broadband emission, the better and more faithfully the conversion into electric signals can be obtained (WHITTINGHAM 1999a). In principle, however, short pulses suffer attenuation to a greater extent and are characterized by less penetration than long pulses.

The simplest way to increase penetration of short pulses is to increase the acoustic power of the ultrasound beam, because signal from deeper tissue regions can be recorded over the noise threshold. However, concerns about potential and undesirable side effects, in particular related to acoustic cavitation, set limits on the possibility of overcoming the frequency-dependent attenuation by increasing peak acoustic amplitudes of the waves probing the tissue. Moreover, low amplitudes are mandatory

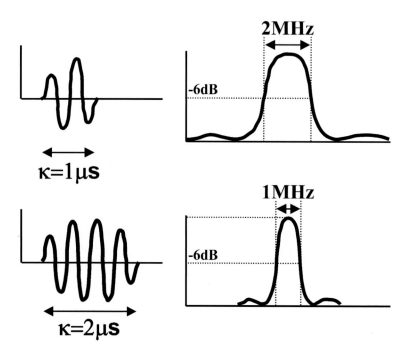

Fig. 1.1. Relationship between spatial pulse length and frequency spectrum. Intensity versus time diagrams (*left illustrations*) illustrate two pulses with different length κ of 1 μs and 2 μs, respectively, and the corresponding spectrum of frequency of 2 MHz and 1 MHz, respectively. The longer pulse (2 μs) generates a narrower bandwidth (1 MHz). (The bandwidth is measured between the 6 dB points of each side of the spectrum)

when pulses for contrast-specific non-destructive modes are designed, in order to limit microbubble destruction.

A substantial effort has been made by the different manufacturers of ultrasound machines to overcome limitations of peak acoustic amplitude by using long wideband transmitting sequences and compression techniques on the receiver side. Basically all use coded transmitted signals and employ correlation and averaging of the echoes on reception (Fig. 1.2).

Coded transmission offers two major advantages over conventional ultrasound beam forming. Coded pulses can be readily recognized from random noise, and pulses with increased average power can be driven within the tissue without increasing the peak acoustic amplitude. As a consequence, a significant improvement of the signal-to-noise ratio is obtained, and frequency-dependent attenuation is reduced. Higher ultrasound frequencies can be used for ultrasound imaging both with abdominal and small-part applications, enclosing penile imaging (Fig. 1.3) leading to increased spatial and contrast resolution (NOWICKI et al. 2004).

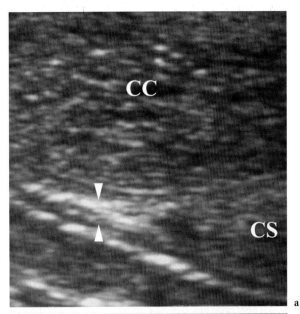

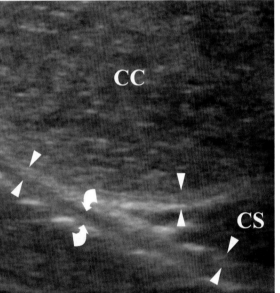

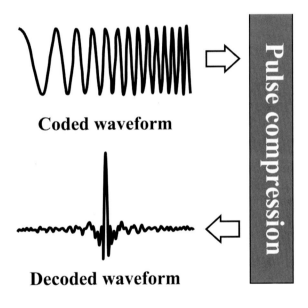

Fig. 1.2. Illustration of coding principle. A broadband coherent code is used to drive a temporally extended pulse. The received signal is decoded to produce an imaging pulse that is characterized by improved signal-to-noise ratio, resulting from the increased bandwidth and higher average power in the elongated excitation. The pressure peak driven within the tissue with the coded pulse is lower than that of the decoded imaging pulse, resulting in a reduced risk of biological effects

Fig. 1.3a,b. Advantages in ultrasound technology. Axial scan of the same portion of a penile shaft obtained using two transducers with different bandwidth and different beam-forming technologies. **a** Using a 5-12-MHz transducer (L12-5, HDI500, Philips), the tunica albuginea (*arrowheads*) of the right corpus cavernosum (*CC*) can be recognized. **b** A much better resolution is obtained using a transducer with wider bandwidth and coded transmission (L17-5, iU22, Philips), which allows better evaluation of the tunica albuginea of the right corpus cavernosum and of the corpus spongiosum (*CS*). Also the Buck's fascia is recognized as a separate layer (*curved arrows*)

1.4
Multiple-Frequency and Wideband Imaging

In broadband transducers the high-frequency components of the spectrum tend to increase the intensity of the ultrasound beam in the most superficial regions and in the focal zone, whereas the low-frequency components extend the penetration depth (WHITTINGHAM 1999a). In multiple-frequency imaging, the available broad bandwidth is subdivided into multiple frequency steps for transmission and reception of sound waves: these transducers enable selection of the optimal frequency range in a given scanning plane as though two or more independent transducers, each with a different center frequency, were available (Fig. 1.4).

Other systems use the entire transducer bandwidth for the transmitted pulse and then adjust the receiver bandwidth to lower frequencies as deeper depths are sampled. These systems give increased flexibility to the ultrasound examination, enabling the same transducer to change the image acquisition parameters during scanning based on the desired clinical information.

1.5
Focusing

Reducing the width and thickness of the ultrasound beam has definite advantages in terms of contrast and spatial resolution. In modern linear-array transducers focusing is produced electronically by activating a series of elements in the array with appropriate delays, so that the trigger pulses to the inner elements are delayed with respect to the pulses to the outer ones. In this way a curved wavefront results from constructive interference bringing the ultrasound beam toward a focus. By adjusting the values of the delays applied to the trigger pulses, the curvature of the wavefront and, therefore, the focal depth can be changed dynamically.

An important factor influencing the lateral resolving power of the system is the dynamic aperture: this is achieved by activating variable numbers of elements dynamically to optimize focusing at many depths.

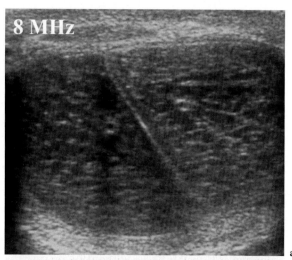
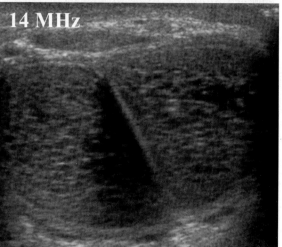

Fig. 1.4a,b. Multiple-frequency transducers. **a,b** Axial images of the penile shaft obtained with an 8–5 MHz multiple frequency transducer (15L8, Sequoia, Siemens) by setting the center frequency at **a** 8 MHz and **b** 14 MHz, respectively. Shifting the frequency band upward, a more defined echotexture is appreciated as a result of an increased resolution

1.6
Transducer Selection and Handling

A variety of linear-array transducers is currently available in the frequency range used for penile imaging. Selection of the most appropriate transducer primarily depends on the frequency, but is also related to other factors. Compared with small transducers, for instance, larger probes tend to have a large near-field beam width leading to a poor lateral resolution at shallow depths.

During penile ultrasound examination probe handling requires maximum stability over the region of interest; compression is not required, and the mobility of the probe to cover the entire shaft is considerably less than in other studies. Because pathologic findings may be very small in size and are evaluated by placing the probe over a curvilinear surface, stability of the transducer is a key factor for high-quality examinations. In our experience, the best grip to obtain probe stability can be obtained by placing the ulnar fingers (long, ring, little) directly on the patient's skin while holding the probe with the radial fingers (so that the probe hangs between the thumb and the index finger). This grip allows easy translation of the probe along its short axis at a given angle minimizing rotational changes.

1.7
New Imaging Modalities

Recent technologic innovations in ultrasound have resulted in improved diagnostic performance for the evaluation of superficial structures. Some of them have a role for penile imaging as well, in particular, wideband Doppler imaging and spatial compounding. Other innovations such as extended field-of-view and 3D rendering or reconstruction can be useful in selected cases.

1.7.1
Advances in Doppler Imaging

The introduction of broadband Doppler technology has led to some advantages in imaging small penile vessels such as collaterals of the cavernosal arteries. Unlike conventional Doppler systems broadband Doppler technology makes use of short pulses to obtain wideband transmission. This creates a significant improvement in the frame rate and axial resolution. Using broadband Doppler technology a more defined display of all penile vessels is obtained, as a consequence of increased spatial resolution of color signal, with limited color "over-writing" on gray-scale structures. Also Doppler sensitivity increases, and temporal resolution improves. Appropriate waveform shaping and coded transmission ensure penetration of a wider band of frequencies and limits signal attenuation with depth.

1.7.2
Spatial Compounding

Careful evaluation of the normal tunica albuginea and of its changes is essential in virtually all penile pathologies. Major problems exist, however, to accomplish this task because of a series of artifacts produced by the ultrasound beam, such as specular reflection artifacts, speckle and shadowing.

Specular reflections produce discontinuities of curved interfaces, such as the tunica albuginea, which appear echogenic only when insonated at perpendicular angles. Speckle results from interference of the coherent waves produced by the elements of the transducer. It appears as subtle brightness fluctuations and small discontinuities of reflecting interfaces such as the tunica albuginea and large calcifications. Shadowing from attenuation of the penile septum reduces visibility of the dorsal aspect of the tunica albuginea, where Peyronie's plaques are more often recognized.

Spatial compound imaging is highly effective to overcome these limitations. This relatively new technique allows combining echoes obtained from ultrasound beams oriented along different directions. Electronic steering is used to image the same tissue multiple times from different directions; then the echoes from these multiple acquisitions are averaged together into a single composite image (ENTREKIN et al. 2001; HANGIANDREOU 2003). Spatial compounding is possible in real-time, although the frame rate is slightly lower than that of conventional imaging.

When imaging the penis spatial compounding improves image quality in different ways. Since a synthetic image is obtained from frames collected at different angles, larger portions of curved interfaces are insonated perpendicularly, and specular reflection artifacts are reduced. This is particularly evident when imaging the tunica albuginea. Moreover, several images (up to nine) are averaged to obtain the compound image resulting in improved signal-to-noise ratio compared with the single frames.

Since speckle artifacts depend on the direction of the ultrasound beam, frames obtained from different view angles have different speckle patterns, which average out when combined in the compound image.

Finally, acoustic shadowing is less evident in the compound image, concentrated behind the attenuating structures. As a consequence, in penile imaging visualization of the dorsal aspect of the tunica albuginea is improved (Fig. 1.5).

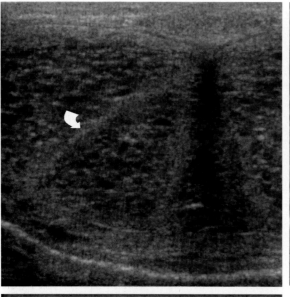
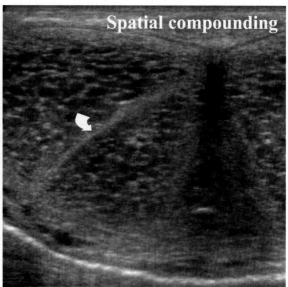
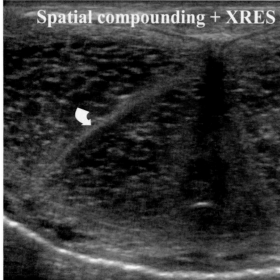

Fig. 1.5a–c. Advantages of spatial compounding and adaptive filtering on image quality. Axial scan of the same penis obtained with the same transducer (L17-5, iU22, Philips). a Conventional grey-scale image showing an intracavernosal pillar (*curved arrow*). b Spatial compounding. Visualization of the pillar and of the sinusoidal spaces improves significantly as a consequence of increased signal-to-noise ratio and reduced speckle artifacts. c Spatial compounding associated with XRES. Visualization of the pillars and of the sinusoidal spaces improves further

1.7.3 Frequency Compounding

Since speckle depends also on the frequency of the ultrasound beam, imaging modalities have been developed that use simultaneous emission of two different bands of frequencies instead of one to decorrelate speckle and improve the signal-to-noise ratio (OKTAR et al. 2003). Some equipment allows for simultaneous use of both spatial and frequency compounding.

1.8 Image Equalization Algorithms

There is a variety of post-equalization algorithm processing modalities that have been developed to make ultrasound images more uniform. Digital imaging optimization (Toshiba), for instance, automatic tissue optimization (GE), iSCAN (Philips), and TEQ (Siemens) provide automatic equalization of images in real time. Other algorithms such as iFOCUS (Philips) are available to automatically control focusing.

1.9
Adaptive Filtering

Real-time image-processing algorithms can be introduced to refine the ultrasound images by emphasizing patterns within the tissue texture and de-emphasizing artifacts and noise. XRES processing (Philips) is one of the latest commercially available algorithms involving adaptive image analysis and enhancement techniques. XRES is designed both to suppress artifacts and to enhance interfaces and margins. Image processing is adapted automatically to the nature of the target. During an analysis phase both real tissue structures and ultrasound artifacts are identified, while in the following enhancement phase the structures are enhanced and the artifacts suppressed. Filters applied during the enhancement phase depend on the characteristics of the images and on their changes over time from image to image. Smoothing, for instance, is applied along an interface to improve continuity, whereas edge enhancement is applied in the perpendicular direction to improve spatial resolution. Smoothing is applied equally in all directions to suppress speckle and noise in regions containing minimal structure or texture.

Preliminary clinical studies have shown that XRES is effective to improve delineation of borders and tissue contrast on images and to reduce the amount of noise without degradation of diagnostic informative contents of images (MEUWLY et al. 2003). As regards penile imaging, depiction of the tunica albuginea and of subtle anatomical features such as boundaries of the sinusoidal spaces and intracavernous pillars is improved (Fig. 1.5).

1.10
Extended Field of View

Ultrasound images have a field of view that is limited by the probe width. During the study, the examiner moves the probe over the area of interest to acquire information on large volumes of tissue and reconstructs in his/her mind the spatial relationships within the scanned area by memorizing many frames (WENG et al. 1997). This is a distinct disadvantage of ultrasound compared to other imaging methods and is a major drawback in conveying the information of the study to clinicians. The extended field-of-view technique has been developed to overcome these limitations. It allows the reconstruction of wide images by progressive addition of data during a hand sweep in real time with a conventional probe (Fig. 1.6).

As regards penile imaging, extended-field acquisition can be useful especially to depict anatomical variations, in trauma patients to depict large hematomas and in patients with severe Peyronie's disease to improve evaluation of plaque extension and provide the urologist with a panoramic view of the albugineal involvement.

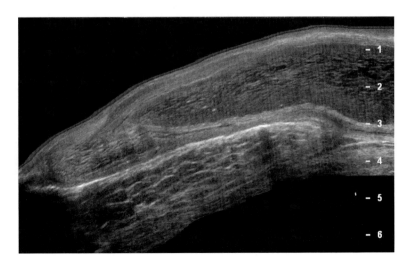

Fig. 1.6. Extended field of view. Panoramic image obtained with a conventional transducer (L17-5, iU22, Philips) showing a large portion of the penile shaft

1.11
Three-Dimensional (3D) Rendering

Software programs for 3D rendering are now available in many scanners, involving capture of a series of sequential power Doppler images while the transducer is translated manually without the necessity for specific hardware (BRANDL et al. 1999). Only spatial rendering of the penile vasculature is obtained with this method; true 3D reconstructions cannot be achieved because effective movements of the transducer are not recorded. Since no external spatial references are present and the reconstruction software assumes that the probe has moved with continuous and uniform translation, scanning must be carried out with extreme accuracy. Variations in translation speed and rotations result in deformed vascular map. Dynamic motion filters, higher wall filters and lower power gain should be used to reduce tissue artifacts and improve 3D rendering (BERTOLOTTO and NEUMAIER 1999).

Although some inaccuracies occur if the motion is not uniform, the complex vascular anatomy of the penis can be better understood using 3D reconstructions (Fig. 1.7). In particular, 3D rendering allows better depiction of helicine arteries and their branches both in normal and in pathological conditions (MONTORSI et al. 1998; SARTESCHI et al. 1998).

1.12
Three-Dimensional (3D) Imaging

The improvement in fast digital computer processing and memory storage capacity has recently improved the possibility of applying 3D technology to ultrasound (CLAUDON et al. 2002). Three-dimensional acquisition can be achieved using either 2D conventional transducers equipped with a small electromagnetic positional sensor or dedicated transducers. Following volume scan acquisition, the monitor displays reconstructed slices according to longitudinal, transverse and coronal planes (Fig. 1.8). Each plane can be oriented within the volume block for detailed analysis by parallel or rotational shifting around any of the three spatial axes. Data can also be displayed as true 3D images using various rendering algorithms, including maximum intensity projection (MIP), transparent, surface and Doppler rendering (BRANDL et al. 1999). Recently, volume transducers in the frequency range suitable for evaluation of the penis have been introduced, opening new interesting perspectives for evaluation of patients with penile malformation, traumas and severe Peyronie's disease.

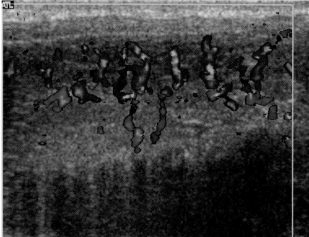
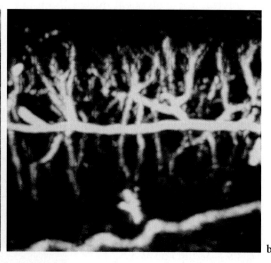

Fig. 1.7a,b. Three-dimensional (3D) rendering. **a** Sagittal color Doppler image showing the helicine arterioles branching from the cavernosal artery. **b** 3D rendering of the penile vasculature obtained from a sequential series of sagittal power Doppler images while the transducer is translated manually along the shaft. An excellent depiction of the cavernosal artery and of the helicine arterioles is obtained up to the more distal branches

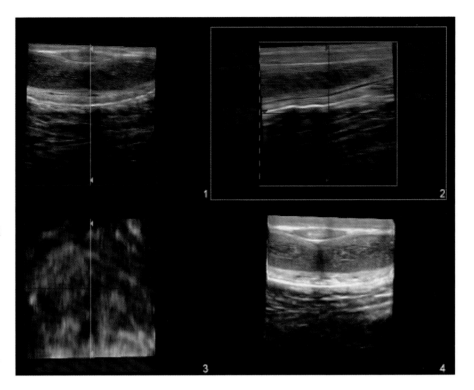

Fig. 1.8. Three-dimensional (3D) imaging. 3D volume acquisition over the penile shaft. Conventional ultrasound scan (*upper-left image*) reveals an axial view of the corpora cavernosa and of the corpus spongiosum. From the 3D data set reconstructed sagittal (*upper right*), coronal (*lower left*) and MIP (*lower right*) images can be obtained

1.13
Contrast-Specific Modes

As illustrated in Chapter 21, high-performance contrast-specific modes are now available to image superficial structures as well. While relatively low insonation frequencies of approximately 4–5 MHz have been initially used in small-part probes to collect signal from a larger percent of resonating bubbles, transducers operating with frequencies of 7 MHz or higher are now available for clinical use (COSGROVE 2004).

References

Bertolotto M, Neumaier CE (1999) Penile sonography. Eur Radiol 9 [Suppl 3]:S407–412

Brandl H, Gritzky A, Haizinger M (1999) 3D ultrasound: a dedicated system. Eur Radiol 9 [Suppl 3]:S331–333

Claudon M, Tranquart F, Evans DH et al (2002) Advances in ultrasound. Eur Radiol 12:7–18

Cosgrove D (2004) Future prospects for SonoVue and CPS. Eur Radiol 14 [Suppl 8]:P116–124

Entrekin RR, Porter BA, Sillesen HH et al (2001) Real-time spatial compound imaging: application to breast, vascular, and musculoskeletal ultrasound. Semin Ultrasound CT MR 22:50–64

Hangiandreou NJ (2003) AAPM/RSNA physics tutorial for residents. Topics in US: B-mode US: basic concepts and new technology. Radiographics 23:1019–1033

Jedrzejewicz T (1999) System architecture for various image reconstruction and processing techniques. Eur Radiol 9 [Suppl 3]:S334–337

Meuwly JY, Thiran JP, Gudinchet F (2003) Application of adaptive image processing technique to real-time spatial compound ultrasound imaging improves image quality. Invest Radiol 38:257–262

Montorsi F, Sarteschi M, Maga T et al (1998) Functional anatomy of cavernous helicine arterioles in potent subjects. J Urol 159:808–810

Nowicki A, Secomski W, Trots I, Litniewski J (2004) Extending penetration depth using coded ultrasonography. Bull Pol Ac Tech 52:215–220

Oktar SO, Yucel C, Ozdemir H et al (2003) Comparison of conventional sonography, real-time compound sonography, tissue harmonic sonography, and tissue harmonic compound sonography of abdominal and pelvic lesions. AJR Am J Roentgenol 181:1341–1347

Oralkan O, Ergun AS, Johnson JA et al (2002) Capacitive micromachined ultrasonic transducers: next-generation arrays for acoustic imaging? IEEE Trans Ultrason Ferroelectr Freq Control 49:1596–1610

Sarteschi LM, Montorsi F, Fabris FM et al (1998) Cavernous arterial and arteriolar circulation in patients with erectile dysfunction: a power Doppler study. J Urol 159:428–432

Weng L, Tirumalai AP, Lowery CM et al (1997) US extended-field-of-view imaging technology. Radiology 203:877–880

Whittingham TA (1999a) Broadband transducers. Eur Radiol 9 [Suppl 3]:S298-303

Whittingham TA (1999b) An overview of digital technology in ultrasonic imaging. Eur Radiol 9 [Suppl 3]:S307–311

Penile Anatomy

Anthony J. Bella, William O. Brant, and Tom F. Lue

CONTENTS

2.1 Skin and Fascia 11
2.2 Tunica Albuginea 11
2.3 Corpora Cavernosa 12
2.4 Associated Musculature 12
2.5 Vascular Anatomy 12
2.6 Lymphatics 14
2.7 Innervation 14
 References 14

2.1 Skin and Fascia

The penis is essentially a tripartite structure, with bilateral corpora cavernosa and the midline ventral corpus spongiosum/glans, all three of which are surrounded by loose subcutaneous tissue and skin that can be moved freely over the erect organ (Fig. 2.1).

The corpora cavernosa function as the main erectile bodies, while the corpus spongiosum contains the urethra. The length of the penis is highly variable, especially in the flaccid state, since it is dependent on the degree of contraction of the cavernosal smooth muscle tissue. There is considerably less variation in length of the fully erect penis, with one study demonstrating a good correspondence between erect length and stretched penile length, as measured from the pubopenile junction to the meatus (Wessells et al. 1996). This length was found to be an average of 12.4 cm. Penile skin is continuous with that of the lower abdominal wall and continues over the glans penis; there it folds back on itself and attaches at the coronal sulcus. The folded portion is known as the prepuce.

There are two fascial layers. The more superficial is the dartos fascia, continuous with Scarpa's fascia of the abdomen. It continues caudally as the dartos fascial layer of the scrotum and Colles' fascia in the perineum. The deeper fascial layer is Buck's fascia, which covers the corpora cavernosa and the corpus spongiosum in separate compartments, including coverage of the deep dorsal vein as well as the dorsal neurovascular bundles. Buck's fascia attaches to the perineal membrane proximally and to the coronal sulcus distally, where it fuses with the tips of the corpora. The fundiform and suspensory ligaments attach to the pubic symphysis and Buck's fascia, and allow the erect penis to achieve a horizontal or greater angle.

2.2 Tunica Albuginea

The corpora are surrounded by tunica albuginea, a strong structure of heterogenous thickness and anatomy, the purpose of which is to both provide rigidity of the erectile bodies as well as to function in the venoocclusive mechanism.

The tunica albuginea consists of two layers, the outer of which is oriented longitudinally and the inner layer consisting of circular fibers. The inner layer contains struts that course the cavernosal space and

A. J. Bella, MD, FRCS(C)
Department of Surgery and Associate Scientist (Neuroscience), University of Ottawa, The Ottawa Hospital, 1053 Carling Avenue, Ottawa, K1Y 4E9, Canada
W. O. Brant, MD
PO Box 40,000, Vail, CO 81658, USA
T. F. Lue, MD
400 Parnassus Ave, A633, San Francisco, CA 94143-0738, USA

serve to augment the support provided by the intracavernosal septum. The corpus spongiosum lacks both the outer layer as well as the struts.

There is variability in albugineal thickness and strength in various locations. Thickness ranges from approximately 0.8 mm at the 5:00 and 7:00 position (just lateral to the corpus spongiosum) to 2.2 mm at the 1:00 and 11:00 positions (Hsu et al. 1994).

2.3 Corpora Cavernosa

The paired corpora cavernosa originate separately underneath the ischiopubic rami, then merge as they pass under the pubic arch. The septum between them is incomplete in humans, although complete in some other species. They are supported by several fibrous structures, including the surrounding tunica albuginea, the intracavernous struts radiating from the inner layer of tunica albuginea, and perineural/periarterial fibrous sheaths.

The spongy inner portion of the corpora consists mainly of interconnected sinusoids separated by smooth muscle trabeculae, which are surrounded by collagen and elastic fibers. These sinusoids are larger centrally and smaller towards the periphery. The corpus spongiosum and its distal termination in the glans penis are similar in internal structure to the corpora cavernosa except that the sinusoids are larger, and there is a lack of outer layer of tunica albuginea that is absent in the glans.

2.4 Associated Musculature

The bulbospongiosal muscle originates at the central perineal tendon, covers the urethral bulb and corpus spongiosum, and inserts into the midline. The paired ischiocavernosus muscles originate from the ischial tuberosisty, cover the proximal corpora, and insert into the inferiomedial surface of the corpora.

2.5 Vascular Anatomy

The main source of blood supply to the penis (Fig. 2.2a) is usually through the internal pudendal artery, a branch of the internal iliac artery. In many instances, however, accessory arteries arise from the external iliac, obturator, vesical, and/or femoral arteries, and may occasionally become the dominant or only arterial supply to the corpus cavernosum (Breza et al. 1989). Damage to these accessory arteries during radical prostatectomy or cystectomy may result in vasculogenic erectile dysfunction (ED) after surgery (Aboseif et al. 1994; Kim et al. 1994).

The internal pudendal artery becomes the common penile artery after giving off a branch to the perineum. The three branches of the penile artery are the dorsal, bulbourethral, and cavernous arteries. The cavernous artery is responsible for tumescence

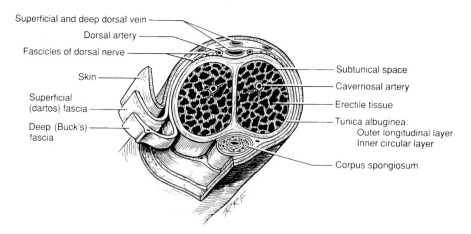

Fig. 2.1. Cross-sectional anatomy of the penis. Used with permission from the American Urological Association from AUA Update Series, vol 13, lesson 2, 1994

of the corpus cavernosum and the dorsal artery for engorgement of the glans penis during erection. The bulbourethral artery supplies the bulb and corpus spongiosum. The cavernous artery enters the corpus cavernosum at the hilum of the penis, where the two crura merge. Distally, the three branches join to form a vascular ring near the glans. Along its course, the cavernous artery gives off many helicine arteries, which supply the trabecular erectile tissue and the sinusoids. These helicine arteries are contracted and tortuous in the flaccid state and become dilated and straight during erection.

The venous drainage from the three corpora (Fig. 2.2b,c) originates in tiny venules leading from the peripheral sinusoids immediately beneath the tunica albuginea. These venules travel in the trabeculae between the tunica and the peripheral sinusoids to form the subtunical venular plexus before exiting as the emissary veins.

Outside the tunica albuginea the skin and subcutaneous tissue drain through multiple superficial veins that run subcutaneously and unite near the root of the penis to form a single (or paired) superficial dorsal vein, which in turn drains into the saphenous veins. Occasionally, the superficial dorsal vein may also drain a portion of the corpora cavernosa.

In the pendulous penis, emissary veins from the corpus cavernosum and spongiosum drain dorsally to the deep dorsal, laterally to the circumflex, and ventrally to the periurethral veins. Beginning at the coronal sulcus, the prominent deep dorsal vein is the main venous drainage of the glans penis, corpus spongiosum, and distal two thirds of the corpora cavernosa. Usually, a single vein, but sometimes more than one deep dorsal vein, runs upward behind the symphysis pubis to join the periprostatic venous plexus.

Emissary veins from the infrapubic penis drain the proximal corpora cavernosa and join to form cavernous and crural veins. These veins join the periurethral veins from the urethral bulb to form the internal pudendal veins.

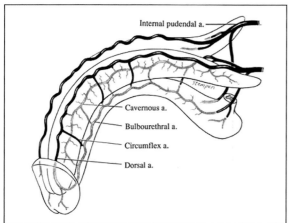

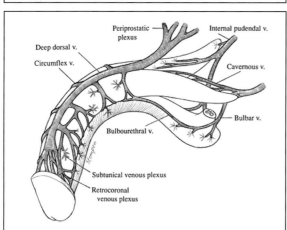

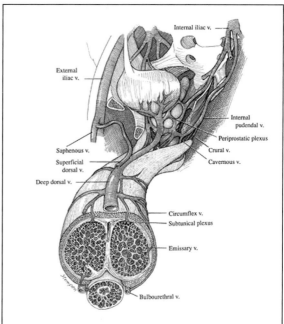

Fig. 2.2a–c. Arterial (a) and venous (b,c) anatomy of the penis. Used with permission of Male sexual function, 2nd edn, ed. Mulcahy (Humana, New Jersey, 2006)

2.6
Lymphatics

Lymphatics of the prepuce and penile shaft converge dorsally, and then drain into both right- and left-sided superficial inguinal lymph nodes via channels alongside superficial external pudendal vessels. Lymphatics of the glans and penile urethra pass deep to Buck's fascia and drain into both superficial and deep inguinal nodes.

2.7
Innervation

The penis is supplied by both somatic and autonomic nerves. The somatic dorsal nerves provide sensory innervation (as well as provide some degree of autonomic function) for the penile skin and glans, and approximately follow the course of the dorsal penile arteries, eventually becoming the pudendal nerve (after joining with other nerves) and entering the spinal cord via S2–4 nerve roots. Sympathetic autonomic fibers derive from the hypogastric plexus and join parasympathetic autonomic fibers from S2–4 in the pelvic plexus. Cavernous nerves represent the penile branches of the pelvic plexus that ramify once piercing the corporal bodies, and thus contain both sympathetic and parasympathetic fibers.

References

Aboseif S, Shinohara K, Breza J et al (1994) Role of penile vascular injury in erectile dysfunction after radical prostatectomy. Br J Urol 73:75–82

Breza J, Aboseif SR, Orvis BR et al (1989) Detailed anatomy of penile neurovascular structures: surgical significance. J Urol 141:437–443

Hsu GL, Brock G, Martinez-Pineiro L et al (1994) Anatomy and strength of the tunica albuginea: its relevance to penile prosthesis extrusion. J Urol 151:1205–1208

Kim ED, Blackburn D, McVary KT (1994) Post-radical prostatectomy penile blood flow: assessment with color flow Doppler ultrasound. J Urol 152:2276–2279

Wessells H, Lue TF, McAninch JW (1996) Penile length in the flaccid and erect states: guidelines for penile augmentation. J Urol 156:995–997

Physiology of Penile Erection and Pathophysiology of Erectile Dysfunction

Anthony J. Bella, William O. Brant, and Tom F. Lue

CONTENTS

3.1 Physiology of Erection 15
3.1.1 Vascular Events 15
3.1.2 Nervous Events 15
3.2 Classification and Epidemiology 16
3.3 Pathophysiology 17
References 19

3.1 Physiology of Erection

Penile erection is primarily a neurovascular event modulated by psychological and hormonal status. Sexual stimulation causes a release of neurotransmitters from the cavernous nerve terminals and relaxing factors from the endothelial cells in the penis, resulting in relaxation of smooth muscle in the arteries and arterioles supplying the erectile tissue.

3.1.1 Vascular Events

As discussed in Chapter 2, a several-fold increase in blood flow occurs with a concomitant increase in compliance of the sinusoids from relaxed cavernous smooth muscle, facilitating rapid filling and expansion of the sinusoidal system against the tunica albuginea. The subtunical venular plexuses are thus compressed between the trabeculae and the tunica albuginea, resulting in almost complete occlusion of venous outflow (Fournier et al. 1987; Banya et al. 1989). Blood is trapped within the corpora cavernosa, which raises the flaccid penis to an erect state. Intracavernous pressures are increased to approximately 100 mmHg (the full erection phase).

During sexual activity, the bulbocavernosus reflex is triggered, thus causing the ischiocavernosus muscles to forcefully compress the base of the blood-filled corpora cavernosa and the penis. The penis becomes very rigid, with an intracavernous pressure reaching several hundred mmHg (the rigid erection phase). During this phase, inflow and outflow temporarily cease. Detumescence can be the result of three separate activities: sympathetic discharge during ejaculation, breakdown of second messengers by phosphodiesterases, or cessation of erectile neurotransmitter release. The venous channels open with contraction of the trabecular smooth muscle, therefore expelling the trapped blood and restoring flaccidity.

3.1.2 Nervous Events

The penis is innervated by autonomic and somatic nerves. The somatic component is controlled by the pudendal nerve, which is responsible for penile sensation and the contraction and relaxation of the bulbocavernosus and ischiocavernosus striated muscles. Blood flow during erection and detumescence is regulated via the cavernous nerves, consisting of sympathetic and parasympathetic nerve fibers, which merge to form these nerves in the pelvis.

The principal neurotransmitter for penile erection is nitric oxide, which is released from nonad-

---

A. J. Bella, MD, FRCS(C)
Department of Surgery and Associate Scientist (Neuroscience), University of Ottawa, The Ottawa Hospital, 1053 Carling Avenue, Ottawa, K1Y 4E9, Canada
W. O. Brant, MD
PO Box 40,000, Vail, CO 81658, USA
T. F. Lue, MD
400 Parnassus Ave, A633, San Francisco, CA 94143-0738, USA

renergic-noncholinergic neurotransmission of the cavernous nerves and the endothelium (LUE 2000). Nitric oxide activates soluble guanylyl cyclase raising intracellular concentrations of cyclic guanosine monophosphate (cGMP). cGMP in turn activates a cGMP-specific protein kinase, which phosphorylates certain proteins and ion channels, resulting in opening of the potassium channels and hyperpolarization, sequestration of intracellular calcium by the endoplasmic reticulum, and inhibition of calcium channels, blocking calcium influx. The consequence is a drop in cytosolic calcium and smooth muscle relaxation/erection. During the return to the flaccid state, cGMP is hydrolyzed to guanosine monophosphate by phosphodiesterase type 5. Other phosphodiesterases are also found in the corpus cavernosum, but they do not appear to play an important role in detumescence.

3.2 Classification and Epidemiology

Erectile dysfunction may be classified as psychogenic, organic (neurogenic, hormonal, arterial, cavernosal and drug-induced), and mixed. Mixed erectile dysfunction is most commonly encountered having both a psychogenic and organic component (Table 3.1). Several pathophysiologic states, such as diabetes mellitus, may have detrimental effects upon erectile capacity via multiple pathways.

Many epidemiologic studies have described the relationship between erectile dysfunction and increasing age, with a reported prevalence of 40% at age 40, compared to 70% by 70 years of age; for severe erectile dysfunction, rates triple from 5% to 15% for men aged 40 compared to 70 (FELDMAN et al. 1994).

Table 3.1. Classification and common causes of erectile dysfunction

Category of erectile dysfunction	Common disorders	Pathophysiology
Neurogenic	Stroke or Alzheimer's disease, spinal cord injury, radical pelvic surgeries, diabetic neuropathy, pelvic injury	Interrupted neuronal transmission, failure to initiate nerve impulse
Psychogenic	Depression, psychological stress, performance anxiety, relationship problems	Impaired nitric oxide (NO) release, over-inhibition of NO release, loss of libido
Hormonal	Hypogonadism, hyperprolactinemia	Loss of libido, inadequate NO release
Vasculogenic (arterial and venogenic)	Hypertension, atherosclerosis, diabetes mellitus, trauma, Peyronie's disease	Impaired veno-occlusion, inadequate arterial inflow
Drug-induced	Antihypertensives, antiandrogens, antidepressants, alcohol abuse, cigarette smoking	Central suppression, decreased libido, alcoholic neuropathy, vascular insufficiency
Systemic diseases	Normal aging, diabetes mellitus, chronic renal failure, coronary heart disease	Multifactorial neuronal and vascular dysfunction

Although more than 70% of men over 65 years are sexually active, 40% are dissatisfied with their sex life (BRAUN et al. 2000; ROSEN et al. 2003). In one large multinational survey, less than 25% of men and women felt that "older people no longer want sex," and over 60% of men and women supported the idea of the elderly using medical treatments to aid in sexual enjoyment (NICOLOSI et al. 2004).

Longitudinal studies within a large cohort demonstrate a non-linear decline for most aspects of sexual function as age increases, with a more pronounced decline in older groups (ARAUJO et al. 2004). As the latent period between sexual stimulation and erection increases, erections are less turgid, ejaculation is less forceful, ejaculatory volume decreases, and the refractory period between erections lengthens. There is also a decrease in penile sensitivity to tactile stimulation, a decrease in serum testosterone concentration, and an increase in cavernous muscle tone (KAISER et al. 1988; ROWLAND et al. 1989; CHRIST et al. 1990). While relational, psychological, and organic issues are important contributors to erectile dysfunction across age groups, organic issues tend to play a more pronounced role as men age (CORONA et al. 2004).

3.3 Pathophysiology

Although psychogenic erectile dysfunction was historically considered to be the most common cause, mixed disorders are most common. Psychogenic erectile dysfunction can be caused by performance anxiety, strained interpersonal relationships, lack of sexual arousability, and overt psychiatric disorders such as depression and schizophrenia. Several studies have confirmed the strong relationship between depression and sexual dysfunction (ARAUJO et al. 1998; SHABSIGH et al. 1998).

Erectile dysfunction is noted in patients with neurological disorders such as Parkinson's and Alzheimer's diseases, stroke, and cerebral trauma, often secondary to a decrease in libido or inability to initiate the erectile process. Spinal cord injury patients have varying degrees of erectile dysfunction largely dependent on the location and extent of the lesion. Sensory input from the genitalia is essential to achieve and maintain reflexogenic erection, and this input becomes more important as the effect of psychological stimuli abates with age. Other common causes of neurogenic erectile dysfunction are surgeries that affect the cavernous nerves, such as radical prostatectomy.

Androgen deficiency results in a decrease in both nocturnal erections and libido. Although testosterone levels do not correspond to severity of erectile dysfunction, in those patients with reduced libido there are lower levels of testosterone as compared to other patients (CORONA et al. 2004). However, erection in response to visual sexual stimulation is preserved in men with hypogonadism, suggesting that androgen is not absolutely essential for erections, due to multiple pathways (BANCROFT and WU 1983; ANGULO et al. 2005). Due to the inhibitory action of prolactin on central dopaminergic activity and the resultant decrease in gonadotropin-releasing hormone secretion, hyperprolactinemia of any cause results in both reproductive and sexual dysfunction (via secondary hypogonadotropic hypogonadism).

Vascular pathology may involve lesions of the inflow or outflow mechanisms of penile erection. Erectile dysfunction may be a manifestation of generalized atherosclerosis and may even be its initial presentation. Common risk factors associated with generalized penile arterial insufficiency include hypertension, hyperlipidemia, cigarette smoking, diabetes mellitus, and pelvic irradiation (ROSEN et al. 1991). Less commonly, local stenosis of the common penile artery may occur in men who have sustained blunt pelvic or perineal trauma (LEVINE et al. 1990).

Dysfunction of the venoocclusive mechanism that normally allows maintenance of erection can cause erectile dysfunction (RAJFER et al. 1988) and may be the result of degenerative changes affecting the penis such as general aging, Peyronie's disease, and diabetes mellitus. Peyronie's disease is more common in middle age, but may be present in the aging male although it tends to be underdiagnosed, especially if there has been a long period without rigid erection. Although generally caused by global penile tissue degeneration, venoocclusive dysfunction may also be the result of congenital or trauma-induced formation of large venous channels draining the corpora cavernosa. Venous leak can be seen in anxious men with excessive adrenergic tone causing structural alterations of the cavernous smooth muscle and endothelium and insufficient trabecular smooth muscle relaxation (CHRIST et al. 1990). Finally, venous leak can be seen in patients with acquired shunts that result from the operative correction of priapism.

A variety of commonly used medications have been reported to cause erectile dysfunction. Central neurotransmitter pathways, including serotonergic, noradrenergic, and dopaminergic pathways involved in sexual function, may be disturbed by antipsychotics, antidepressants, and antihypertensive drugs. Although any antihypertensive agent could theoretically cause erectile dysfunction by decreasing the availability of blood to the corporal arteries (i.e., a pressure-head phenomenon), differences are noted between various classes of medications, with less erectile dysfunction associated with angiotensin-converting enzyme inhibitors and selective beta-adrenergic blocking drugs (Grimm et al. 1997; Papatsoris and Korantzopoulos 2006; Shiri et al. 2006). Non-selective beta-adrenergic blocking drugs may cause erectile dysfunction by potentiating alpha-1 adrenergic activity in the penis as well as by a possible central mechanism (Horowitz and Goble 1979). Thiazide diuretics have been reported to cause erectile dysfunction by an unknown mechanism (Chang et al. 1991). Spironolactone, acting as an anti-androgen, can cause a decrease in libido and gynecomastia as well as causing erectile dysfunction. Cimetidine, a histamine-H2 receptor antagonist, has been reported to decrease libido and cause erectile failure; it acts as an anti-androgen and can cause hyperprolactinemia (Wolfe 1979). Other drugs known to cause erectile dysfunction are estrogens and drugs with anti-androgenic action such as ketoconazole and cyproterone acetate.

In many disease states, the associated erectile dysfunction may be due to multiple causes. About 50 percent of men with chronic diabetes mellitus are reported to have erectile dysfunction. In addition to the disease's effect on small vessels, it may also affect the cavernous nerve terminals and endothelial cells, resulting in a deficiency of erectogenic neurotransmitter release. Additionally, in diabetics, corporal smooth muscle relaxation in response to neuronal- and endothelial-derived nitric oxide (NO) is impaired and may be secondary to the accumulation of glycosylation products (Saenz De Tejada et al. 1989; Seftel et al. 1997; Cartledge et al. 2001; Angulo et al. 2003). The pathophysiology of erectile dysfunction in DM is multifactorial, consisting of vascular, neurological, endothelial, and hormonal insults. The penile microvasculature is very sensitive to insults that affect other sites in the vascular system. DM is associated with atherosclerosis of both large and small penile vessels. Several studies point to corporal and pudendal arterial insufficiency as a common finding on both Doppler ultrasound and angiographic studies (Herman et al. 1978; Wang et al. 1993). DM affects a variety of nerve fibers, and histologic studies in animals and humans have demonstrated quantitative and qualitative changes in penile nerves (Faerman et al. 1974; Italiano et al. 1993; Morano 2003). On a cellular level, neurotransmitter abnormalities have been found in both human diabetics as well as in experimental animal models (Ehmke et al. 1995; Vernet et al. 1995). In diabetics, corporal smooth muscle relaxation in response to neuronal- and endothelial-derived nitric oxide (NO) is impaired and may be due to the accumulation of glycosylation products (Saenz De Tejada et al. 1989; Seftel et al. 1997; Cartledge et al. 2001; Angulo et al. 2003). Although the data are somewhat conflicting, there may also be decreased production of NO (Ehmke et al. 1995). Additionally, animal and human studies have demonstrated hypogonadism in diabetics, which may contribute to both erectile dysfunction and decreased libido; however, this tends to be mild and likely does not play as great a role as the neuronal and vascular injuries (Murray et al. 1987; Murray et al. 1992). Reduced libido may also be a significant etiology for ED in DM, although this has not been studied in conjunction with testosterone levels (Nakanishi et al. 2004).

Chronic renal failure is also frequently associated with diminished erectile function, impaired libido, and infertility. The mechanism is probably multifactorial: low serum testosterone concentrations, diabetes mellitus, vascular insufficiency, multiple medications, autonomic and somatic neuropathy, and psychological stress. Men with angina, myocardial infarction, or heart failure may have erectile dysfunction from anxiety, depression, or concomitant penile arterial insufficiency.

Social drugs including cigarettes and alcohol also affect erectile function. Cigarette smoking may acutely induce vasoconstriction and penile venous leakage because of its contractile effect on the cavernous smooth muscle (Juenemann et al. 1987); more importantly, chronic use may accelerate atherosclerotic changes in the penile microvasculature. Alcohol in small amounts may improve erections and increases libido because of its vasodilatory effect and the suppression of anxiety; however, large amounts can cause central sedation, decreased libido, and transient erectile dysfunction. Chronic alcoholism may cause hypogonadism and polyneuropathy, which may affect penile nerve function (Miller and Gold 1988).

As physicians, we may cause erectile dysfunction through the medications we prescribe and the surgeries we perform. Pelvic surgeries, particularly radical prostatectomies, frequently cause erectile dysfunction; analogous to diabetes mellitus, as described above, the erectile dysfunction may be the result of multiple pathophysiologies despite one underlying insult. Despite surgical advances in preservation of the cavernous nerves (Walsh and Donker 1982), only 20% of patients return to pre-procedural erectile function a year after prostatectomy (Hu et al. 2004). Even in nerve-sparing procedures, postoperative neuropraxia results in a cascade of events including loss of nocturnal erections, smooth muscle apoptosis, increased fibrosis, and eventual anatomic changes leading to venous leakage (Mulhall et al. 2002; Leungwattanakij et al. 2003; Iacono et al. 2005).

Erectile dysfunction may be the first manifestation of many diseases including diabetes mellitus, coronary artery disease, hyperlipidemia, hypertension, spinal-cord compression, pituitary tumors, and pelvic malignancies. For example, a recent prevalence study found that men with erectile dysfunction were twice as likely to have DM and concluded that erectile dysfunction may be used as an early marker for DM. This relationship was particularly strong in the younger age groups, in which the odds ratio of having DM was 3 (Sun et al. 2006). Two earlier studies found that 11% (Maatman et al. 1987) and 12% (Deutsch and Sherman 1980) of impotent men were found to have previously undiagnosed DM.

References

Angulo J, Cuevas P, Fernandez A et al (2003) Diabetes impairs endothelium-dependent relaxation of human penile vascular tissues mediated by NO and EDHF. Biochem Biophys Res Commun 312: 1202–1208

Angulo J, Cuevas P, Gabancho S et al (2005) Enhancement of both EDHF and NO/cGMP pathways is necessary to reverse erectile dysfunction in diabetic rats. J Sex Med 2: 341–346

Araujo AB, Durante R, Feldman HA et al (1998) The relationship between depressive symptoms and male erectile dysfunction: cross-sectional results from the Massachusetts Male Aging Study. Psychosom Med 60: 458–465

Araujo AB, Mohr BA, McKinlay JB (2004) Changes in sexual function in middle-aged and older men: longitudinal data from the Massachusetts Male Aging Study. J Am Geriatr Soc 52: 1502–1509

Bancroft J, Wu FC (1983) Changes in erectile responsiveness during androgen replacement therapy. Arch Sex Behav 12: 59–66

Banya Y, Ushiki T, Takagane H et al (1989) Two circulatory routes within the human corpus cavernosum penis: a scanning electron microscopic study of corrosion casts. J Urol 142: 879–883

Braun M, Wassmer G, Klotz T et al (2000) Epidemiology of erectile dysfunction: results of the Cologne Male Survey. Int J Impot Res 12: 305–311

Cartledge JJ, Eardley I, Morrison JF (2001) Advanced glycation end-products are responsible for the impairment of corpus cavernosal smooth muscle relaxation seen in diabetes. BJU Int 87: 402–407

Chang SW, Fine R, Siegel D et al (1991) The impact of diuretic therapy on reported sexual function. Arch Intern Med 151: 2402–2408

Christ GJ, Maayani S, Valcic M et al (1990) Pharmacological studies of human erectile tissue: characteristics of spontaneous contractions and alterations in alpha-adrenoceptor responsiveness with age and disease in isolated tissues. Br J Pharmacol 101: 375–381

Corona G, Mannucci E, Mansani R et al (2004) Aging and pathogenesis of erectile dysfunction. Int J Impot Res 16: 395–402

Deutsch S, Sherman L (1980) Previously unrecognized diabetes mellitus in sexually impotent men. JAMA 244: 2430–2432

Ehmke H, Junemann KP, Mayer B et al (1995) Nitric oxide synthase and vasoactive intestinal polypeptide colocalization in neurons innervating the human penile circulation. Int J Impot Res 7: 147–156

Faerman I, Glocer L, Fox D et al (1974) Impotence and diabetes. Histological studies of the autonomic nervous fibers of the corpora cavernosa in impotent diabetic males. Diabetes 23: 971–976

Feldman HA, Goldstein I, Hatzichristou DG et al (1994) Impotence and its medical and psychosocial correlates: results of the Massachusetts Male Aging Study. J Urol 151: 54–61

Fournier GR, Jr., Juenemann KP, Lue TF et al (1987) Mechanisms of venous occlusion during canine penile erection: an anatomic demonstration. J Urol 137: 163–167

Grimm RH, Jr., Grandits GA, Prineas RJ et al (1997) Long-term effects on sexual function of five antihypertensive drugs and nutritional hygienic treatment in hypertensive men and women. Treatment of Mild Hypertension Study (TOMHS). Hypertension 29: 8–14

Herman A, Adar R, Rubinstein Z (1978) Vascular lesions associated with impotence in diabetic and nondiabetic arterial occlusive disease. Diabetes 27: 975–81

Horowitz JD, Goble AJ (1979) Drugs and impaired male sexual function. Drugs 18: 206–217

Hu JC, Elkin EP, Pasta DJ et al (2004) Predicting quality of life after radical prostatectomy: results from CaPSURE. J Urol 171: 703–707; discussion 707–708

Iacono F, Giannella R, Somma P et al (2005) Histological alterations in cavernous tissue after radical prostatectomy. J Urol 173: 1673–1676

Italiano G, Petrelli L, Marin A et al (1993) Ultrastructural analysis of the cavernous and dorsal penile nerves in experimental diabetes. Int J Impot Res 5: 149–160

Juenemann KP, Lue TF, Luo JA et al (1987) The effect of cigarette smoking on penile erection. J Urol 138: 438–441

Kaiser FE, Viosca SP, Morley JE et al (1988) Impotence and aging: clinical and hormonal factors. J Am Geriatr Soc 36: 511–519

Leungwattanakij S, Bivalacqua TJ, Usta MF et al (2003) Cavernous neurotomy causes hypoxia and fibrosis in rat corpus cavernosum. J Androl 24: 239–245

Levine FJ, Greenfield AJ, Goldstein I (1990) Arteriographically determined occlusive disease within the hypogastric-cavernous bed in impotent patients following blunt perineal and pelvic trauma. J Urol 144: 1147–1153

Lue TF (2000) Erectile dysfunction. N Engl J Med 342: 1802–1813

Maatman TJ, Montague DK, Martin LM (1987) Erectile dysfunction in men with diabetes mellitus. Urology 29: 589–592

Miller NS, Gold MS (1988) The human sexual response and alcohol and drugs. J Subst Abuse Treat 5: 171–177

Morano S (2003) Pathophysiology of diabetic sexual dysfunction. J Endocrinol Invest 26: 65–69

Mulhall JP, Slovick R, Hotaling J et al (2002) Erectile dysfunction after radical prostatectomy: hemodynamic profiles and their correlation with the recovery of erectile function. J Urol 167: 1371–1375

Murray FT, Johnson RD, Sciadini M et al (1992) Erectile and copulatory dysfunction in chronically diabetic BB/WOR rats. Am J Physiol 263: E151–157

Murray FT, Wyss HU, Thomas RG et al (1987) Gonadal dysfunction in diabetic men with organic impotence. J Clin Endocrinol Metab 65: 127–135

Nakanishi S, Yamane K, Kamei N et al (2004) Erectile dysfunction is strongly linked with decreased libido in diabetic men. Aging Male 7: 113–119

Nicolosi A, Laumann EO, Glasser DB et al (2004) Sexual behavior and sexual dysfunctions after age 40: the global study of sexual attitudes and behaviors. Urology 64: 991–997

Papatsoris AG, Korantzopoulos PG (2006) Hypertension, antihypertensive therapy, and erectile dysfunction. Angiology 57: 47–52

Rajfer J, Rosciszewski A, Mehringer M (1988) Prevalence of corporeal venous leakage in impotent men. J Urol 140: 69–71

Rosen MP, Greenfield AJ, Walker TG et al (1991) Cigarette smoking: an independent risk factor for atherosclerosis in the hypogastric-cavernous arterial bed of men with arteriogenic impotence. J Urol 145: 759–763

Rosen R, Altwein J, Boyle P et al (2003) Lower urinary tract symptoms and male sexual dysfunction: the multinational survey of the aging male (MSAM-7). Eur Urol 44: 637–649

Rowland DL, Greenleaf W, Mas M et al (1989) Penile and finger sensory thresholds in young, aging, and diabetic males. Arch Sex Behav 18: 1–12

Saenz de Tejada I, Goldstein I, Azadzoi K et al (1989) Impaired neurogenic and endothelium-mediated relaxation of penile smooth muscle from diabetic men with impotence. N Engl J Med 320: 1025–1030

Seftel AD, Vaziri ND, Ni Z et al (1997) Advanced glycation end products in human penis: elevation in diabetic tissue, site of deposition, and possible effect through iNOS or eNOS. Urology 50: 1016–1026

Shabsigh R, Klein LT, Seidman S et al (1998) Increased incidence of depressive symptoms in men with erectile dysfunction. Urology 52: 848–852

Shiri R, Koskimaki J, Hakkinen J et al (2006) Cardiovascular drug use and the incidence of erectile dysfunction. Int J Impot Res 19: 208–212

Sun P, Cameron A, Seftel A et al (2006) Erectile dysfunction–an observable marker of diabetes mellitus? A large national epidemiological study. J Urol 176: 1081–1085; discussion 1085

Vernet D, Cai L, Garban H et al (1995) Reduction of penile nitric oxide synthase in diabetic BB/WORdp (type I) and BBZ/WORdp (type II) rats with erectile dysfunction. Endocrinology 136: 5709–5717

Walsh PC, Donker PJ (1982) Impotence following radical prostatectomy: insight into etiology and prevention. J Urol 128: 492–497

Wang CJ, Shen SY, Wu CC et al (1993) Penile blood flow study in diabetic impotence. Urol Int 50: 209–212

Clinical Evaluation of Erectile Dysfunction in the Era of PDE-5 Inhibitors: The Residual Role of Penile Color Doppler US

Emanuele Belgrano, Stefano Bucci, Giovanni Liguori, and Carlo Trombetta

CONTENTS

4.1 Definition 21
4.2 Clinical Features 21
4.3 Diagnosis of Erectile Dysfunction 21
4.4 Color Doppler Ultrasonography 22
4.4.1 Trauma Patients 22
4.4.2 Peyronie's Disease 22
4.4.3 Silent Coronary Artery Disease 22

References 23

4.1
Definition

Erectile dysfunction has been defined by the National Institute of Health (NIH) as the inability to achieve and/or maintain an erection for satisfactory sexual intercourse. Discordant data have been reported on erectile dysfunction epidemiology with prevalence ranging from 12% to 52%. A recent study reported a prevalence of 12.8% in Italy (Foresta et al. 2005). French epidemiological studies estimate that the prevalence of erectile dysfunction is between 11% and 44%. Prevalence surveys show a correlation with age: the relative risk of erectile dysfunction increases by a factor of 2 to 4 between the ages of 40 and 70 years (Costa et al. 2005).

4.2
Clinical Features

Erectile dysfunction is a multi-factorial disorder and a common presentation for several systemic illnesses, particularly vascular occlusive diseases such as diabetes, arterial hypertension, and atherosclerosis. Few patients consult their doctor, and only a small proportion of them receive treatment. Only few doctors take the initiative to discuss the question of their patients' sex life (Costa et al. 2005). In fact, the clinician must be familiar with the pathophysiologic mechanisms of erectile dysfunction, its associations with other systemic diseases, the indications for specialist referral, and the role of specialized testing to diagnose and treat this disorder effectively (Lobo and Nehra 2005).

The andrologist's cultural baggage must include the ability to identify the pathology that can determine erectile dysfunction and the capacity to program a specific diagnostic workup (Foresta et al. 2005). Demonstration of erectile disorders represents an excellent opportunity to conduct a general workup. In fact, management of erectile dysfunction is an integral part of preventive medicine since more than one-third of patients ignores their underlying health problem (Costa et al. 2005).

4.3
Diagnosis of Erectile Dysfunction

Baseline diagnostic evaluation for erectile dysfunction can identify the underlying pathological conditions and associated risk factors in 80% of patients. Such screening may diagnose reversible causes of erectile dysfunction and also unmasks medical conditions that manifest with erectile dysfunction as the first symptom (Hatzichristou et al. 2002).

E. Belgrano, Professor and Chairman; S. Bucci, MD; G. Liguori, MD; C. Trombetta, MD, Associate Professor
Department of Urology, University of Trieste, Ospedale di Cattinara, Strada di Fiume 449, Trieste, 34149, Italy

The clinical evaluation of patients with erectile dysfunction should be thorough and systematic, with attention to the appropriate use of sexual symptom questionnaires and symptom scales, detailed medical and sexual history, physical examination, and basic screening laboratory tests. Still open is the question of which specific tests such as tumescence and rigidity measurements, intracavernous administration of vasoactive drugs and color/duplex Doppler sonography are required for adequate clinical assessment.

4.4 Color Doppler Ultrasonography

In the field of erectile dysfunction, penile vascular imaging modalities have diminished in importance over the past 10 years with the introduction of new effective oral medications and recognition that surgical treatment of both penile venous leak and arterial insufficiency has poor long-term clinical outcomes.

Moreover, the introduction of phosphodiesterase-5 (PDE5) inhibitors has revolutionized the therapy of erectile dysfunction and radically changed the way in which patients are investigated (SPEEL et al. 2001). Documentation of a good quality erection in response to a PDE5-inhibiting drug confirms grossly adequate arterial inflow and effective veno-occlusive mechanisms. However, Doppler interrogation of penile vessels continues to have a role in the evaluation of specific patients presenting with erectile dysfunction, in particular, in trauma patients and in patients with Peyronie's disease.

4.4.1 Trauma Patients

Detailed evaluation of the penile vascular supply is mandatory to plan intervention in patients with postraumatic erectile dysfunction who are candidates for penile revascularization surgery. These patients are frequently young, have often suffered traumatic straddle injuries to the pelvis and may be unresponsive to oral and intracavernosal therapy (GOLIJANIN et al. 2007a; GOLIJANIN et al. 2007b).

4.4.2 Peyronie's Disease

As erectile dysfunction occurs in a considerable percentage of patients with Peyronie's disease (RALPH et al. 1992; AHMED et al. 1998; KADIOGLU et al. 2000), evaluation of the penile vessels with Doppler techniques is useful to distinguish different causes for impotence and is critical for detecting subclinical abnormalities of penile hemodynamics that may have a role in postoperative erectile dysfunction (MONTORSI et al. 2000).

In fact, any therapeutic intervention for Peyronie's disease may have some adverse impact upon erectile function; documentation of the baseline erectile function is therefore imperative, from both the medical and the medico-legal perspective. Moreover, in patients with normal erection, either shortening or lengthening procedures can be undertaken, whereas in patients with coexistent erectile dysfunction shortening procedures or prosthesis implantation should be considered the treatment of choice (AHMED et al. 1998; HAKIM 2002).

4.4.3 Silent Coronary Artery Disease

An increasing role of Doppler techniques is now recognized in identification of patients without symptomatic peripheral vascular disease and with silent coronary artery disease presenting with erectile dysfunction (BARRETT-CONNOR 2004). In fact, erectile dysfunction is now being recognized as one of the earliest manifestations of endothelial dysfunction and peripheral vascular disease. In patients with significant risk factors for cardiovascular disease, such as hypertension, smoking, trauma, hyperlipidemia, diabetes mellitus, obesity and inactivity, decrease in sexual ability is regarded as one of the first clinical parameters of increased risk of significant coronary artery and peripheral vascular disease (GOLDSTEIN 2000; EL-SAKKA et al. 2004; SHAMLOUL et al. 2004; GOLIJANIN et al. 2007a; GOLIJANIN et al. 2007b). Doppler interrogation of the penile vasculature can be used in these patients to assess the need for further cardiac or peripheral vascular assessment.

References

Ahmed M, Chilton CP, Munson KW et al (1998) The role of colour Doppler imaging in the management of Peyronie's disease. Br J Urol 81:604–606

Barrett-Connor E (2004) Cardiovascular risk stratification and cardiovascular risk factors associated with erectile dysfunction: assessing cardiovascular risk in men with erectile dysfunction. Clin Cardiol 27:I8–13

Costa P, Grivel T, Giuliano F et al (2005) [Erectile dysfunction: a sentinel symptom?]. Prog Urol 15:203–207

El-Sakka AI, Morsy AM, Fagih BI, Nassar AH (2004) Coronary artery risk factors in patients with erectile dysfunction. J Urol 172:251–254

Foresta C, Caretta N, Palego P et al (2005) Diagnosing erectile dysfunction: flow-chart. Int J Androl 28 Suppl 2:64–68

Goldstein I (2000) The mutually reinforcing triad of depressive symptoms, cardiovascular disease, and erectile dysfunction. Am J Cardiol 86:41F–45F

Golijanin D, Singer E, Davis R et al (2007a) Doppler evaluation of erectile dysfunction-part 1. Int J Impot Res 19:37–42

Golijanin D, Singer E, Davis R et al (2007b) Doppler evaluation of erectile dysfunction-part 2. Int J Impot Res 19:43–48

Hakim LS (2002) Peyronie's disease: an update. The role of diagnostics. Int J Impot Res 14:321–323

Hatzichristou D, Hatzimouratidis K, Bekas M et al (2002) Diagnostic steps in the evaluation of patients with erectile dysfunction. J Urol 168:615–620

Kadioglu A, Tefekli A, Erol H et al (2000) Color Doppler ultrasound assessment of penile vascular system in men with Peyronie's disease. Int J Impot Res 12:263–267

Lobo JR, Nehra A (2005) Clinical evaluation of erectile dysfunction in the era of PDE-5 inhibitors. Urol Clin North Am 32:447–455, vi

Montorsi F, Salonia A, Maga T et al (2000) Evidence based assessment of long-term results of plaque incision and vein grafting for Peyronie's disease. J Urol 163:1704–1708

Ralph DJ, Hughes T, Lees WR, Pryor JP (1992) Pre-operative assessment of Peyronie's disease using colour Doppler sonography. Br J Urol 69:629–632

Shamloul R, Ghanem HM, Salem A et al (2004) Correlation between penile duplex findings and stress electrocardiography in men with erectile dysfunction. Int J Impot Res 16:235–237

Speel TG, Bleumer I, Diemont WL et al (2001) The value of sildenafil as mode of stimulation in pharmaco-penile duplex ultrasonography. Int J Impot Res 13:189–191

US Anatomy of the Penis:
Common Findings and Anatomical Variations

MICHELE BERTOLOTTO, ANDREA LISSIANI, RICCARDO PIZZOLATO, and MICHELINE DJOUGUELA FUTE

CONTENTS

5.1 Background 25
5.2 Evaluation Technique 25
5.3 Grey-Scale Ultrasound Anatomy 26
5.4 Color Doppler Ultrasound Anatomy 28
5.4.1 Cavernosal Arteries 28
5.4.2 Dorsal Arteries 29
5.4.3 Bulbar and Urethral Arteries 29
5.4.4 Vascularization of the Penile Tip 29
5.4.5 Arterial Communications 31
5.4.6 Helicine Arterioles 31
5.4.7 Cavernosal-Spongiosal Communications 32
5.4.8 Penile Veins 33

5.5 Duplex Doppler Interrogation 34
5.5.1 Cavernosal Arteries 34
5.5.2 Dorsal Arteries 34
5.5.3 Arterial Communications 34
5.5.4 Helicine Arterioles 34
5.5.5 Cavernosal-Spongiosal Communications 36

References 37

5.1 Background

Because it is a superficial structure, the penis is ideally suited to ultrasound imaging. In fact, improved spatial resolution and increased color Doppler sensitivity provided by the latest generation of ultrasound equipment allow an excellent evaluation of normal and pathological penile structures. Ultrasound evaluation of the penis, however, requires a good knowledge of penile anatomy to identify subtle changes that can be appreciated in pathological conditions.

In this chapter the normal appearance of penile anatomical structures at ultrasound will be described, both while flaccid and during erection. Specific topics discussed will be ultrasound appearance of the corporal bodies and penile envelopes, visibility of normal penile vessels at color Doppler ultrasonography and normal changes of Doppler spectra during the onset of erection.

5.2 Evaluation Technique

Penile sonography should be performed using high frequency linear probes with the patient in the supine position and the penis scanned from its ventral surface using longitudinal and transverse views. No standoff pad is required when the latest sonographic equipment is used. Evaluation should be carried out while the penis is flaccid and after intracavernosal injection of vasoactive drugs (DOUBILET et al. 1991). Prostaglandin E1 injection at the dosage of 10 µg is usually adequate to obtain a suitable erectile response in potent patients (BERTOLOTTO and NEUMAIER 1999). Some authors, however, routinely

M. BERTOLOTTO, MD; R. PIZZOLATO, MD; M. DJOUGUELA FUTE, MD
Department of Radiology, University of Trieste, Ospedale di Cattinara, Strada di Fiume 447, Trieste, 34124, Italy
A. LISSIANI, MD
Department of Urology, University of Trieste, Ospedale di Cattinara, Strada di Fiume 447, Trieste, 34124, Italy

use 20 μg. A lower initial dosage of 5 μg is recommended in young patients in order to limit the risk of prolonged and painful erection (Lin and Bradley 1985). Injection of other intracorporeal vasoactive agents such as papaverin is nowadays considered only in selected cases due to the high risk of iatrogenic prolonged erection.

Color Doppler interrogation and spectral analysis is performed with slow flow settings that are tuned during the examination on minimal PRF values that do not determine aliasing. Color gain is tuned just under the noise threshold of the system. Spectral interrogation of the cavernosal arteries is obtained at the base of the penis under the guidance of color Doppler signal, and the angle correction cursor is adjusted to match the correct axis of flow. Steering is used to obtain a good angular correction.

5.3
Grey-Scale Ultrasound Anatomy

The different anatomical features of the penis are better evaluated during tumescence and erection (Lue et al. 1985). In the flaccid state, the corporal bodies present at ultrasonography as cylindrical structures with intermediate echogenicity and homogeneous echotexture.

The corpus spongiosum and the glans are more echogenic than the corpora cavernosa. When collapsed, the urethra appears as a transverse line. The echogenicity of the corpora cavernosa progressively decreases during tumescence starting from the region surrounding the cavernosal arteries because of sinusoids dilatation. During maximal penile rigidity, a fine echogenic network is appreciable in the corpora cavernosa due to sinusoidal interfaces. Sinusoidal spaces at the base of the penis are normally larger that in the remaining portions of the shaft. Blood entrapped within the sinusoids often appears slightly corpusculated (Fig. 5.1).

The Colles' fascia is barely visible in normal patients. The tunica albuginea and the Buck's fascia are stuck together and appear as a thin echogenic line surrounding the corpora, which became thinner during erection. Two distinct layers become appreciable only when fluid extravasation accumulates between them or very high frequency transducers are used. Vascular structures, however, may provide a suitable interface to separate small portions of the Buck's fascia from the underlying tunica albuginea in normal penises as well. In particular, the Buck's fascia becomes visible at ultrasound near dilated circumflex veins, and a subtle echogenic line representing the Buck's fascia is usually recognized in the dorsal aspect of the penis dividing the plane of the deep vessels from that of the superficial vessels (Lue and Tanagho 1987; Mueller and Lue 1988) and near the corpus spongiosum (Fig. 5.2).

The penile septum appears as an echogenic structure with back attenuation dividing the corpora cavernosa that can hamper visualization of the tunica albuginea in the dorsal aspect of the penis (Fig. 5.2).

The intracavernous pillars are recognizable on transverse scans as straight echogenic lines thicker than the sinusoidal walls, which run from one side to the other of the tunica albuginea. The distal penile ligament, an aggregation of the outer longitudinal layer of the tunica albuginea that acts as a buttress for the glans penis (Hsu et al. 2004; Hsu et al. 2005), is recognized at ultrasound as a linear structure more echogenic than the surrounding glanular tissue located centrally within the glans dorsal to the distal urethra (Fig. 5.3).

Several penile vessels can be identified at grey-scale ultrasound as well. In particular, the cavernosal arteries appear as a pair of dots located slightly medially in each corpus cavernosum. On longitudinal scans they present as narrow tubular structures with echogenic wall (Quam et al. 1989). The diameter of the normal cavernosal arteries ranges from 0.3 to 05 mm in the flaccid state and increases to 0.6–1.0 mm after an intracavernosal injection of vasoactive agents (Fig. 5.4).

During the onset of erection, cavernosal artery pulsation is evident in normal subjects (Lee et al. 1993; Kim 2002). The dorsal arteries are visible in the dorsal aspect of the shaft as anechoic structures with a similar diameter to the cavernosal arteries. As occurs for the cavernosal arteries, also the diameter of the dorsal arteries increases during erection, but to a lesser extent compared with the cavernosal arteries (Lee et al. 1993). Dorsal veins present with less echogenic wall compared to the arteries.

US Anatomy of the Penis: Common Findings and Anatomical Variations

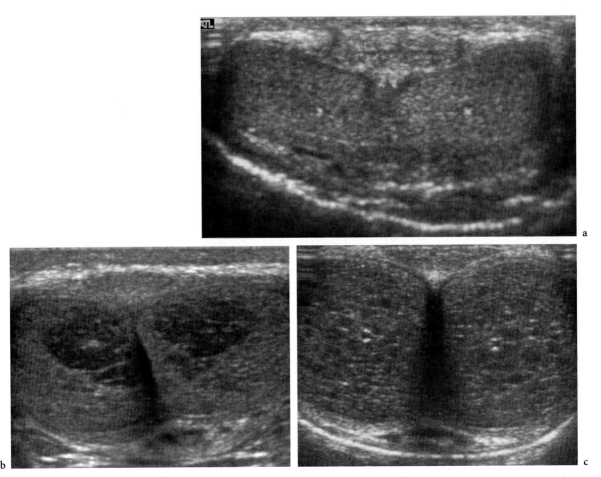

Fig. 5.1a–c. Normal grey-scale ultrasound anatomy. Axial scans. **a** In the flaccid state, the penile bodies present with intermediate echogenicity and homogeneous echotexture. **b** During the first minutes after cavernosal injection distension of the cavernosal sinusoids begins in the central portion of the corpora cavenosa, which appears less echogenic that the outer portion. **c** When complete erection is achieved a fine echogenic network is appreciable within the corpora cavernosa

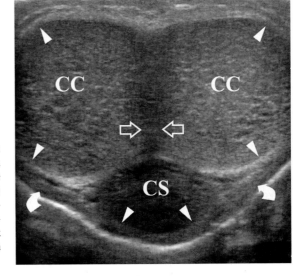

Fig. 5.2. Normal grey-scale ultrasound anatomy. Axial scan on the dorsal aspect of the penis showing the paired corpora cavernosa (*CC*), the corpus spongiosum (*CS*) and the penile septum (*open arrows*). The tunica albuginea (*arrowheads*) appears as a thin echogenic line surrounding the penile bodies. The Buck's fascia is visualized near the corpus spongiosum (*curved arrows*) while in the remaining portions is stuck on the tunica albuginea. The penile septum appears as an echogenic structure with back attenuation

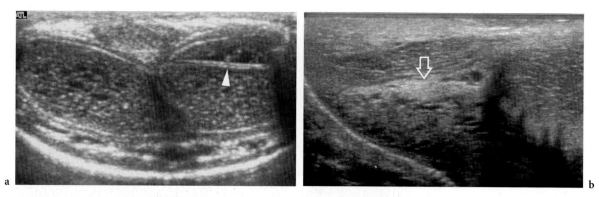

Fig. 5.3a,b. Normal grey-scale ultrasound anatomy. Axial **a** and longitudinal **b** scans obtained on the ventral aspect of the penis. **a** Intracavernous pillar (*arrowhead*) appearing as an echogenic line running from the lateral to the medial aspect of the tunica albuginea. **b** The distal penile ligament (*open arrow*) is recognized as a linear echogenic structure located centrally within the glans

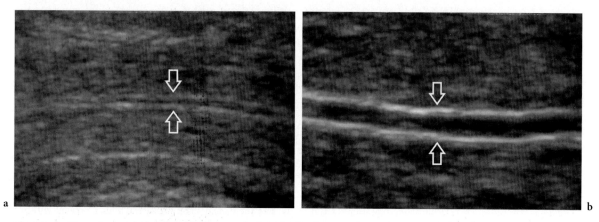

Fig. 5.4a,b. Normal grey-scale ultrasound anatomy. Longitudinal scans obtained on the ventral aspect of the penis showing the cavernosal artery (*open arrows*) while flaccid **a** and during the onset or erection **b**. The artery presents as a narrow tubular structure with echogenic wall whose diameter increases during erection

5.4
Color Doppler Ultrasound Anatomy

A full evaluation of penile arteries is obtained during the onset of erection. In this phase it is possible to study the pathway of the cavernosal, dorsal and urethral arteries and to identify the presence of anatomical variations and vascular communications. Conversely, depiction of penile veins increases during detumescence.

Variations in penile arterial anatomy are observed in up to 83% of patients (Jarow et al. 1993) and are commonly recognized at color Doppler ultrasonography (Chiou et al. 1999). Power Doppler investigation can be useful to improve depiction of small vessels with slow flow.

5.4.1
Cavernosal Arteries

Common anatomical variations of penile arteries include asymmetry, bifurcated cavernosal artery, multiple cavernosal arteries, presence of recurrent branches, unilateral origin of all cavernosal branches, accessory cavernosal branches, and aberrant origin from the dorsal artery (Fig. 5.5). Occasionally the cavernosal artery consists of multiple short, rapidly tapering segments, periodically reconstituted by perforating vessels from the dorsal penile artery (Juskiewenski et al. 1982; Wahl et al. 1997).

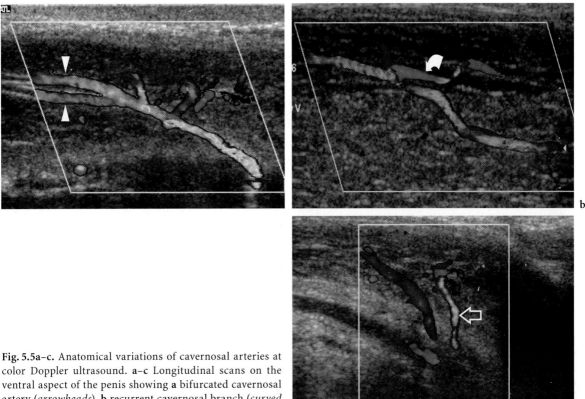

Fig. 5.5a–c. Anatomical variations of cavernosal arteries at color Doppler ultrasound. a–c Longitudinal scans on the ventral aspect of the penis showing **a** bifurcated cavernosal artery (*arrowheads*), **b** recurrent cavernosal branch (*curved arrow*), and **c** accessory cavernosal artery (*open arrow*)

5.4.2
Dorsal Arteries

Variations of the arterial vascular supply to the corpus spongiosum, to the urethra and glans are common. Asymmetry of the dorsal arteries is often recognized (Fig. 5.6), in which one artery is well developed, while the other is small, or even atrophic (CHIOU et al. 1999).

5.4.3
Bulbar and Urethral Arteries

At color Doppler ultrasound multiple branches of variable location are recognized feeding the bulb of the corpus spongiosum (KISHORE et al. 2005). Visualization of a main trunk entering the bulb is inconstant.

Often no urethral arteries are recognized at color Doppler interrogation at the midshaft and in the distal portion of the penis, reflecting anatomical results showing that these vessels are inconstant (JUSKIEWENSKI et al. 1982). When present, two urethral arteries are usually identified running within the corpus spongiosum for a variable tract (Fig. 5.7). Aberrant origin from the cavernous or from the dorsal artery may be recognized.

5.4.4
Vascularization of the Penile Tip

The arrangement of the distal portion of the dorsal arteries is variable (JUSKIEWENSKI et al. 1982). Occasionally, small dorsal collaterals feeding the corpora cavernosa, particularly near the tip, may be identified. When both dorsal arteries are well developed, they usually communicate behind the glans through a transverse anastomosis from which anterior branches arise feeding the glans. When one of the dorsal arteries is small or atrophic, the arterial vascular supply to the glans arises mostly from the dominant vessel (Fig. 5.8).

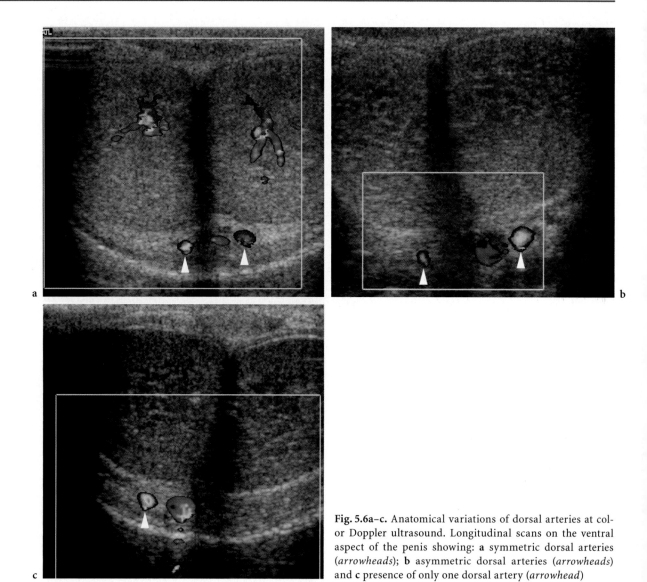

Fig. 5.6a–c. Anatomical variations of dorsal arteries at color Doppler ultrasound. Longitudinal scans on the ventral aspect of the penis showing: **a** symmetric dorsal arteries (*arrowheads*); **b** asymmetric dorsal arteries (*arrowheads*) and **c** presence of only one dorsal artery (*arrowhead*)

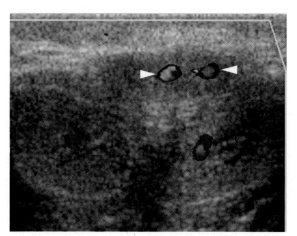

Fig. 5.7. Color Doppler ultrasound appearance of urethral arteries. Axial scan on the ventral aspect of the penis showing the paired urethral arteries (*arrowheads*) running within the corpus spongiosum

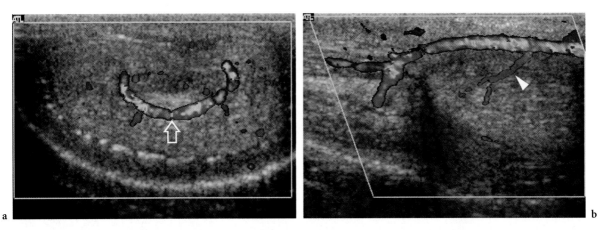

Fig. 5.8a,b. Color Doppler ultrasound anatomy. Arrangement of the distal portion of the dorsal arteries. **a** Axial scan showing communication of the dorsal arteries behind the glans through a transverse anastomosis (*open arrow*). **b** Longitudinal scan showing a small dorsal collateral (*arrowhead*) feeding the corpus cavernosum

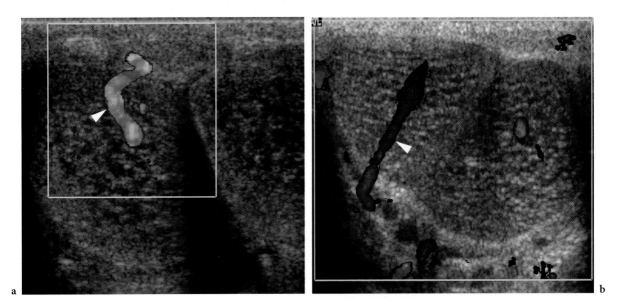

Fig. 5.9a,b. Color Doppler appearance of arterial communications (*arrowheads*) among the penile arteries. Axial scans on the ventral aspect of the penis. **a** Communication between the right cavernosal and urethral artery. **b** Communication between the right dorsal and cavernosal artery

5.4.5 Arterial Communications

A variety of arterial communications is appreciable among the different arteries of the penis. In particular, communications between the cavernosal arteries are identified in virtually all patients. Arterial communications between the cavernosal and the urethral artery, between the cavernosal artery and the arteries of the bulb of the corpus spongiosum, and dorsal penile-cavernosal perforators are less common (Fig. 5.9).

5.4.6 Helicine Arterioles

The morphological features of helicine arterioles can be investigated using power Doppler ultrasonography (MONTORSI et al. 1998). These vessels cannot be identified during flaccidity due to insufficient blood flow. They become evident during the onset of erection as small vessels with tortuous course originating from the cavernous arteries that branch in two to three orders of ramifications

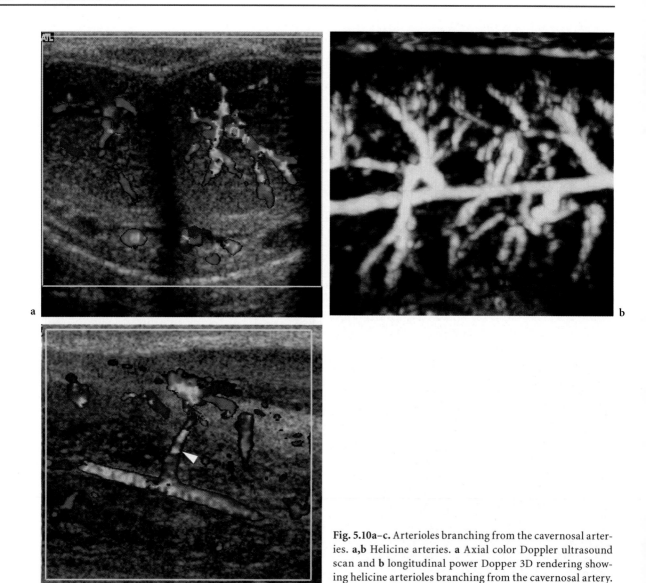

Fig. 5.10a–c. Arterioles branching from the cavernosal arteries. a,b Helicine arteries. a Axial color Doppler ultrasound scan and b longitudinal power Dopper 3D rendering showing helicine arterioles branching from the cavernosal artery. c Cavernosal-spongiosal communication (*arrowhead*) presenting as a straight vessel entering the corpus spongiosum

(Fig. 5.10). When venous occlusion occurs helicine arteries become progressively less visible and disappear with maximum rigidity, reflecting reduction and eventually discontinuance of penile blood inflow.

5.4.7
Cavernosal-Spongiosal Communications

These vessels are either arterovenous shunts connecting the cavernosal arteries with the corpus spongiosum (WAGNER et al. 1982) or, more likely, arterial anastomoses connecting the cavernosal arteries with the submucosal urethral arterial network (JUSKIEWENSKI et al. 1982; DROUPY et al. 1999; GOTTA et al. 2003). Cavernosal-spongiosal communications are recognized at color Doppler ultrasound in virtually all subjects (BERTOLOTTO et al. 2002). The exact role of these vessels has not been elucidated (DROUPY et al. 1999). It is conceivable that they behave as accessory feeding vessels of the intermediate and distal portion of the corpus spongiosum.

At color Doppler ultrasound cavernosal-spongiosal communications are recognized as vessels branching from the cavernosal artery that run towards the ventral aspect of the penile shaft, pass through the tunica albuginea, and enter the corpus spongiosum. Only few cavernosal-spongiosal communications are detected in the flaccid penis, while three to four for each corpus cavernosum are detected during the onset of erection with flow directed toward the corpus spongiosum (Fig. 5.10). No direct communications are appreciable between cavernosal-spongiosal communications and the urethral or bulbar arteries; as a consequence, these vessels are anatomically distinct from obvious cavernosal-spongiosal arterial communications.

5.4.8
Penile Veins

Depiction of penile veins at color Doppler ultrasound is inconstant in normal subjects due to low flow regimen both while flaccid and during erection (Kim et al. 2001). A variety of venous structures, however, can be identified during turgescence and especially during detumescence (Fig. 5.11). One or more superficial veins can be identified. A large vein is often recognized in the ventral aspect of the penis between the corpora cavernosa in patients with normal erection as well. A prominent deep dorsal vein

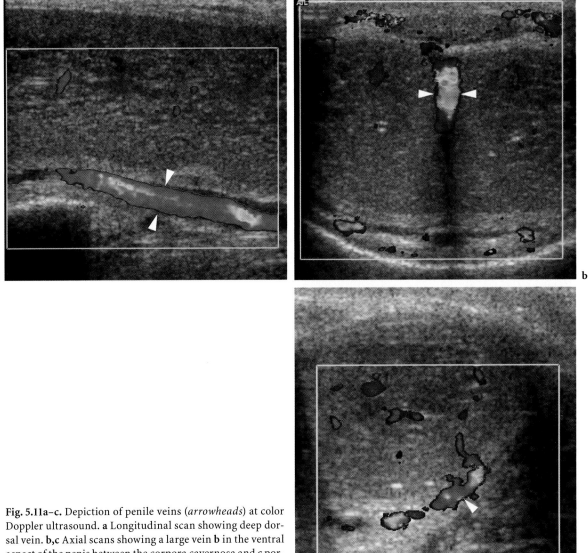

Fig. 5.11a–c. Depiction of penile veins (*arrowheads*) at color Doppler ultrasound. **a** Longitudinal scan showing deep dorsal vein. **b,c** Axial scans showing a large vein **b** in the ventral aspect of the penis between the corpora cavernosa and **c** portions of the emissary and circumflex veins

is commonly depicted and interrogated, but often several veins are recognized in the dorsal aspect of the penis below the Buck's fascia. These color Doppler findings are consistent with a recent anatomical study (Hsu et al. 2003). Visualization of portions of the subalbugineal venous plexus, emissary, and circumflex veins is uncommon.

5.5
Duplex Doppler Interrogation

Different Doppler waveforms are recognized in the cavernosal arteries while flaccid and during erection (Fitzgerald et al. 1991; Schwartz et al. 1991; Kim 2002). Peak systolic velocity varies significantly according to the sampling location. In general, velocity values are highest at proximal sites and decrease progressively at distal sites of measurement (Chiou et al. 1999). As a consequence, standardization of the sampling location is needed to reduce the variability of duplex Doppler interrogation of the cavernosal arteries, which is performed at the origin, where they angle posteriorly toward the crus, and a favourable Doppler angle is obtained (Kim 2002).

5.5.1
Cavernosal Arteries

These vessels present during the onset of erection with characteristic progression of Doppler waveform reflecting blood pressure changes within the cavernosal bodies (Fig. 5.12). Spectral waveform changes have been classified into six phases scored from 0 to 5 (Schwartz et al. 1991). In the flaccid state (phase 0) monophasic waveforms are recognized in the cavernosal arteries with low velocity, high resistance flow, typically of 15–25 cm/s. With the onset of erection (phase 1), there is an increase in systolic and diastolic flows. Peak systolic velocity >35 cm/s and diastolic velocity >8 cm/s are usually recorded in normal subjects in this phase. Peak systolic velocities as high as 80–100 cm/s and diastolic velocities of 20 cm/s or more are often recorded in young patients with normal erections. When the blood pressure within the corpora cavernosa begins to rise, a dicrotic notch appears at end systole, and a progressive decrease of the diastolic flow is observed (phase 2). When the cavernosal pressure equals the diastolic pressure, diastolic flow declines to zero. Holodiastolic flow reversal (phase 4) reflects cavernosal pressure above the diastolic pressure and full erection. During rigid erection the systolic envelope is narrowed and diastolic flow disappears (phase 5). The systolic peak reduces or even disappears, reflecting cavernosal pressure approaching or exceeding blood systolic pressure. Cavernosal phase 5 requires contraction of the bulbocavernous muscles and is not commonly observed after pharmacologically induced erection. The bulbocavernous reflex, however, can be stimulated with compression of the glans penis (Broderick and Arger 1993). During detumescence diastolic flow appears again.

5.5.2
Dorsal Arteries

These vessels are outside the tunica albuginea and therefore are not subjected to the intracorporeal pressure changes with each phase of erection; therefore, even in well-sustained rigidity, anterograde diastolic flow persists (Broderick and Arger 1993). Generally speaking, Doppler spectral pattern and peak systolic velocity of dorsal penile arteries increase from about 20 cm/s while flaccid to 40 cm/s or more during erection (Lee et al. 1993).

5.5.3
Arterial Communications

Doppler waveform changes of anastomotic arterial branches, dorsal-cavernous and cavernous-cavernous arterial communications are quite variable, depending on size and position along the shaft.

5.5.4
Helicine Arterioles

Specific characteristic changes have been identified in the helicine arterioles (Montorsi et al. 1998) reflecting waveform changes within the cavernosal arteries. In particular, an average peak systolic velocity of 21–23 cm/s and a mean diastolic velocitiy of 2–3 cm/s have been recorded in subjects with normal erection during cavernosal phase 1 and phase 2 at the origin of the helicine arterioles. Peak systolic velocity reduces progressively in the distal ramifications of these vessels. During cavernosal phase 3 and phase 4, the mean peak systolic velocity at the ori-

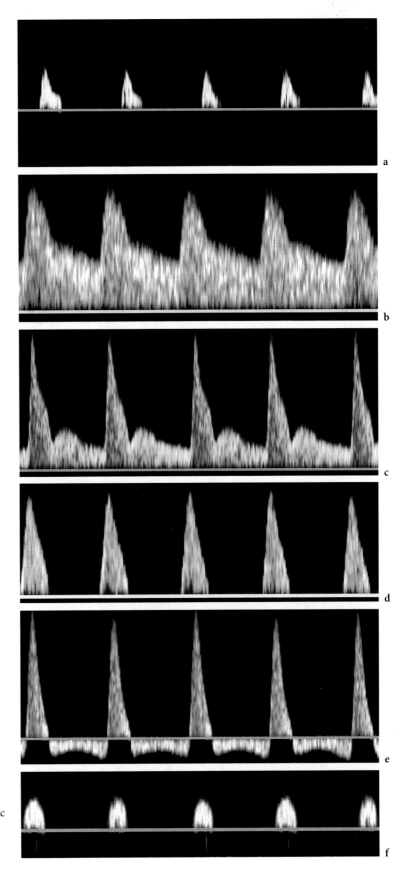

Fig. 5.12a–f. Normal waveform changes in the cavernosal arteries during the onset of erection. **a** Phase 0. Monophasic flow with minimal or no diastolic flow occurring in the flaccid state. **b** Phase 1. Increased systolic and diastolic flow. **c** Phase 2. Dicrotic notch appearance at end systole and progressive decrease of the diastolic flow. **d** Phase 3. End diastolic flow disappearance. **e** Phase 4. Diastolic flow reversal. **f** Phase 5. Reduction of the systolic peak during rigid erection

gin of the helicine arterioles reduces, and diastolic velocity declines to 0. During cavernosal phase 5 helicine arterioles disappear.

5.5.5
Cavernosal-Spongiosal Communications

Also in these vessels characteristic changes are recognized reflecting waveform changes within the cavernosal arteries (BERTOLOTTO et al. 2002). In particular, within the corpus cavernosum cavernosal-spongiosal communications have arterial waveforms, and peak systolic velocity increases from approximately 6 cm/s while flaccid to approximately 10 cm/s during erection. The resistive index progressively increases from cavernosal phase 1 to phase 3. When full erection is reached cavernosal-spongiosal communications tend to close and disappear or, in other cases, their diastolic velocity markedly reduces or declines to 0. A characteristic Doppler spectrum can be appreciable with a positive diastolic flow, which can be due to a steel phenomenon towards the corpus spongiosum and an inverse systolic peak that is likely due to the hydraulic "ram stroke" produced near the occlusion site (Fig. 5.13).

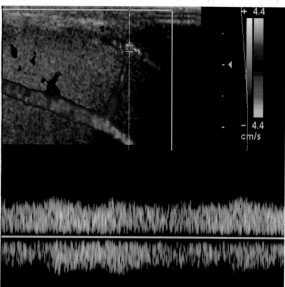

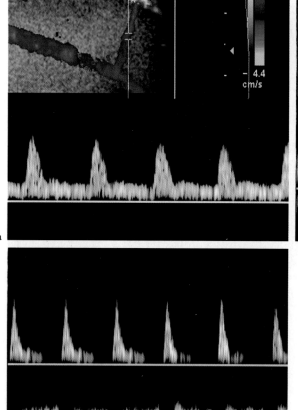

Fig. 5.13a–c. Duplex Doppler interrogation of cavernosal-spongiosal communcations. **a** Within the corpus cavernosum the vessel has an arterial waveform, whereas **b** after the passage of the tunica albuginea a venous waveform is recorded. **c** Doppler interrogation during full erection (cavernosal phase 4) shows diastolic flow disappearance or positive diastolic flow with systolic peak inversion

Immediately after the passage of the tunica albuginea, venous waveforms are recorded in the same vessels or arterial flows with very low vascular resistances.

References

Bertolotto M, Neumaier CE (1999) Penile sonography. Eur Radiol 9 [Suppl 3]:S407–412

Bertolotto M, Neumaier CE, Martinoli C et al (2002) Color Doppler appearance of penile cavernosal-spongiosal communications in patients with normal and impaired erection. Eur Radiol 12:2287–2293

Broderick GA, Arger P (1993) Duplex Doppler ultrasonography: noninvasive assessment of penile anatomy and function. Semin Roentgenol 28:43–56

Chiou RK, Alberts GL, Pomeroy BD et al (1999) Study of cavernosal arterial anatomy using color and power Doppler sonography: impact on hemodynamic parameter measurement. J Urol 162:358–360

Doubilet PM, Benson CB, Silverman SG, Gluck CD (1991) The penis. Semin Ultrasound CT MR 12:157–175

Droupy S, Giuliano F, Jardin A, Benoit G (1999) Caverno-spongious shunts: anatomical study of intrapenile vascular pathways. Eur Urol 36:123–128

Fitzgerald SW, Erickson SJ, Foley WD et al (1991) Color Doppler sonography in the evaluation of erectile dysfunction: patterns of temporal response to papaverine. AJR Am J Roentgenol 157:331–336

Gotta SF, Kassaniou S, Kokoua A, Gnanazan NG (2003) [Anatomic study of arterial and venous cavernospongious shunt in the human penis: surgical findings]. Ann Urol (Paris) 37:135–139

Hsu GL, Hsieh CH, Wen HS et al (2003) Penile venous anatomy: an additional description and its clinical implication. J Androl 24:921–927

Hsu GL, Hsieh CH, Wen HS et al (2004) Anatomy of the human penis: the relationship of the architecture between skeletal and smooth muscles. J Androl 25:426–431

Hsu GL, Lin CW, Hsieh CH et al (2005) Distal ligament in human glans: a comparative study of penile architecture. J Androl 26:624–628

Jarow JP, Pugh VW, Routh WD, Dyer RB (1993) Comparison of penile duplex ultrasonography to pudendal arteriography. Variant penile arterial anatomy affects interpretation of duplex ultrasonography. Invest Radiol 28:806–810

Juskiewenski s, Vaysse P, Moscovici J et al (1982) A study of the arterial blood supply to the penis. Anat Clin 4:101–107

Kim JM, Joh YD, Huh JD, Choi S (2001) Doppler sonography of the penile cavernosal artery: comparison of intraurethral instillation and intracorporeal injection of prostaglandin E1. J Clin Ultrasound 29:273–278

Kim SH (2002) Doppler US evaluation of erectile dysfunction. Abdom Imaging 27:578–587

Kishore TA, Bhat S, John RP (2005) Colour Doppler ultrasonographic location of the bulbourethral artery, and its impact on surgical outcome. BJU Int 96:624–628

Lee B, Sikka SC, Randrup ER et al (1993) Standardization of penile blood flow parameters in normal men using intracavernous prostaglandin E1 and visual sexual stimulation. J Urol 149:49–52

Lin JT, Bradley WE (1985) Penile neuropathy in insulin-dependent diabetes mellitus. J Urol 133:213–215

Lue TF, Hricak H, Marich KW, Tanagho EA (1985) Vasculogenic impotence evaluated by high-resolution ultrasonography and pulsed Doppler spectrum analysis. Radiology 155:777–781

Lue TF, Tanagho EA (1987) Physiology of erection and pharmacological management of impotence. J Urol 137:829–836

Montorsi F, Sarteschi M, Maga T et al (1998) Functional anatomy of cavernous helicine arterioles in potent subjects. J Urol 159:808–810

Mueller SC, Lue TF (1988) Evaluation of vasculogenic impotence. Urol Clin North Am 15:65–76

Quam JP, King BF, James EM et al (1989) Duplex and color Doppler sonographic evaluation of vasculogenic impotence. AJR Am J Roentgenol 153:1141–1147

Schwartz AN, Lowe M, Berger RE et al (1991) Assessment of normal and abnormal erectile function: color Doppler flow sonography versus conventional techniques. Radiology 180:105–109

Wagner G, Willis EA, Bro-Rasmussen F, Nielsen MH (1982) New theory on the mechanism of erection involving hitherto undescribed vessels. Lancet 1:416–418

Wahl SI, Rubin MB, Bakal CW (1997) Radiologic evaluation of penile arterial anatomy in arteriogenic impotence. Int J Impot Res 9:93–97

US Evaluation of Erectile Dysfunction

Pietro Pavlica, Massimo Valentino, and Libero Barozzi

CONTENTS

6.1 Background 39
6.2 Preliminary Clinical Assessment 39
6.3 Ultrasonography 42
6.3.1 Environment 42
6.3.2 Transducers 42
6.3.3 Vasoactive Drug Delivery 43
6.3.3.1 Intracavernosal Injection 43
6.3.3.2 Transurethral Drug Delivery 44
6.3.3.3 Transdermal Drug Delivery 44
6.3.4 Scanning 44
6.3.5 Timing 45
6.4 Ultrasound Imaging Findings in Erectile Dysfunction 45
6.4.1 Grey-Scale Ultrasound Findings 45
6.4.2 Color Doppler Imaging 46
6.4.3 Spectral Doppler Imaging 48
6.5 Other Imaging Modalities 51
6.6 Complications 52
References 52

6.1 Background

Grey-scale and color-Doppler ultrasonographies are the most widely used, non-invasive and readily available imaging modalities for diagnostic purposes in studying erectile dysfunction (Lehmann et al. 1996). In fact, after clinical examination, it is the first tool in imaging algorithms used for the evaluation of the anatomic and functional status of the penis and of the penile vessels in patients who complain of erectile problems (NIH 1993).

P. Pavlica, MD; M. Valentino, MD; L. Barozzi, MD
Department of Radiology, University Hospital S. Orsola-Malpighi, Via Massarenti 9, Bologna, 40138, Italy

The examination should be goal-oriented, depending on the clinical problem at hand. Although the anatomy and acoustic structure of the corpora cavernosa may be informative, the functional characteristics after pharmacological stimulation are more important and are performed in real time ultrasound (Bertolotto and Neumaier 1999). Diagnosis is usually performed during scanning, on the basis of both structural and functional data (Meuleman et al. 1992b). When performing the exam a standard set of images is mandatory for general survey and special views can be indicated to detect particular lesions (Lue 1993).

6.2 Preliminary Clinical Assessment

Prior to instrumental or invasive procedures, patient-reported assessment should be performed. Patient self report, administered questionnaires, event logs or simple patient diaries are commonly used for the diagnosis of erectile dysfunction (Rosen et al. 2006).

The International Index of Erectile Function (IIEF) questionnaire (Table 6.1) can be used to measure the erectile function (Rosen et al. 1997). It simplifies the preliminary assessment and can help to evaluate and define the cause of the erectile dysfunction and identify the underlying vascular issue. Even though the IIEF questionnaire was originally proposed to evaluate the results of treatments, it can also be used in clinical practice to evaluate the erectile function in all patients attending ultrasound investigation. The questionnaire has been shown to be highly versatile and can be employed in all patients with erectile dysfunction regardless of the cause, co-morbidities and cultural background.

Table 6.1. International Index of Erectile Function (IIEF)

Q1	How often were you able to get an erection during sexual activity? 0 = no sexual activity; 1 = almost never or never; 2 = a few times (less than half the time); 3 = sometimes (about half the time); 4 = most times (more than half the time); 5 = almost always or always
Q2	When you had erections with sexual stimulation, how often were your erections hard enough for penetration? 0 = no sexual activity; 1 = almost never or never; 2 = a few times (less than half the time); 3 = sometimes (about half the time); 4 = most times (more than half the time); 5 = almost always or always
Q3	When you attempted intercourse, how often were you able to penetrate (enter) your partner? 0 = did not attempt intercourse; 1 = almost never or never; 2 = a few times (less than half the time); 3 = sometimes (about half the time); 4 = most times (more than half the time); 5 = almost always or always
Q4	During sexual intercourse, how often were you able to maintain your erection after you had penetrated (entered) your partner? 0 = did not attempt intercourse; 1 = almost never or never; 2 = a few times (less than half the time); 3 = sometimes (about half the time); 4 = most times (more than half the time); 5 = almost always or always
Q5	During sexual intercourse, how difficult was it to maintain your erection to completion of intercourse? 0 = did not attempt intercourse; 1 = extremely difficult; 2 = very difficult; 3 = difficult; 4 = slightly difficult; 5 = not difficult
Q6	How many times have you attempted sexual intercourse? 0 = no attempts; 1 = 1 to 2 attempts; 2 = 3 to 4 attempts; 3 = 5 to 6 attempts; 4 = 7 to 10 attempts; 5 = ≥11 attempts
Q7	When you attempted sexual intercourse, how often was it satisfactory for you? 0 = did not attempt intercourse; 1 = almost never or never; 2 = a few times (less than half the time); 3 = sometimes (about half the time); 4 = most times (more than half the time); 5 = almost always or always
Q8	How much have you enjoyed sexual intercourse? 0 = no intercourse; 1 = no enjoyment at all; 2 = not very enjoyable; 3 = fairly enjoyable; 4 = highly enjoyable; 5 = very highly enjoyable
Q9	When you had sexual stimulation or intercourse, how often did you ejaculate? 0 = no sexual stimulation or intercourse; 1 = almost never or never; 2 = a few times (less than half the time); 3 = sometimes (about half the time); 4 = most times (more than half the time); 5 = almost always or always
Q10	When you had sexual stimulation or intercourse, how often did you have the feeling of orgasm or climax? 1 = almost never or never; 2 = a few times (less than half the time); 3 = sometimes (about half the time); 4 = most times (more than half the time); 5 = almost always or always
Q11	How often have you felt sexual desire? 1 = almost never or never; 2 = a few times (less than half the time); 3 = sometimes (about half the time); 4 = most times (more than half the time); 5 = almost always or always
Q12	How would you rate your level of sexual desire? 1 = very low or none at all; 2 = low; 3 = moderate; 4 = high; 5 = very high
Q13	How satisfied have you been with your overall sex life? 1 = very dissatisfied; 2 = moderately dissatisfied; 3 = equally satisfied and dissatisfied; 4 = moderately satisfied; 5 = very satisfied
Q14	How satisfied have you been with your sexual relationship with your partner? 1 = very dissatisfied; 2 = moderately dissatisfied; 3 = equally satisfied and dissatisfied; 4 = moderately satisfied; 5 = very satisfied
Q15	How do you rate your confidence that you could get and keep an erection? 1 = very low or none at all; 2 = low; 3 = moderate; 4 = high; 5 = very high

A simplified and reduced version has been developed (Table 6.2), called the Sexual Health Inventory for Men (SHIM), and is used in clinical practice as a valid method to evaluate the severity of erectile dysfunction (Rosen et al. 2002). The SHIM score also allows the efficacy of treatment to be monitored.

These two indices give a global evaluation of erectile function, but do not assess other sexual disorders since they do not provide information regarding the causes of erectile dysfunction, which can be organic or psychological or secondary to other health issues (diabetes, cardiovascular disease, drugs, neurological disease, etc.).

Another important issue in the initial medical and sexual history of the patient regards the erection hardness, which is fundamentally key to erectile function. An Evaluation Hardness Grading Scale (EHGS) can be used (Table 6.3), consisting of a self-reported measure that classifies erection hardness on a four-point scale (Mulhall et al. 2006). This evaluation is very simple and quick to perform and gives important clinical information of patient satisfaction of his erectile function.

Table 6.2. Sexual Health Inventory for Men (SHIM)

Over the past 6 months						
1. How do you rate your confidence that you could get and keep an erection?		Very low 1	Low 2	Moderate 3	High 4	Very high 5
2. When you had erections with sexual stimulation, how often were your erections hard enough for penetration (entering your partner)?	No sexual activity 0	Almost never or never 1	A few times (much less than half the time) 2	Sometimes (about half the time) 3	Most times (much more than half the time) 4	(Almost always or always 5
3. During sexual intercourse, how often were you able to maintain your erection after you had penetrated (entered) your partner?	Did not attempt intercourse 0	Almost never or never 1	A few times (much less than half the time) 2	Sometimes (about half the time) 3	Most times (much more than half the time) 4	(Almost always or always) 5
4. During sexual intercourse, how difficult was it to maintain your erection to completion of intercourse?	Did not attempt intercourse 0	Extremely difficult 1	Very difficult 2	Difficult 3	Slightly difficult 4	Not difficult 5
5. When you attempted sexual intercourse, how often was it satisfactory for you?	Did not attempt intercourse 0	Almost never or never 1	A few times (much less than half the time) 2	Sometimes (about half the time) 3	Most times (much more than half the time) 4	Almost always or always 5

Add the numbers corresponding to questions 1-5 to obtain the SHIM score. The Sexual Health Inventory for Men further classifies erectile dysfunction (ED) with the following breakpoints: 1-7 severe ED; 8-11 moderate ED; 12-16 mild to moderate ED; 17-21 mild ED

Table 6.3. Erection Hardness Grading Scale (EHGS)

Grade	Definition of erection hardness
1	Increase in size of penis, but not hardness (rigidity)
2	Increase in size and slight increase in hardness (rigidity), but insufficient for sexual intercorse
3	Increase in hardness (rigidity), sufficient for sexual intercourse, but not fully hard (rigid)
4	Fully hard rigid erection

6.3
Ultrasonography

Ultrasound evaluation of patients with erectile dysfunction should be performed in the appropriate environment, respecting the privacy of the patient. Good quality equipment and transducers suited to evaluation of superficial structures must be used.

6.3.1
Environment

The sonographic examination of the patient with erectile dysfunction cannot be considered corresponding to a conventional ultrasound scanning, but requires some basic rules of privacy, avoiding all the negative factors depending on the environment, which can interfere dangerously with the erectile phenomenon (BRODERICK 1998).

An independent and dedicated ultrasound laboratory supplied with the technical requirements that can amplify or improve the action of the drugs used to induce the erection is desirable, even if not mandatory. In any case the laboratory where the examination is performed must be locked, and nobody should be allowed to enter during the examination time. Low lighting is preferable and the presence of a maximum of two medical staff. Avoiding the presence of nurses is recommended with the exclusion of the preliminary phases to reduce the negative influence of psychological factors. After the intracavernosal drug injection, the patients can be left alone before the Doppler measurements on both cavernosal arteries are performed. Once the evaluated parameters become stable, but the erection obtained is insufficient or absent, the patient is usually left alone for some minutes and invited to stimulate the penis manually. If the degree of the rigidity obtained is less than the best spontaneous erection referred by the patient during normal sexual activity, a second dose of prostaglandin can be injected. When a venous erectile dysfunction is suspected, it is useful to ask the patient to stand and invite him to walk, because this will increase the erection and reduce the examination time. The increased erection obtained is psychologically important for the patient.

To improve the drug response, audiovisual sexual stimulation has been proposed to promote smooth muscle relaxation during penile color Doppler examination. Audiovisual stimulation is performed with commercially available virtual glasses with tridimensional capabilities and stereophonic headphones. The device allows the patient to be cut off from the surrounding environment without increasing test-related stress and anxiety. This type of induced arousal suggests the possibility of performing the dynamic evaluation with a reduced dose of the drug or with simple oral agents in place of intracavernosal injection (PESCATORI et al. 2000; PARK et al. 2002). The clinical results are suggestive, but the method is not in very widespread use and needs more extensive confirmation.

6.3.2
Transducers

Technical requirements for grey-scale and color Doppler ultrasonography of the penis are described in detail in Chapter 1. In particular, high frequency small-parts transducers are mandatory, preferably with high density crystals so that an elevated spatial resolution is possible both at grey-scale and color-Doppler ultrasound (BERTOLOTTO and NEUMAIER 1999).

Gain and power settings should be optimized so that all structures of the penis are appreciable. Harmonic imaging and 3D reconstruction techniques can be used, if available, but they are not mandatory for the diagnosis even though they can offer a more detailed image of the small post-cavernosal arteries, which are frequently compromised in subjects with diabetes or systemic arterial disease.

6.3.3
Vasoactive Drug Delivery

A variety of techniques have been suggested for delivery of vasoactive drugs in patients with erectile dysfunction undergoing color Doppler evaluation. While the most commonly used method is intracavernosal injection, other modalities such as transurethral and transdermal drug delivery have been considered, in the attempt to reduce the invasive character of the study, and risk of possible complications.

6.3.3.1
Intracavernosal Injection

Intracavernosal injection of vasoactive substances (dynamic penile ultrasonography) is one of the most important phases in the examination of patients with erectile dysfunction (CORMIO et al. 1996). This minimally invasive procedure is associated with anxiety and apprehension that may negatively influence the erectile response and cause false-positive results.

The substances used in the clinical practice vary in composition, dose and mechanism of action (MEULEMAN et al. 1992a). Sometimes they can be used simultaneously in the same mixture. Currently, the most diffuse product is prostaglandin E1 (PGE1), which is used at doses varying from 5 mcg to 20 mcg. It is a product with a high level of security and safety, because it seldom induces a persistent priapism that requires medical or surgical interventions.

The employed dose is selected on the basis of the preliminary clinical assessment, which allows the patients to be divided into two main groups. The first includes subjects who still have nocturnal erections and some preserved sexual activity; in this group a single dose of 5 or 10 mcg can be sufficient, but, if an incomplete erection is obtained, a second injection can be performed after 30 min to differentiate a real organic erectile dysfunction from an insufficient response to a low dose of the drug (LEHMANN et al. 1999; CHEN et al. 2000). The second group includes those who report short erections, generally insufficient to perform a complete intercourse. In this case a 20-mcg dose of PGE1 is preferred (LEHMANN et al. 1999). Prostaglandins can be responsible for a long-standing erection that lasts 3–4 h associated with pain, which generally disappears spontaneously probably as a consequence of the complete metabolic consumption by the intracavernosal enzymes.

Papaverine is the second most used drug to stimulate erections at a dose ranging from 10 to 40 mg. A great individual variability in the response to the same dose has been observed and the time of erection is usually longer than that obtained with PGE1 (FITZGERALD et al. 1991). The most common systemic signs are secondary to peripheral vasodilatation with a sense of heat and occasionally hypotension. These effects are sometimes not tolerated by the patients performing self-injection at home. Focal fibrosis of the erectile tissue or diffuse corporeal fibrosis have been frequently observed and are the consequence of focal or diffuse ischemia of the erectile tissue. For these reasons papaverine is currently not used systematically even though its erectile effect is more intense and the rigidity more evident than with other vasoactive products.

The relaxation of the erectile tissue and the vasodilatation obtained with papaverine are generally more evident, probably because of the higher quantity of nitric oxide (NO) involved. The action of the NO is essentially an arterial vasodilatation, while the effect on the cavernosal musculature is less evident.

Other drugs used are phentolamine and phenoxybenzamine, alpha-lytic drugs that produce relaxation of the smooth muscle of the arterial wall and of the erectile tissue. Some authors have proposed the use of a mixture of all three vasoactive substances, whose action is similar, but probably follow different biochemical pathways: papaverine, phentolamine and prostaglandin.

The erectile response observed in patients without arteriogenic erectile dysfunction is usually intense and the incidence of priapism frequent. The association called "Trimix" shows a high incidence of complications, and the individual dose is difficult to define (GOVIER et al. 1995).

The intracavernosal injection is performed on the lateral aspect of the penis at the proximal or medial third of the shaft (Fig. 6.1). Commonly, a 30-G needle is used and the puncture is performed away from the dorsal nerves of the penis. Intraspongiosal or intraurethral injection should be carefully avoided. Incorrect puncture can produce pain, particularly if performed near the dorsal nerves, or urethral pain/heat, if the product has been injected into the corpus spongiosum. Subcutaneous injections cause less pain and local swelling, but no erection. These complications are more frequently observed in patients at the beginning of self-injection.

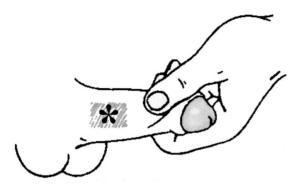

Fig. 6.1. Schematic drawing showing the elective site on the lateral surface of the penis (*) where to perform intracavernosal drug injection

6.3.3.2
Transurethral Drug Delivery

In place of intracavernosal injection to examine patients with erectile dysfunction intraurethral instillation of prostaglandin E1 at the dose of 0.5 mg has been proposed as an alternative method to reduce the distress connected to the direct injection (TAM et al. 1998). Although the urethral mucosa is not the best route of drug transfer, its anatomical structure with numerous submucosal veins that communicate between the corpus spongiosum and the corpora cavernosa can be considered an alternative way to induce erection. Color Doppler parameters and specifically peak systolic velocity (PSV) measured the increase statistically, and in about 65% erections sufficient for intercourse were obtained. The transurethral administration of prostaglandin E1 has shown a positive effect in the treatment of a substantial proportion of men with chronic erectile dysfunction, but the procedure is not suitable to define the nature and the severity of it (PADMA-NATHAN et al. 1997).

6.3.3.3
Transdermal Drug Delivery

Some authors have studied the possibility to deliver prostaglandin E1 using transdermal liposomal formulations through the foreskin in men with erectile dysfunction secondary to spinal cord injury or with mild arterial insufficiency (FOLDVARI et al. 1998).

Topical applications of drugs can increase PSV by 15 to 22 cm/s (KIM and MCVARY 1995). Also the mean cavernosal artery diameter has been reported to increase by 0.9 to 1.1 mm. The highest flow velocity is archived at 45 min after the application of the product, but the results are variable and inconstant, and the method cannot be proposed to evaluate the nature of the erectile dysfunction.

6.3.4
Scanning

Ultrasound examination of the penis in patients with erectile dysfunction is performed with scans at rest, before induced erection and in the erection/tumescence phases. After intracorporeal drug injection scans are usually performed after 5, 10, 15 and 20 min at the level of both cavernosal arteries. Scanning is preferably made on the ventral surface, especially when the erection is obtained, because the probe orientation is particularly favorable to study the cavernosal flow. The basal study generally has a low diagnostic yield and can be omitted if a preliminary clinical evaluation has been performed. After drug injection grey-scale scanning is performed that allows a good detection of the cavernosal arteries and evaluation of the cavernosal tissue distension. The septum and the tunica albuginea are well depicted.

Afterwards color imaging is performed using a reduced field of view to maintain a high frame rate. Pulse repetition frequency (PRF) values of 1,000–1,500 Hz are employed with a low wall filter. Longitudinal scans on the cavernosal arteries are performed with steering of the color box so that a good definition of the blood flow is acquired. The cavernosal arteries have a parallel course to the linear probe with a non-favorable Doppler angle, because of being perpendicular to the direction of flow. The sample volume size is about 1 mm, which is the corresponding measure of the diameter of the cavernosal vessels. Color imaging allows an easy detection of the arteries from the base of the penis down to the retrobalanic zone. Grey-scale and color Doppler anatomy of the penis has been described in Chapter 5. Briefly, anatomical variations of the cavernosal arteries are present in 20–30% of the patients with double or triple arterial vessels. They can have the same outer diameter or can be different in size and length. The blood velocities measured are dependent of their diameter (MANCINI et al. 1996). The helicine arterioles and their branches can be easily detected because of their perpendicular course in respect to the probe. The 3D reconstruction of the intracorporeal vessels allows defining the spatial distribution of the small vessels and a semiquantitative evaluation of the vascular density and of the size of the helicine arterioles, which are frequently compromised in patients with diabetes or systemic vascular pathology.

Following identification at color Doppler ultrasound, the cavernosal vessels are interrogated. Pulse-wave (PW) duplex Doppler is turned on putting the sample volume on the cavernosal arteries. The spectral analysis is preferably performed at the base of the penis where the Doppler angle is particularly favorable (between 30° and 50°) and the flow velocity shows major reproducibility and correctness (MILLS and SETHIA 1996). The flow velocity must be measured repeatedly (at least three times) at the same level and the mean value reported. Functional studies have shown a progressive decrease of blood velocity in the cavernosal arteries from the base to the glans penis

6.3.5
Timing

The time necessary to obtain an erection after pharmacostimulation varies greatly from one patient to another. For this reason continuous monitoring is necessary up to 30–40 min. In some subjects a rapid erection is observed after 5 min, but in the majority of the examinations it is necessary to wait 15–20 min to have a stable erection. If the erection does not realize after 20 min, it is good practice to prolong the test to 30–40 min to exclude late responses. To reduce the time to erection the patient can be invited to stand up and to walk in the ultrasound laboratory. Sexual visual stimulation can be employed with good results (ERBAGCI et al. 2002). All these maneuvers increase the erection firmness especially in patients with venous leakage because of the increase of the venous pressure in the superficial and deep venous network of the penis (PESCATORI et al. 2000; PARK et al. 2002).

6.4
Ultrasound Imaging Findings in Erectile Dysfunction

Several changes are detected in patients with erectile dysfunction that are useful to differentiate among different underlying causes for this condition. In particular, anatomical and vascular alterations can be evaluated at grey-scale and color Doppler ultrasound, as well as pathological spectral changes in the cavernosal arteries and in other penile vessels.

6.4.1
Grey-Scale Ultrasound Findings

The morphological aspects to define with grey-scale ultrasonography are the presence of calcifications and kinking of the cavernosal arteries; diameter and size changes of the cavernosal arteries before and after pharmacological injection; distension and texture of the erectile tissue evaluated before and during erection.

In older patients, and in those suffering from diabetes or chronic renal failure, microcalcifications in the wall of the cavernosal arteries are frequently detectable and are the expression of calcium deposits in atheromatous endothelial plaques (Fig. 6.2) or in the tunica media as observed in subjects on chronic hemodialysis (Fig. 6.3).

Measurement of the diameter changes in the cavernosal arteries after drug injection is clinically more useful since it expresses the stiffness of the arterial wall. In normal subjects there is normally a 75 to 120% increase in size of the vessels whose diameter is of 0.5–0.7 mm at rest and 1–1.2 mm after stimulation. This measurement is performed using the maximum electronic magnification of the scanner to reduce errors due to incorrect positioning of the electronic calipers (CHIOU et al. 1999).

The size increase of the arteries in patients with arteriogenic ED is usually less than 75%. The functional response of the vessels to the drug is non-specific and not always expression of stenosis or obstruction, but can be secondary to a reduced elasticity or contraction of the muscular wall. A normal vascular response is considered when the increase in size is of 100% or more with respect to the basal values.

The measurement of the diameter changes of the corpora cavernosa during the different phases of erection is another parameter that has been used. The distension can be asymmetric because of reduced relaxation of the cavernosal tissue on one site due to structural changes (fibrosis) or secondary to unilateral reduced flow because of unilateral arterial obstruction (Fig. 6.4).

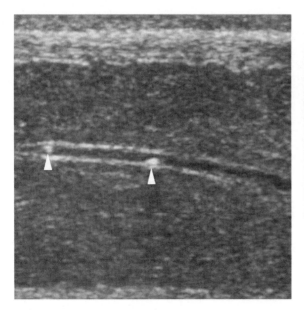

Fig. 6.2. Longitudinal scan. Thickening of the cavernosal artery wall with calcifications (*arrowheads*) in a patient with diabetes

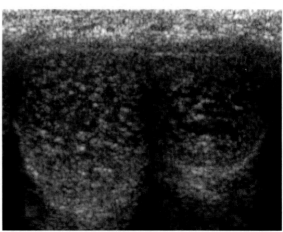

Fig. 6.4. Transversal scan. Asymmetric distension of the corpora cavernosa secondary to obstruction of the left cavernosal artery

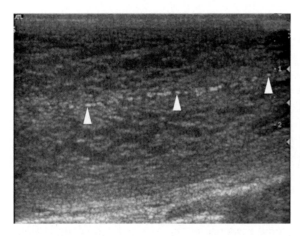

Fig. 6.3. Longitudinal scan. Diffuse small calcifications of the cavernosal arteries (*arrowheads*) in a patient in chronic hemodialysis

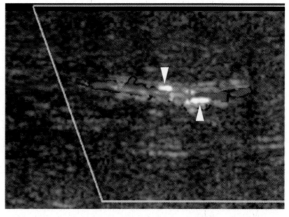

Fig. 6.5. Longitudinal scan. Reduced distension with calcifications (*arrowheads*) and stenosis of the cavernosal artery in severe arteriogenic erectile dysfunction

The measurement of the area of the corpora cavernosa in the transversal scan is simple using the electronic facilities of the ultrasound equipment. It is possible to calculate immediately the area delimitated with the trackball. Actually these measurements are rarely used in the clinical practice because penile changes in size and rigidity are well evaluated clinically and manually (NELSON and LUE 1989).

6.4.2
Color Doppler Imaging

Color imaging is fundamental to identify the cavernosal arteries and to detect the presence and direction of flow, especially in patients with reduced distension of the vessel (Fig. 6.5) after drug stimulation (MANCINI et al. 2000). The vessel kinkings, stenosis or obstruction are easily identified (Fig. 6.6). Obstructions appear as non-colored segments (Fig. 6.7) of the arteries, while stenoses are associated with areas of increased velocity and post-stenotic turbulence. Color Doppler imaging is useful to detect flow in the cavernoso-dorsal (Fig. 6.8) and cavernoso-urethral anastomoses, which are common in patients with arteriogenic erectile dysfunction.

Because of extensive arterial lesions, the flow in the elicine arteries is reduced (Fig. 6.9), and sometimes the distal part of the cavernosal arteries is not visualized because of reduced flow velocity (Sarteschi et al. 1998). Power Doppler imaging (Fig. 6.10) and the 3D rendering techniques (Fig. 6.11) are proposed to detect the arterial wall lesions and the distribution of the elicine arteries in subjects with diffuse lesions of the small intracorporeal vessels as observed in diabetics (Montorsi et al. 1998; Klingler et al. 1999).

In patients with venous occlusive erectile dysfunction the cavernosal flow is elevated and easily detected. The vessels show an increased diameter and can be followed for a long course in the center of the corpus cavernosum. The helicine arterioles are numerous and visible up to the tunica albuginea

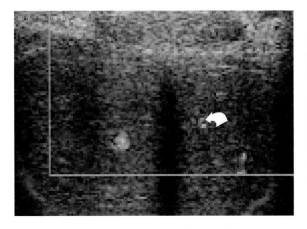

Fig. 6.6. Color Doppler in transversal scan after pharmacostimulation showing differences in size between the cavernosal arteries. The left artery (*curved arrow*) is smaller in diameter with reduced flow velocity

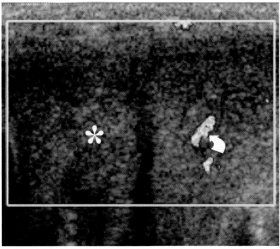

Fig. 6.7. Transversal scan. Complete obstruction of the right cavernosal artery with no flow detectable (*). Normal-appearing left cavernosal artery (*curved arrow*)

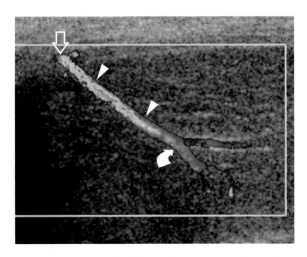

Fig. 6.8. Cavernoso-dorsal arterial anastomosis in a patient with erectile dysfunction. Color Doppler imaging shows a vessel (*arrowheads*) connecting the dorsal artery (*open arrow*) to the cavernosal artery (*curved arrow*)

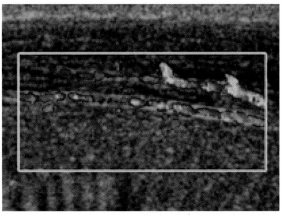

Fig. 6.9. Longitudinal scan. Double cavernosal artery showing wall stiffness and a marked reduction of visibility of helicine arterioles

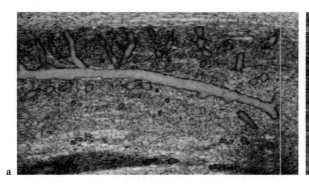
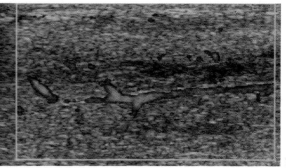

Fig. 6.10a,b. Power Doppler images in longitudinal scans showing the differences between the number and distribution of the elicine arteries in a normal subject (**a**) and in a diabetic patient (**b**)

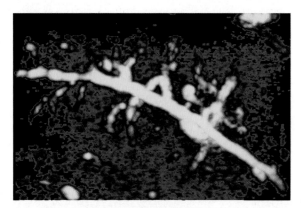

Fig. 6.11. Longitudinal scan. 3D rendering obtained from power Doppler images showing poor visibility and irregularity of helicine arterioles

(HAMPSON et al. 1992). Venous leakage pathways are patent (Fig. 6.12).

6.4.3
Spectral Doppler Imaging

Spectral analysis is the most important parameter used to characterize the severity and the nature of the erectile dysfunction (KNISPEL and ANDRESEN 1992). It is possible to calculate semiquantitatively the penile perfusion and indirectly to calculate the intracorporeal pressure, which are the main factors that influence the validity and duration of the erection (SHABSIGH et al. 1989).

There is a general agreement that the peak systolic velocity (PSV) measured at the level of the peno-scrotal junction is the best parameter for a clinical judgment of the arterial perfusion (OATES et al. 1995). PSV above 35 cm/s is considered the expression of a normally functioning arterial tree, even though arteriography can detect atheromatous parietal lesions that are hemodynamically non-significant. When the Doppler examination reveals a PSV less than 25 cm/s, the erectile dysfunction is considered of arteriogenic origin (Fig. 6.13) with a sensitivity of about 100% and a specificity of 95% as shown by the arteriographic studies that correlated flow data with arteriographic images (VALJI and BOOKSTEIN 1993).

Much more complex is the clinical evaluation of patients who show PSV values between 25 and 35 cm/s. This range of values is commonly observed in older subjects with mild erectile dysfunction (Fig. 6.14). Probably they have a stiffness of the arterial walls with intimal thickening and reduced response to PGE1 stimulation, secondary to an endothelial lesion and reduced NO production. In these patients stenosis or obstruction of the precavernosal arteries can be suspected and the flow study of these larger vessels should be performed. The terminal branches of the internal pudendal artery can be explored with a high linear frequency probe positioned in the perineal area under the scrotum.

The flow detected at the level of the cavernosal arteries can be asymmetric, and when the difference of PSV is greater than 10 cm/s a unilateral arterial insufficiency must be suspected with secondary flow impairment (Fig. 6.15).

When the arterial obstruction is complete, color Doppler imaging can show flow inversion in the cavernosal artery, easily detected in the longitudinal and transversal scans because of the different color of flow (Fig. 6.16). At spectral analysis the flow is reversed in the proximal portion of the artery and normally directed in the distal part. The curve obtained is of low amplitude with increased time to peak. The

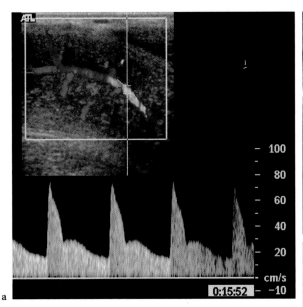
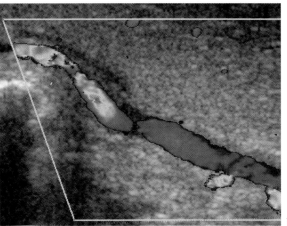
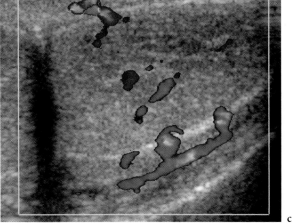

Fig. 6.12a–c. Venous occlusive erectile dysfunction. **a** Doppler interrogation of the cavernosal artery during maximum penile turgidity after cavernosal injection of 20 μg of prostaglandin E1 shows high-velocity cavernosal artery flows of 77 cm/s and persistent end diastolic velocity of 18 cm/s. **b,c** Evidence of blood flow within the dorsal vein (**b**) and within the perforant and circumflex veins (**c**). (Reprinted with permission from: Bertolotto M, Gasparini C, Calderan L, Lissiani A, Cova MA (2005) Color Doppler ultrasonography of the penis: state of the art. Giornale Italiano di Ecografia 8: 113–127)

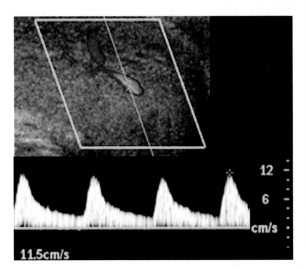

Fig. 6.13. Longitudinal scan. Arteriogenic erectile dysfunction with PSV of 11.5 cm/s measured at the base of the penis

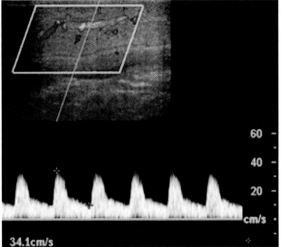

Fig. 6.14. Longitudinal scan. Erectile dysfunction in a subject with PSV of 34 cm/s. These borderline values are clinically common. The origin of erectile dysfunction is difficult to define

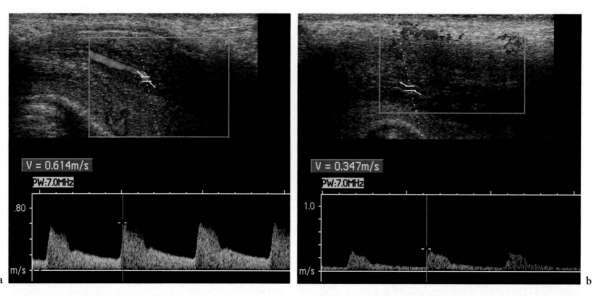

Fig. 6.15a,b. Differences in PSV between the two cavernosal arteries in a patient with mild erectile dysfunction. **a** On the right side 61 cm/s are measured, while **b** on the left 34 cm/s are measured consistent with unilateral arterial damage

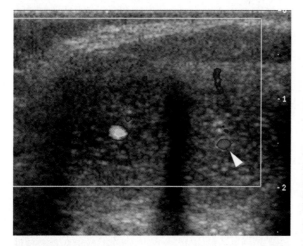

Fig. 6.16. Transversal scan. Color Doppler image showing flow inversion in the left cavernosal artery (*arrowhead*) consistent with arterial obstruction and retrograde recanalization. (Reprinted with permission from: Bertolotto M, Gasparini C, Calderan L, Lissiani A, Cova MA (2005) Color Doppler ultrasonography of the penis: state of the art. Giornale Italiano di Ecografia 8: 113–127)

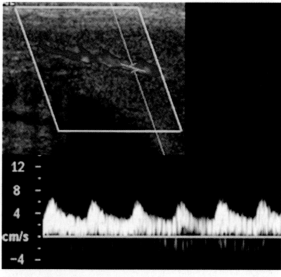

Fig. 6.17. Longitudinal scan. Mixed type of erectile dysfunction with low systolic flow (<10 cm/s) and persistent diastolic flow measured at the base of the penis

blood flows from the contralateral patent cavernous artery or from the dorsal artery through transeptal or dorso-cavernosal anastomoses (Wegner et al. 1995). Cavernosal-spongiosal communications with reversed flow can refill the cavernosal artery retrogradely as well.

Spectral curve in patients with arteriogenic erectile dysfunction is characterized by the absence of typical phase variations that can be observed in normal subjects. The flow is reduced and unchanged during the whole scanning time.

Valid erections can sometimes be observed in patients with extensive arteriogenic lesions and PSV below 25 cm/s, but with a preserved and active veno-occlusive mechanism that compensates for the reduced arterial inflow. In these cases the beginning of the erection is delayed, but can sometimes be long standing.

Veno-occlusive erectile dysfunction is more common in clinical practice and is usually observed in younger patients without arterial disease. As confirmed by cavernosography and cavernosomanometry (Kropman et al. 1992), the diagnosis is made on the basis of a high and persistent peak systolic velocity, which is superior to the cut-off values of 35 cm/s, and end diastolic velocity (Fig. 6.12) with a sensitivity of 90–94%.

The disappearance or inversion of the diastolic flow is indicative of a correctly functioning veno-occlusive mechanism, and the erectile dysfunction is probably of different origin (hormonal, psychological) (Wespes et al. 1998).

The use of the resistive index (RI) to measure the venous function does not show advantages over the simple end diastolic velocity values. RIs of 0.9–1.0 are indicative of normality, while lower values suggest venous leakage. When the RI is below 0.75 end diastolic velocity is generally higher than 10–12 cm/s in 95% of patients. In these cases the venous leakage is persistent and elevated, and there is no efficacy of oral drugs. The presence of an elevated end diastolic velocity is indicative of low intracavernosal pressure, inadequate to obtain and maintain a rigidity sufficient for normal intercourse (de Meyer and Thibo 1998). Less frequently observed are cases of erectile dysfunction of mixed origin, arteriogenic and venous, showing low systolic velocity and persistent diastolic flow (Fig. 6.17).

The response to pharmacological stimulation in the dorsal penile arteries is completely different from in the cavernosal. They do not show the typical phase changes detected in the cavernosal arteries and secondary to the intracorporeal pressure (Hwang et al. 1991). The flow is elevated even in full rigidity. They provide blood to the glans, and the peak systolic velocity increases to produce an engorgement of the glans vasculature with secondary distension and stiffness of this part of the penis. Lesions of these vessels can be the cause of reduced tumescence of the glans and of a "soft-tip" during erection.

In the deep dorsal vein the flow is always high during all the phases of erection. Commonly it increases after drug injection. The flow velocity measurement is not clinically useful in patients with erectile dysfunction and particularly in those with venous leakage (Virag and Sussman 1998).

Dorsal-cavernosal anastomosis is commonly detected in patients after pharmacologically induced erection, independently of the nature of the erectile dysfunction. The flow direction is normally from the dorsal artery to the cavernosal and the end diastolic velocity is always high and not influenced by the intracorporeal pressure.

6.5
Other Imaging Modalities

Arteriography of the pudendal artery (using the transfemoral or transbrachial approach) and cavernosography have been used before the introduction of color Doppler imaging to detect the nature of the erectile dysfunction (Delcour et al. 1986; Bookstein 1987; Rosen et al. 1991). At present the role of these techniques is limited to selected cases with specific clinical problems already studied with sonography.

The study of the arterial tree can be performed using the traditional arterial approach, but CT angiography is today the first line procedure using a multislice machine and multiplanar or 3D reconstructions, which allow a complete depiction of the pudendal and cavernous arteries.

The exam is employed in young patients with acute onset of the erectile dysfunction, with asymmetric flow in the cavernosal arteries or after blunt lower abdominal trauma, where a traumatic lesion or compression of a large artery is suspected. This non-invasive procedure can identify patients who can have advantages from an interventional procedure with restoration of the flow.

Dynamic infusion cavernosography (Fig. 6.18) with vasoactive substance injection (Lue et al. 1986) is currently performed in patients with venous leakage before vein ligation. It is used to identify the sites of the veins involved that can be at the level of the deep dorsal vein and the cavernosal vein at the base of the crural vein.

Postoperative potency or increased rigidity has been reported in 60–70% of patients with venogenic erectile dysfunction. Venous leak surgery is a useful treatment modality in subjects with pure venous leakage detected with color Doppler and pharmacocavernosography (Vale et al. 1995). This minor surgical procedure is preferred to implant surgery or to use of vacuum device (Keogan et al. 1996).

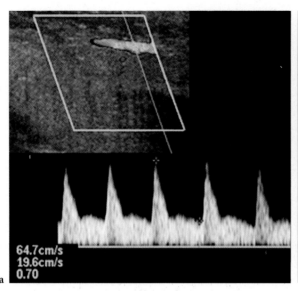 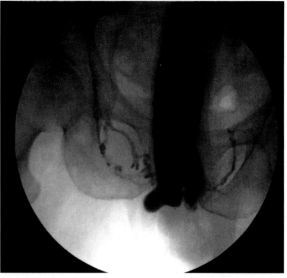

Fig. 6.18a,b. Severe venogenic erectile dysfunction in a young patient. **a** Color Doppler interrogation of the cavernosal arteries shows PSV of 64 cm/s and elevated EDV of 19 cm/s. The RI is 0.70 indicative of venous leakage. **b** Cavernosography performed before venous ligation surgery confirms venous leakage

6.6
Complications

Minor complications following intracavernosal drug injection are common, while major complications are rarely observed. The patient can report modest pain or a burning sensation, followed by a sense of tension or rarely intense pain, especially when rigidity appears. Penile pain is independent of the erection and can be due to albuginea acute distension or the action of the chemical product on the intracorporeal sensitive structures. This form of pain during tumescence/erection is more common in subjects who have no erections (spontaneous or nocturnal) or after prostate surgery, probably due to an acquired stiffness of the cavernous tissue. The pharmacologically induced erection producing a sudden distension is also associated with pain. When the pain is persistent or not tolerated by the patient, the best therapeutic solution is to lie down and to administrate an analgesic or ansiolitic drug. To facilitate detumescence the patient can be invited to void spontaneously because this maneuver opens the bladder neck, which is contracted during erection and promotes detumescence.

Patients with rigid erection at the end of the procedure are invited to wait 90 min for a review. If detumescence has not occurred they are invited to wait another 60 min. If the erection persists with a RI >1.0, it is advisable to inject etilefrin to avoid unpleasant consequences.

When the induced erection is maintained over 4.5 h an ischemic priapism is present, and treatment is mandatory. The patient may be anxious, restless and distressed, complaining of intense penile pain, with rigidity at clinical examination. Color Doppler shows the typical features of low-flow priapism, which are described in Chapter 10. In these cases the first procedure is an intracavernosal injection of etilefrin and direct blood aspiration from the corpora cavarnosa by inserting two 16-18-G needles through the glans penis. It is advisable to perform a superficial anesthesia of the glans with a 0.5 ml of lidocaine at 1% with a 30-G needle in the site where the largest needles will be introduced. Exceptionally, a surgical procedure is necessary. Late complications can be observed after repeated cavernosal self injection with focal or diffuse corporal fibrosis, which are described in Chapter 18.

References

Bertolotto M, Neumaier CE (1999) Penile sonography. Eur Radiol 9 [Suppl 3]:S407–412
Bookstein JJ (1987) Cavernosal venocclusive insufficiency in male impotence: evaluation of degree and location. Radiology 164:175–178

Broderick GA (1998) Evidence based assessment of erectile dysfunction. Int J Impot Res 10 [Suppl 2]:S64–73; discussion S77–69

Chen J, Greenstein A, Matzkin H (2000) Is a second injection of vasoactive medication necessary during color duplex Doppler evaluation of young patients with veno-occlusive erectile dysfunction? Urology 55:927–930

Chiou RK, Alberts GL, Pomeroy BD et al (1999) Study of cavernosal arterial anatomy using color and power Doppler sonography: impact on hemodynamic parameter measurement. J Urol 162:358–360

Cormio L, Bettocchi C, Zizzi V et al (1996) [Penile dynamic color Doppler echography in the diagnosis of erection disorders]. Arch Ital Urol Androl 68:53–55

de Meyer JM, Thibo P (1998) The correlation among cavernous pressure, penile rigidity and resistance index. J Urol 160:63–66

Delcour C, Wespes E, Vandenbosch G et al (1986) Impotence: evaluation with cavernosography. Radiology 161:803–806

Erbagci A, Yagci F, Sarica K et al (2002) Evaluation and therapeutic regulation of erectile dysfunction with visual stimulation test. An objective approach by using the sildenafil citrate test. Urol Int 69:21–26

Fitzgerald SW, Erickson SJ, Foley WD et al (1991) Color Doppler sonography in the evaluation of erectile dysfunction: patterns of temporal response to papaverine. AJR Am J Roentgenol 157:331–336

Foldvari M, Oguejiofor C, Afridi S et al (1998) Liposome encapsulated prostaglandin E1 in erectile dysfunction: correlation between in vitro delivery through foreskin and efficacy in patients. Urology 52:838–843

Govier FE, Asase D, Hefty TR et al (1995) Timing of penile color flow duplex ultrasonography using a triple drug mixture. J Urol 153:1472–1475

Hampson SJ, Cowie AG, Richards D, Lees WR (1992) Independent evaluation of impotence by colour Doppler imaging and cavernosometry. Eur Urol 21:27–31

Hwang TI, Liu PZ, Yang CR (1991) Evaluation of penile dorsal arteries and deep arteries in arteriogenic impotence. J Urol 146:46–49

Keogan MT, Kliewer MA, Hertzberg BS et al (1996) Doppler sonography in the evaluation of corporovenous competence after penile vein ligation surgery. J Ultrasound Med 15:227–233

Kim ED, McVary KT (1995) Topical prostaglandin-E1 for the treatment of erectile dysfunction. J Urol 153:1828–1830

Klingler HC, Kratzik C, Pycha A, Marberger M (1999) Value of power Doppler sonography in the investigation of erectile dysfunction. Eur Urol 36:320–326

Knispel HH, Andresen R (1992) Color-coded duplex sonography in impotence: significance of different flow parameters in patients and controls. Eur Urol 21:22–26

Kropman RF, Schipper J, van Oostayen JA et al (1992) The value of increased end diastolic velocity during penile duplex sonography in relation to pathological venous leakage in erectile dysfunction. J Urol 148:314–317

Lehmann K, John H, Kacl G et al (1999) Variable response to intracavernous prostaglandin E1 testing for erectile dysfunction. Urology 54:539–543

Lehmann K, Kacl G, Hagspiel K, Hauri D (1996) [The value of color-coded duplex ultrasound as standard assessment in erectile dysfunction]. Urologe A 35:456–461; discussion 461–452

Lue TF (1993) Erectile dysfunction: problems and challenges. J Urol 149:1256–1257

Lue TF, Hricak H, Schmidt RA, Tanagho EA (1986) Functional evaluation of penile veins by cavernosography in papaverine-induced erection. J Urol 135:479–482

Mancini M, Bartolini M, Maggi M et al (1996) The presence of arterial anatomical variations can affect the results of duplex sonographic evaluation of penile vessels in impotent patients. J Urol 155:1919–1923

Mancini M, Bartolini M, Maggi M et al (2000) Duplex ultrasound evaluation of cavernosal peak systolic velocity and waveform acceleration in the penile flaccid state: clinical significance in the assessment of the arterial supply in patients with erectile dysfunction. Int J Androl 23:199–204

Meuleman EJ, Bemelmans BL, Doesburg WH et al (1992a) Penile pharmacological duplex ultrasonography: a dose-effect study comparing papaverine, papaverine/phentolamine and prostaglandin E1. J Urol 148:63–66

Meuleman EJ, Bemelmans BL, van Asten WN et al (1992b) Assessment of penile blood flow by duplex ultrasonography in 44 men with normal erectile potency in different phases of erection. J Urol 147:51–56

Mills RD, Sethia KK (1996) Reproducibility of penile arterial colour duplex ultrasonography. Br J Urol 78:109–112

Montorsi F, Sarteschi M, Maga T et al (1998) Functional anatomy of cavernous helicine arterioles in potent subjects. J Urol 159:808–810

Mulhall JP, Levine LA, Junemann KP (2006) Erection hardness: a unifying factor for defining response in the treatment of erectile dysfunction. Urology 68:17–25

Nelson RP, Lue TF (1989) Determination of erectile penile volume by ultrasonography. J Urol 141:1123–1126

NIH Consensus Conference (1993) Impotence. NIH Consensus Development Panel on Impotence. JAMA 270:83–90

Oates CP, Pickard RS, Powell PH et al (1995) The use of duplex ultrasound in the assessment of arterial supply to the penis in vasculogenic impotence. J Urol 153:354–357

Padma-Nathan H, Hellstrom WJ, Kaiser FE et al (1997) Treatment of men with erectile dysfunction with transurethral alprostadil. Medicated Urethral System for Erection (MUSE) Study Group. N Engl J Med 336:1–7

Park K, Kwon DD, Oh BR et al (2002) Efficacy of virtual glasses in audio-visual sexual stimulation during penile color duplex Doppler ultrasonography. Eur Urol 41:62–65

Pescatori ES, Silingardi V, Galeazzi GM et al (2000) Audiovisual sexual stimulation by virtual glasses is effective in inducing complete cavernosal smooth muscle relaxation: a pharmacocavernosometric study. Int J Impot Res 12:83–88; discussion 88–90

Rosen MP, Schwartz AN, Levine FJ, Greenfield AJ (1991) Radiologic assessment of impotence: angiography, sonography, cavernosography, and scintigraphy. AJR Am J Roentgenol 157:923–931; discussion 932–924

Rosen RC, Althof SE, Giuliano F (2006) Research instruments for the diagnosis and treatment of patients with erectile dysfunction. Urology 68:6–16

Rosen RC, Cappelleri JC, Gendrano N, 3rd (2002) The International Index of Erectile Function (IIEF): a state-of-the-science review. Int J Impot Res 14:226–244

Rosen RC, Riley A, Wagner G et al (1997) The international index of erectile function (IIEF): a multidimensional scale for assessment of erectile dysfunction. Urology 49:822–830

Sarteschi LM, Montorsi F, Fabris FM et al (1998) Cavernous arterial and arteriolar circulation in patients with erectile dysfunction: a power Doppler study. J Urol 159:428–432

Shabsigh R, Fishman IJ, Quesada ET et al (1989) Evaluation of vasculogenic erectile impotence using penile duplex ultrasonography. J Urol 142:1469–1474

Tam PY, Keller T, Poppiti R et al (1998) Hemodynamic effects of transurethral alprostadil measured by color duplex ultrasonography in men with erectile dysfunction. J Urol 160:1321–1324

Vale JA, Feneley MR, Lees WR, Kirby RS (1995) Venous leak surgery: long-term follow-up of patients undergoing excision and ligation of the deep dorsal vein of the penis. Br J Urol 76:192–195

Valji K, Bookstein JJ (1993) Diagnosis of arteriogenic impotence: efficacy of duplex sonography as a screening tool. AJR Am J Roentgenol 160:65–69

Virag R, Sussman H (1998) [Exploration of the deep dorsal vein of the penis using pulsed Doppler ultrasonography. Preliminary study]. J Mal Vasc 23:195–198

Wegner HE, Andresen R, Knispel HH et al (1995) Evaluation of penile arteries with color-coded duplex sonography: prevalence and possible therapeutic implications of connections between dorsal and cavernous arteries in impotent men. J Urol 153:1469–1471

Wespes E, Raviv G, Vanegas JP et al (1998) Corporeal veno-occlusive dysfunction: a distal arterial pathology? J Urol 160:2054–2057

Peyronie's Disease: Etiology and Treatment

William O. Brant, Anthony J. Bella, and Tom F. Lue

CONTENTS

7.1 Introduction and Presentation 55
7.2 Epidemiology and Natural History 55
7.3 Etiology 56
7.4 Evaluation 56
7.5 Treatment: Medical 57
7.6 Treatment-Surgical 58
References 58

7.1
Introduction and Presentation

In 1743, François Gigot de la Peyronie described the fibrous penile plaques that we now associate with his name. These plaques have been characterized histologically (Brock et al. 1997), ultrastructurally (Hirano et al. 1997), and, to some degree, molecularly (El-Sakka et al. 1997b; Hirano et al. 1997; Magee et al. 2002). Although there is no universal consensus on the definition, most authors describe Peyronie's disease as some combination of penile pain, deformity, and/or palpable plaque (Mulhall et al. 2004; Zargooshi 2004). In general, the penile deformity adopts a dorsal curvature although the manifestation may be protean. One series described 46% dorsal curvature, 29% lateral, and 9% ventral, with the remained being mixed or a combination of curvatures (Kadioglu et al. 2002). Although curvature is the most common deformity, other malformations can occur, including penile shortening, hinging, and indentations or bottle-neck configurations. Additionally, erectile dysfunction is a common (20–40%) associated finding; this may be generalized or localized (i.e., flaccidity limited to distal to the lesion). Patients often present because of difficult or painful (for the patient and/or the partner) intromission, erectile dysfunction, or penile shortening.

7.2
Epidemiology and Natural History

Despite the well-described histology and variety of deformities, the epidemiology remains relatively vague and the etiology even more elusive. The reported prevalence of the condition varies widely. Lindsay et al. reported 0.4% (1991), and Devine et al. 1% (1997). Sommer et al. (2002), analyzing over 4,000 respondents to a questionnaire, reported a prevalence of 3.2%, with Peyronie's disease defined as a palpable plaque. La Pera et al. (2001) reported a prevalence of 7%. In general, these studies have relied on questionnaires. More recently, Mulhall et al. (2004) reported on physician-identified penile plaques found during a screening program for prostate cancer. Peyronie's disease, defined as a palpable penile plaque, was found in 9%. In this population, a relatively high number (1/3) were found to have the plaque, but denied any penile deformity. The high prevalence found in this study may result from the fact that (1) the population screened consisted of older men compared to other studies and (2) a physician performed the exams,

W. O. Brant, MD
PO Box 40,000, Vail, CO 81658, USA
A. J. Bella, MD, FRCS(C)
Department of Surgery and Associate Scientist (Neuroscience), University of Ottawa, The Ottawa Hospital, 1053 Carling Avenue, Ottawa, K1Y 4E9, Canada
T. F. Lue, MD
400 Parnassus Ave, A633, San Francisco, CA 94143-0738, USA

thus discovering masses that the patients may not be aware of. It is not commented on in their study whether the 1/3 without deformity were aware that they had a penile mass. It is likely that this higher prevalence (up to 9%) is partially due to more men pursuing treatment for erectile dysfunction, since men may not recognize deviation or other deformities in the flaccid state.

Peyronie's disease may be associated with other fibrotic disorders such as Dupuytren's contracture or Lederhosen syndrome. Its association with vascular comorbidities is controversial (Kadioglu et al. 2002; Mulhall et al. 2004; Usta et al. 2004), as is the role of overt trauma such as penile fracture (Zargooshi 2004).

Often, the disease state may be divided into an acute (or inflammatory) phase and a chronic phase. During the former, there may be penile pain, even when flaccid, and there are often dynamic changes of the penile malformation. During the latter, pain (at least without intromission) resolves, and the malformation becomes stable in its characteristics. Contemporary series have reported a disappointing 13% or less rate of spontaneous regression without intervention (Gelbard et al. 1990; Kadioglu et al. 2002).

7.3
Etiology

Despite historic suggestions that Peyronie's disease might be the result of incest or intercourse with an uninterested partner (Dunsmuir and Kirby 1996), Peyronie's plaques appear histologically and biochemically to result from inflammation (El-Sakka et al. 1997b). This has been used to support the longstanding clinical suspicion that penile trauma plays a major, if not exclusive, role in the development of the plaques. Based on pathologic studies, Smith (1966) defined the cause of Peyronie's plaques as tunical scarring resulting from vascular inflammation between the tunica and the corporal tissue. Structurally, the tunica consists of an outer, longitudinally oriented layer with an inner, circularly oriented layer (Brock et al. 1997). Fibers radiate from this inner layer and act as struts to augment the septum and provide support. With even minimal trauma, insertions of these struts may separate, with resultant bleeding and inflammation. Devine postulated that, in older men, this process was more likely to occur, since tissues are less elastic and thereby more prone to disruption (Devine and Horton 1988). In addition, edema resulting from trauma may prevent egress of cytokines and related inflammatory mediators, thus perpetuating the local injury (Lue 2002). The inflammatory process and aberrant wound healing lead to fibrosis, loss of elastic tissues, and excessive collagen deposition, which may account for the initial pain and subsequent penile plaque and deformity. In Peyronie's disease there is increased collagen, with a higher ratio of collagen type III to I than in normal tunica albuginea, a loss of elastic fibers, and increased fibrin deposits (Akkus et al. 1997; Brock et al. 1997). There are increased numbers of fibroblasts as well as infiltration of inflammatory cells, particularly early in the disease. In chronic disease, calcification may be noted in up to 1/3 of cases. Several potential biochemical pathways have been identified, including transforming growth factor beta (TGFb) (El-Sakka et al. 1997a; El-Sakka et al. 1997b), plasminogen activator inhibitor type 1 (Davila et al. 2005), and osteoblast-stimulating factor 1 (Lue 2002).

In general, the plaques are found peripherally, usually on the dorsal aspect of the penis. However, the abnormal tissue may extend beyond the palpable lesion (Iacono et al. 1993; Somers and Dawson 1997), or even into the corporal tissue or intercavernosal septum (Brant et al. 2007). An area of relative inelasticity and contracture results in both loss of length and ipsilateral deviation, as the normally elastic fibers are replaced by relatively noncompliant collagen-rich tissue. The inelasticity of the plaques may also impede the normal vasoocclusive mechanism of erection and thus leads to venous leak (Hellstrom and Bivalacqua 2000).

7.4
Evaluation

Patients are usually given a preliminary diagnosis of Peyronie's disease when they present with classic symptoms of the disease: penile mass, curvature, or pain. Objectively, clinicians may measure penile length, plaque size, penile curvature, and possibly induce an artificial erection in clinic with vasoactive intracorporal injections. Various imaging modalities have also been used (Andresen et al. 1998);

we routinely perform ultrasonography due to its easy availability, low risk, and ability to image and quantify both calcified and soft tissue elements of Peyronie's disease as well as assess vascular status if a reconstructive procedure is being considered. Possible associated disorders (e.g., Dupuytren's contractures or vascular disease) and inciting events (e.g., trauma or genitourinary instrumentation) should be evaluated. It is important to establish the psychological effect of Peyronie's disease on the patient as well as determine the extent of associated erectile dysfunction. It is often helpful to have the patient take photographs of the erect penis at home to characterize the deformity; if the patient cannot or will not do this, an office pharmacoerection should be performed.

7.5
Treatment: Medical

It has been well recognized that the variety of treatment options for Peyronie's disease is in proportion to their overall disappointing results. Few of these agents have been found to be completely efficacious and almost all studies are epidemiologically hampered by low patient numbers, lack of control groups, lack of reproducibility, and an inability to distinguish efficacy from spontaneous improvement of the disease process, especially with regard to pain where spontaneous resolution is generally the rule. Nonetheless, early medical intervention at the stage of evolving disease is likely to be more efficacious than intervention when the disease is stable.

Although vitamin E is likely the most commonly used agent for PD, controlled studies have not supported its superiority over placebo (GELBARD et al. 1990). However, it may have a role in combined therapy (PRIETO CASTRO et al. 2003).

Potassium para-aminobenzoate (POTOBA) is an antifibrotic agent that has been used in a variety of disease states, and at least one placebo controlled study demonstrated superiority in terms of decreased plaque size with treatment (WEIDNER et al. 2005). However, the medication is very difficult to take, with a poor taste and the potential for gastrointestinal side effects.

Colchicine is another antifibrotic agent, with excellent support from basic science and animal model investigations of Peyronie's disease. Controlled studies in humans have given mixed results (PRIETO CASTRO et al. 2003; SAFARINEJAD 2004). Similar to POTOBA, gastrointestinal side effects are relatively common. Additionally, it may cause bone marrow suppression. Due to the difficulties in taking these medications, POTOBA and colchicine are no longer commonly used in contemporary management of Peyronie's disease.

Pentoxifylline has been used in humans in a variety of inflammatory and fibrotic conditions. The mechanism is not fully known; pentoxifylline blocks the TGF-beta 1-mediated pathway of inflammation, prevents deposition of collagen type I, and acts as a non-specific PDE inhibitor. VALENTE et al. (2003) have demonstrated that both sildenafil and pentoxifylline reduce the plaque size in tunical fibrosis induced by injection of transforming growth factor (TGF) beta-1. Encouraged by pentoxifylline's observed suppression of collagen production in Peyronie's cells in tissue culture as well as its efficacy in other human fibrotic disorders, we have been offering patients treatment with pentoxifylline as an option for Peyronie's disease since 2002 (unpublished data).

Verapamil, a calcium-channel blocker, has been used successfully when injected directly into the lesion, although poorer effects were noted when the drug was injected subcutaneously (BRAKE et al. 2001) or used as a topical ointment (MARTIN et al. 2002). Although it has been difficult to perform controlled studies due to the invasive nature of the treatment, a small controlled study did demonstrate improvement in curvature, plaque volume, and erectile function (REHMAN et al. 1998). Verapamil has also been given via an electromotive transdermal system.

Interferon alpha-2b has also been given as an intralesional injection. Uncontrolled studies have had mixed results, but at least one controlled trial showed improvement in curvature, plaque size, pain, and blood flow (DANG et al. 2004; HELLSTROM et al. 2006). Unfortunately, the injections are expensive and can cause flu-like symptoms.

Extracorporeal shockwave lithotripsy has been generally disappointing and a recent, novel approach to perform a placebo-controlled trial demonstrated possible improvement in pain, but no improvement in penile curvature (HATZICHRISTODOULOU et al. 2006). Radiation has also been disappointing and also may compromise erectile function (INCROCCI et al. 2000). Contemporary evidence does not support either of these two approaches for treatment of Peyronie's disease.

7.6
Treatment-Surgical

Although it is beyond the scope of this chapter to discuss the specifics of reconstructive surgery for Peyronie's disease, several general points should be made. It is imperative to wait until the disease has reached a stable phase prior to contemplating surgical intervention. Surgical approaches generally fall into three categories: plication, grafting, and prosthesis. The three most important preoperative criteria are: (1) patient erectile function, (2) ability to penetrate (i.e., the extent of the deformity, including hinging and curvature), and (3) patient expectations.

Three general procedures are available for correction: (1) for a penis of adequate length and adequate erectile function, perform a straightening procedure, either non-incisional or incisional; (2) for a very short penis or one with an deformity (such as an hourglass or severe indentation) with good erectile function, apply a biologic graft (either autograft or xenograft); (3) for curvature associated with severe erectile dysfunction, place an inflatable prosthesis and perform associated procedures (grafting, plication, or modeling) if the prosthesis alone does not provide adequate straightening. A grafting procedure, using either autologous or xenograft material, may help the patient regain some degree of penile length lost from the underlying fibrosis, but there is an attendant risk of de novo erectile dysfunction. Patients, especially those with baseline erectile dysfunction, must be aware of this, and should always be counseled regarding the option of a penile prosthesis. We inform patients that a prosthesis may be placed at a later date, should the need arise. In high risk patients, it may even be preferable to perform a two-stage procedure, as the substantial increase in operative time if both grafting and prosthesis are performed at the same setting may carry a higher risk of perioperative prosthetic infection.

An additional important factor in preoperative counseling is to address patient expectations about postoperative penile length. Many patients are understandably distraught about the penile shortening that often accompanies Peyronie's disease. However, they often have an unrealistic recollection of their past erectile length, and we rarely can demonstrate this in any objective fashion, since we seldom have premorbid penile measurements available. The stretched penile length is routinely documented in the patient record, and he is made aware that the grafting procedure is usually limited to adding 1/2 to 1 inch to the stretched flaccid length. Patients need to be educated that a simple plication surgery may result in a straight erection, but will not restore any length, and thus overall length is lost; a grafting procedure may restore some length, but cannot exceed more than 1 inch above the stretched length of the penis.

References

Akkus E, Carrier S, Baba K et al (1997) Structural alterations in the tunica albuginea of the penis: impact of Peyronie's disease, ageing and impotence. Br J Urol 79:47–53

Andresen R, Wegner HE, Miller K, Banzer D (1998) Imaging modalities in Peyronie's disease. An intrapersonal comparison of ultrasound sonography, X-ray in mammography technique, computerized tomography, and nuclear magnetic resonance in 20 patients. Eur Urol 34:128–134; discussion 135

Brake M, Loertzer H, Horsch R, Keller H (2001) Treatment of Peyronie's disease with local interferon-alpha 2b. BJU Int 87:654–657

Brant WO, Bella AJ, Garcia MM et al (2007) Isolated septal fibrosis or hematoma-atypical Peyronie's disease? J Urol 177:179-182; discussion 183

Brock G, Hsu GL, Nunes L et al (1997) The anatomy of the tunica albuginea in the normal penis and Peyronie's disease. J Urol 157:276–281

Dang G, Matern R, Bivalacqua TJ et al (2004) Intralesional interferon-alpha-2B injections for the treatment of Peyronie's disease. South Med J 97:42–46

Davila HH, Magee TR, Zuniga FI et al (2005) Peyronie's disease associated with increase in plasminogen activator inhibitor in fibrotic plaque. Urology 65:645–648

Devine CJ Jr, Horton CE (1988) Peyronie's disease. Clin Plast Surg 15:405–409

Devine CJ, Jr., Somers KD, Jordan SG, Schlossberg SM (1997) Proposal: trauma as the cause of the Peyronie's lesion. J Urol 157:285–290

Dunsmuir WD, Kirby RS (1996) Francois de LaPeyronie (1978-1747): the man and the disease he described. Br J Urol 78:613–622

El-Sakka AI, Hassoba HM, Chui RM et al (1997a) An animal model of Peyronie's-like condition associated with an increase of transforming growth factor beta mRNA and protein expression. J Urol 158:2284–2290

El-Sakka AI, Hassoba HM, Pillarisetty RJ et al (1997b) Peyronie's disease is associated with an increase in transforming growth factor-beta protein expression. J Urol 158:1391–1394

Gelbard MK, Dorey F, James K (1990) The natural history of Peyronie's disease. J Urol 144:1376–1379

Hatzichristodoulou G, Meisner C, Liske P et al (2006) Efficacy of extracorporeal shock wave therapy (ESWT) in patients with Peyronie's disease (PD)-first results of a prospective, randomized, placebo-controlled, single-blind study. J Urol 175:320

Hellstrom WJ, Bivalacqua TJ (2000) Peyronie's disease: etiology, medical, and surgical therapy. J Androl 21:347–354

Hellstrom WJ, Kendirci M, Matern R et al (2006) Single-blind, multicenter, placebo controlled, parallel study to assess the safety and efficacy of intralesional interferon alpha-2B for minimally invasive treatment for Peyronie's disease. J Urol 176:394–398

Hirano D, Takimoto Y, Yamamoto T et al (1997) Electron microscopic study of the penile plaques and adjacent corpora cavernosa in Peyronie's disease. Int J Urol 4:274–278

Iacono F, Barra S, De Rosa G et al (1993) Microstructural disorders of tunica albuginea in patients affected by Peyronie's disease with or without erection dysfunction. J Urol 150:1806–1809

Incrocci L, Hop WC, Slob AK (2000) Current sexual functioning in 106 patients with Peyronie's disease treated with radiotherapy 9 years earlier. Urology 56:1030–1034

Kadioglu A, Tefekli A, Erol B et al (2002) A retrospective review of 307 men with Peyronie's disease. J Urol 168:1075–1079

La Pera G, Pescatori ES, Calabrese M et al (2001) Peyronie's disease: prevalence and association with cigarette smoking. A multicenter population-based study in men aged 50–69 years. Eur Urol 40:525–530

Lindsay MB, Schain DM, Grambsch P et al (1991) The incidence of Peyronie's disease in Rochester, Minnesota, 1950 through 1984. J Urol 146:1007–1009

Lue TF (2002) Peyronie's disease: an anatomically-based hypothesis and beyond. Int J Impot Res 14:411–413

Magee TR, Qian A, Rajfer J et al (2002) Gene expression profiles in the Peyronie's disease plaque. Urology 59:451–457

Martin DJ, Badwan K, Parker M, Mulhall JP (2002) Transdermal application of verapamil gel to the penile shaft fails to infiltrate the tunica albuginea. J Urol 168:2483–2485

Mulhall JP, Creech SD, Boorjian SA et al (2004) Subjective and objective analysis of the prevalence of Peyronie's disease in a population of men presenting for prostate cancer screening. J Urol 171:2350–2353

Prieto Castro RM, Leva Vallejo ME, Regueiro Lopez JC et al (2003) Combined treatment with vitamin E and colchicine in the early stages of Peyronie's disease. BJU Int 91:522–524

Rehman J, Benet A, Melman A (1998) Use of intralesional verapamil to dissolve Peyronie's disease plaque: a long-term single-blind study. Urology 51:620–626

Safarinejad MR (2004) Therapeutic effects of colchicine in the management of Peyronie's disease: a randomized double-blind, placebo-controlled study. Int J Impot Res 16:238–243

Smith BH (1966) Peyronie's disease. Am J Clin Pathol 45:670–678

Somers KD, Dawson DM (1997) Fibrin deposition in Peyronie's disease plaque. J Urol 157:311–315

Sommer F, Schwarzer U, Wassmer G et al (2002) Epidemiology of Peyronie's disease. Int J Impot Res 14:379–383

Usta MF, Bivalacqua TJ, Jabren GW et al (2004) Relationship between the severity of penile curvature and the presence of comorbidities in men with Peyronie's disease. J Urol 171:775–779

Valente EG, Vernet D, Ferrini MG et al (2003) L-arginine and phosphodiesterase (PDE) inhibitors counteract fibrosis in the Peyronie's fibrotic plaque and related fibroblast cultures. Nitric Oxide 9:229–244

Weidner W, Hauck EW, Schnitker J (2005) Potassium para-aminobenzoate (POTABA) in the treatment of Peyronie's disease: a prospective, placebo-controlled, randomized study. Eur Urol 47:530–535; discussion 535–536

Zargooshi J (2004) Trauma as the cause of Peyronie's disease: penile fracture as a model of trauma. J Urol 172:186–188

US Evaluation of Patients with Peyronie's Disease

Michele Bertolotto, Matteo Coss, and Carlo E. Neumaier

CONTENTS

8.1 Background 61
8.2 Evaluation Technique 61
8.3 Grey-Scale Ultrasonography 62
8.3.1 Evaluation of the Tunica Albuginea 62
8.3.2 Echogenicity of the Plaques 63
8.3.3 Calcifications 64
8.3.4 Position, Extent and Morphology of the Plaques 64
8.3.5 Involvement of Adjacent Structures 64
8.4 Doppler Ultrasonography 66
8.5 Differential Diagnosis 67
8.6 Diagnostic Role of Other Imaging Modalities 68
References 69

8.1
Background

Peyronie's disease is characterized by formation of fibrous tissue plaques within the tunica albuginea causing penile pain, deformity, and shortening. As illustrated in Chapter 7, the diagnosis is based on medical history, autophotography, and a clinical examination with plaque palpation. Ultrasound and other imaging modalities are confirming and allow accurate evaluation of disease extent and assessment of associated erectile dysfunction.

8.2
Evaluation Technique

Ultrasound evaluation of patients with Peyronie's disease requires pharmacologically induced erection. After careful palpation of the penile shaft while flaccid, prostaglandin E1 is injected within the corpora cavernosa, usually at a dose of 10 µg, followed by a further 10 µg if there is a suboptimal erectile response.

Careful ultrasound evaluation of the tunica albuginea is obtained along longitudinal and transverse planes with high-frequency linear probes. In general, the higher the ultrasound frequencies, the better detail is obtained. Use of real time spatial compounding and of adaptive image-processing technique may be useful to reduce artifacts and dynamically enhance margins, improving visualization of tissue conspicuity and increasing diagnostic confidence in evaluation of the tunica albuginea and of the plaques (Fig. 8.1).

After plaque assessment, Doppler interrogation of all visible vessels should be done, and the erectile response of the patient should be evaluated. Doppler spectra are recorded on both cavernosal arteries un-

M. Bertolotto, MD; M. Coss, MD
Department of Radiology, University of Trieste, Ospedale di Cattinara, Strada di Fiume 447, Trieste, 34124, Italy
C. E. Neumaier, MD
Department of Diagnostic Imaging, National Cancer Institute, Largo Rosanna Benzi 10, Genova, 16132, Italy

der the guidance of color signal measuring peak systolic velocity and end diastolic velocity for at least 30 min after prostaglandin E1 injection. Anatomical variations, arterial vascular communications, and leakage pathways identified along the penile shaft should be interrogated, with specific notice to vessels adjacent to the plaques.

8.3
Grey-Scale Ultrasonography

When suitable transducers are used, an excellent evaluation of the tunica albuginea and of the plaques is obtained. The degree and direction of penile curvature, location, extent, echogenicity, and morphology of the plaques should be considered, as well as the presence of calcifications and involvement of adjacent structures. In patients undergoing medical treatment ultrasound enables us to detect areas of disease progress during the follow-up that would have been missed upon clinical palpation (WEGNER et al. 1997).

8.3.1
Evaluation of the Tunica Albuginea

Subjectively, the tunica albuginea of patients with Peyronie's disease is perceived as globally thickened and more echogenic than in most of the patients with other penile pathologies, even in locations in which no circumscribed plaques are identified. Microcalcifications can be occasionally identified also in regions in which the tunica albuginea does not appear definitely thickened. In this context, circumscribed plaques are identified as more pronounced, measurable, and irregularly thickening (AMIN et al. 1993). In our experience, about 5% of patients with Peyronie's disease do not present with circumscribed plaques, but with measurable thickening of the entire tunica albuginea (Fig. 8.2). These patients usually present with erectile dysfunction, severe penile shortening, and variable degrees of penile bending depending on whether there are circumscribed areas in which diffuse albugineal thickening is more pronounced.

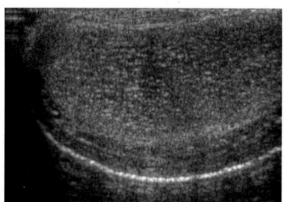
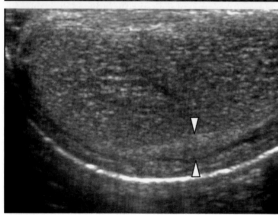

Fig. 8.1a,b. Peyronie's disease. Axial images of the penile shaft obtained on the same section both with conventional grey-scale ultrasonography and with real time spatial compound imaging. **a** Conventional grey-scale ultrasonography shows thickening of the dorsal aspect of the tunica albuginea. **b** Spatial compound imaging identifies a distinct plaque (*arrowheads*) and better delineates its extension

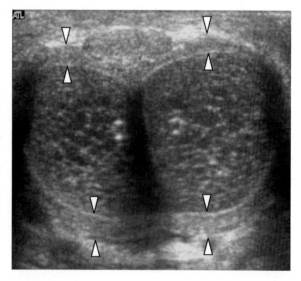

Fig. 8.2. Patient with Peyronie's disease presenting with severe penile shortening and erectile dysfunction. No significant penile bending was appreciable. Grey-scale ultrasonography shows diffuse thickening of the entire tunica albuginea (*arrowheads*)

8.3.2 Echogenicity of the Plaques

The echoes from the tunica albuginea are specular reflections and thus are demonstrated with efficiency only when the ultrasound beam is perpendicular to them. Perpendicular insonation, in particular, is of paramount importance to evaluate the echogenicity of the plaques. In fact, in our experience, the vast majority of non-calcified plaques are isoechoic or slightly hyperechoic compared with the surrounding tunica albuginea. Hypoechoic plaques are rare (Fig. 8.3). Echogenic plaques might appear as hypoechoic due to incorrect insonation in patients with insufficient penile turgidity or when plaque visualization is hampered by artifacts such as acoustic shadow produced by the penile septum (Fig. 8.4) or by extensive albugineal fibrotic changes. In fact, in contrast to the common belief, in our experience hypoechoic appearance of the plaque is usually a consequence of beam attenuation in patients with disease stabilization (Fig. 8.5) rather than a sign of inflammation in the active state of the disease.

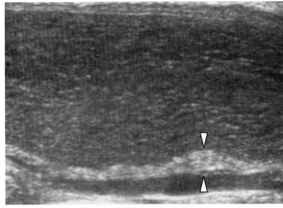
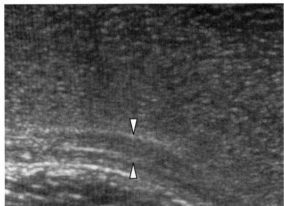
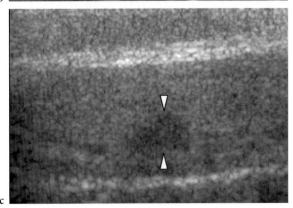

Fig. 8.3a–c. Patients with Peyronie's disease presenting with dorsal plaques of different echogenicity (*arrowheads*). Longitudinal scans on the ventral aspect of the penis. a Hyperechoic plaque. b Isoechoic plaque. c Hypoechoic plaque

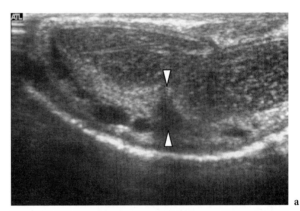
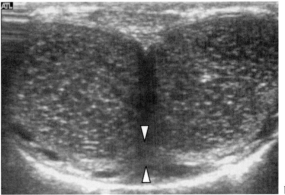

Fig. 8.4a,b. Pitfalls in evaluating echogenicity of the plaque. Grey-scale ultrasonography of a the flaccid and b the erect penis showing images of the same plaque (*arrowheads*). a The plaque appears as hypoechoic while flaccid due to incorrect insonation and artifacts produced by the penile septum. b When maximum erection is reached the plaque appears as hyperechoic

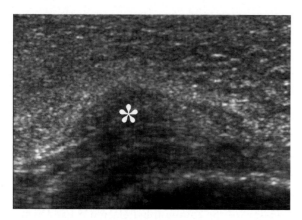

Fig. 8.5. Pitfalls in evaluating echogenicity of the plaque. Patient with a large dorsal plaque showing a relatively hypoechoic area in the region of maximum albugineal thickening (*) produced by attenuation of the ultrasound beam

8.3.3
Calcifications

Detection of plaque calcifications allows diagnosis of disease stabilization and provides information useful to select patients for lithotripsy therapy (WILKINS et al. 2003). Ultrasound shows 100% sensitivity in detecting and measuring gross calcifications of the plaques. The detection rate of microcalcifications increases when the highest frequency probes and real time spatial compounding are used (Fig. 8.6). Acoustic shadowing produced by extensive calcification of the plaques can reduce visibility of associated pathological changes of the corpora cavernosa. These limitations are reduced using careful examination techniques.

8.3.4
Position, Extent and Morphology of the Plaques

Plaque size and location, degree, and direction of the penile curvature (dorsal, ventral, lateral, or some combination) present a considerable concern when deciding on intervention.

Peyronie's plaques are more often located on the dorsal aspect of the penis, but they can also be found ventrally or, less frequently, in other positions (Fig. 8.7). Circumscribed plaques present with focal thickening of the albuginea corresponding to the site of penile bending. Annular plaques produce hourglass deformity: the girth of the corpora cavernosa is reduced at the site of the plaque, compared with the more proximal and distal regions of the shaft. Measurement of the size of the corpora cavernosa in different portions of the penis while erect is useful to assess the severity of the deformity.

8.3.5
Involvement of Adjacent Structures

In patients with Peyronie's disease preoperative recognition of penile septum involvement is important because it contraindicates plaque removal with grafting. Grey scale ultrasonography allows the recognition of plaque involvement of the penile septum when its normal ultrasonographic features are replaced by inhomogeneous tissue with echogenicity similar to the adjacent plaque. Small and large calcifications may be present. This pathological situation is most often observed in patients with large dorsal plaques, but can occur

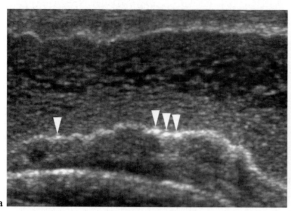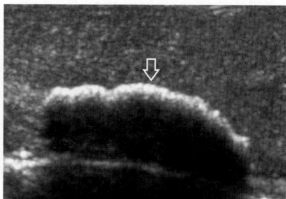

Fig. 8.6a,b. Calcified dorsal plaques. Longitudinal scans on the ventral aspect of the penis. **a** Isoechoic plaque showing small calcifications (*arrowheads*). **b** Extensively calcified plaque (*open arrow*) presenting with back attenuation

also in patients with ventral plaques. The relationships between the plaques and the penile vasculature should be evaluated as well. In particular, in patients with extensive dorsal plaques encasement of the neurovascular bundle can occur (MONTORSI et al. 1994). This condition must be identified before surgical correction of the curvature to minimize the risk of postoperative penile numbness. Plaque encasement of the cavernosal arteries is rare (BERTOLOTTO et al. 2002), but must be identified as a cause of arteriogenic erectile dysfunction (Fig. 8.8).

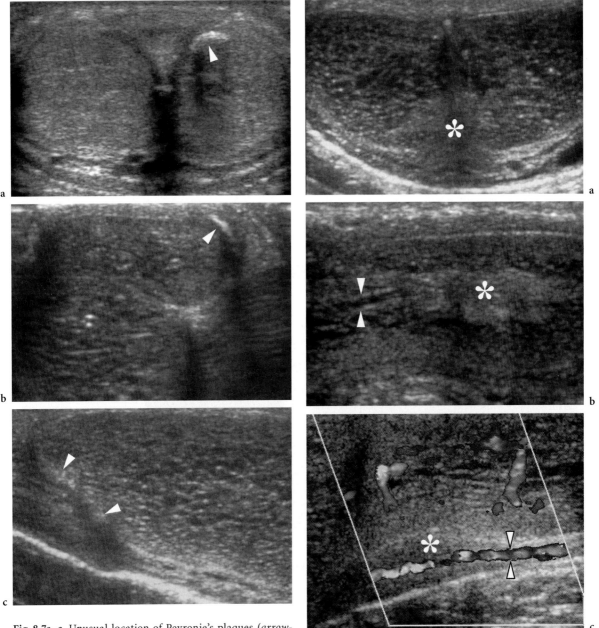

Fig. 8.7a–c. Unusual location of Peyronie's plaques (*arrowheads*). **a** Axial scan on the ventral aspect of the penis showing a partially calcified ventral plaque. **b** Axial scan on the right lateral aspect of the penis showing a partially calcified right-lateral plaque. **c** Longitudinal scan on the distal portion of the penis showing a dorsal plaque on the tip of a corpus cavernosum

Fig. 8.8a–c. Peyronie's plaques (*) involving the adjacent structures. **a** Axial scan showing involvement of the penile septum. **b** Longitudinal scan showing encasement of the cavernosal artery (*arrowheads*). **c** Color Doppler longitudinal scan showing encasement of the dorsal artery (*arrowheads*)

8.4 Doppler Ultrasonography

Color Doppler ultrasonography and duplex Doppler interrogation of the cavernosal arteries provide information on penile arterial inflow and venous outflow, which is useful to plan surgical or medical intervention. In particular, in patients with Peyronie's disease there is a higher incidence of venous leakage than in the age-matched control population (KADIOGLU et al. 2000). While in normal erection venules draining the corpora cavernosa are passively compressed between the expanding corporeal tissue and the tunica albuginea, in patients with Peyronie's disease corporeal compliance is decreased, preventing venous compression (MONTORSI et al. 1994). This mechanism is particularly evident adjacent to large circumscribed plaques producing severe penile bending or hourglass deformity and can result in widespread venous occlusive dysfunction or in localized venous leakage at the site of fibrotic plaque.

Duplex Doppler interrogation of cavernosal arteries allows diagnosis of widespread venous occlusive dysfunction when high velocity, low resistance flows are recorded (MONTORSI et al. 1994). In patients with plaque-related leakage normal cavernosal waveform changes are usually recorded, while leakage pathways are identified at color Doppler ultrasound adjacent to the plaque (Fig. 8.9). Moreover, there is Doppler evidence that in patients with severe Peyronie's disease cavernosal-spongiosal communications near the plaques remain patent with a higher peak systolic velocity and lower resistance index compared to the other cavernosal-spongiosal communications, supporting the hypothesis that blood leakage can occur also through these vessels (BERTOLOTTO et al. 2002).

Although alteration of the venous occlusive mechanism has been claimed to be present in a high percent of Peyronie's patients with erectile dysfunction (WEIDNER et al. 1997), the role of arterial inflow must be investigated. In fact, color Doppler ultrasonography shows associated arterial insufficiency in 30%–50% of these patients (KADIOGLU et

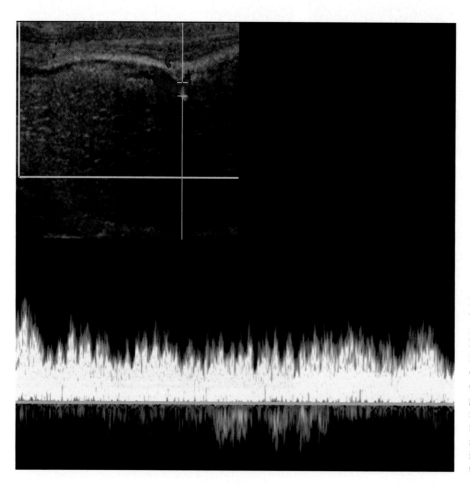

Fig. 8.9. Plaque-related venous leakage. Annular plaque producing hourglass deformity and reduced turgidity in the distal portions of the corpora cavernosa and glans. Doppler interrogation shows venous flows at the level of penile deformation due to incomplete distension of the erectile tissue

al. 2000). As mentioned before, plaque encasement of the cavernosal arteries is rare, but must be considered as a possible cause of arteriogenic erectile dysfunction. A clinically relevant reduction of penile arterial inflow results from bilateral cavernosal artery encasement or from unilateral encasement in men with widespread arterial disease. Doppler interrogation of the involved cavernosal artery distal to the plaque usually shows absence of flows or abrupt reduction of the peak systolic velocity (Ralph et al. 1992; Ahmed et al. 1998). Refilling from distal collaterals can present with cavernosal artery flow reversal.

When evaluating the penis of patients with Peyronie's disease before grafting, perforating collateral vessels should be detected, assessing their relationships with the plaque. In fact, shortening surgical procedures are preferred to correct dorsal curvature in patients with arterial perforating collaterals between the dorsal and the cavernosal arteries in order to preserve these vessels, which if injured might contribute to postoperative erectile dysfunction (Kadioglu et al. 2000).

Some investigators claim that in patients with Peyronie's disease Doppler analysis can reveal hyperperfusion around the plaques as a sign of inflammation in the active state of the disease, while absence of color signals around the plaques should be considered as a sign of disease stabilization (Carbone et al. 1999; Fornara and Gerbershagen 2004). Other investigators, however, failed to confirm these findings. In fact, the presence or absence of flow in microvascular structures cannot be determined with Doppler techniques. In our experience, detection of color signals around the plaques usually results from patency of leakage pathways, from emissary veins passing through the plaque, or from twinkling artifacts produced by calcifications (Fig. 8.10).

8.5 Differential Diagnosis

During ultrasound evaluation of patients referred for Peyronie's disease, other possible causes of penile bending and induration must be considered. The most common conditions that enter in the differential diagnoses include: congenital curvature of the penis, chordee with or without hypospadia, dorsal vein thrombosis (Hakim 2002), albugineal scar and cavernosal fibrosis secondary to local trauma, chronic inflammation, scleroderma (Chen et al. 2001), benign or malignant primary or secondary tumors. In particular, epithelioid sarcoma of the penis is a rare, slowly growing mesenchymal neo-

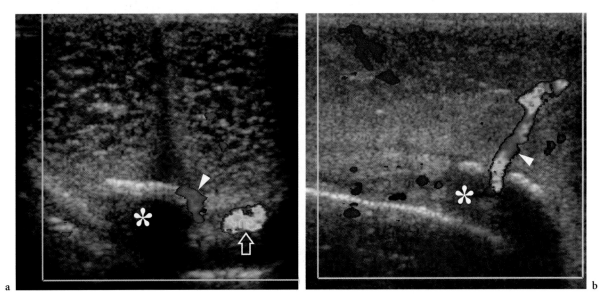

Fig. 8.10a,b. Color Doppler ultrasound scans. Calcified dorsal plaques (*). Normal penile vessels simulating plaque vascularization. a Axial scan showing left dorsal artery (*open arrow*) and an emissary vein passing through the plaque (*arrowhead*). b Communication between the cavernosal and the dorsal artery (*arrowhead*) passing though the plaque

plasm that may manifest as focal induration and mimic Peyronie's disease (SIRIKCI et al. 1999; USTA et al. 2003). Although rare, this lesion should be considered in the differential diagnosis of growing plaques.

Also isolated fibrosis of the penile septum (BRANT et al. 2007) and ventral curvature secondary to fibrosis and scarring of the corpus spongiosum, which can result from urethral instrumentation, should be considered (AFSAR and SOZDUYAR 1992). The ultrasound features of these pathological conditions are described in other chapters.

8.6 Diagnostic Role of Other Imaging Modalities

X-rays in mammography technique and CT are able to detect calcifications of Peyronie plaques and to determine the degree of plaque calcification (ANDRESEN et al. 1998). Non-calcified plaques, however, cannot be shown accurately. The information gained by these methods does not support the use of ionizing radiation for this purpose (FORNARA and GERBERSHAGEN 2004).

Dynamic infusion cavernosometry and cavernosography have been used in the past to evaluate erectile function in patients with Peyronie's disease (JORDAN and ANGERMEIER 1993; HAKIM 2002). This procedure is an effective means to obtain objective information on the presence of abnormal venous drainage that is either diffuse or localized at the site of the plaques, but is no longer performed on Peyronie's disease patients because of its invasiveness and potential risks of severe complications. An excellent correlation was found between the diagnosis of veno-occlusive dysfunction with cavernosometry/cavernosography and with duplex Doppler interrogation of the cavernosal arteries (LOPEZ and JAROW 1993). In fact, in patients with Peyronie's disease enough clinically useful information on erectile function is obtained non-invasively with Doppler techniques.

Magnetic resonance imaging is at least as sensitive as ultrasonography to determine the extent of plaque formation and to assess whether the corpora cavernosa and the penile septum are involved (VOSSOUGH et al. 2002). Moreover, magnetic resonance imaging is more sensitive than grey scale ultrasonography in assessing non-calcified plaques at the penile basis (HAUCK et al. 2003) and can be useful during the follow-up of patients undergoing conservative pharmacologic treatment as an objective measure of therapeutic response.

Plaques appear as thickened and irregular low signal intensity areas on T1- and T2-weighted images in and around the tunica albuginea, which are best seen on T2-weighted images (PRETORIUS et al. 2001). A diffuse, irregular plaque-like thickening of the tunica albuginea can be recognized as well (Fig. 8.11). Extension of the plaque into the corpora cavernosa or penile septum is seen as areas of irregular dark signal intensity.

Several authors suggest that after intravenous gadolinium administration enhancement of the plaque offers information regarding the presence of active inflammation within or around the plaque (ANDRESEN et al. 1998). This procedure could therefore be useful in guiding appropriate therapeutic strategy and timing by depicting the stage of the disease. Magnetic resonance imaging, however, is an expensive imaging modality and is not commonly used in our clinical practice to evaluate patients with Peyronie's disease. In fact, inflammation causes pain. Examination and medical history usually provide enough clinically useful information.

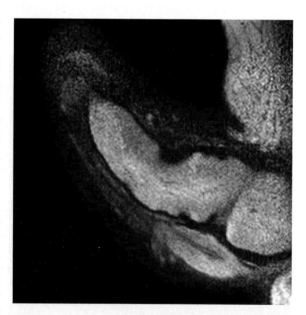

Fig. 8.11. Magnetic resonance imaging appearance of Peyronie's disease. Parasagittal T2-weighted image of the penis obtained after intracavernosal prostaglandin injection shows penile deformation and diffuse, irregular thickening of the tunica albuginea

Moreover, these findings are questionable. While a correlation between plaque enhancement characteristics, pain, and histologically proved inflammation has been demonstrated by some authors (ANDRESEN et al. 1998), other investigators found no correlation between plaque enhancement and pain symptomatology (VOSSHENRICH et al. 1995). Finally, signal from microvessels may be difficult to distinguish from enhancement of larger vessels such as dorsal arteries and veins, especially when the plaque is located dorsally and, as occurs for other organs and lesions, diffusion of gadolinium within fibrotic plaques may result in artifactual enhancement. Evaluation of contrast enhancement curves after gadolinium administration might be useful to differentiate plaque vascularity from late enhancement of fibrous tissue.

References

Afsar H, Sozduyar N (1992) Urethral manipulation syndrome (Kelamy syndrome): acquired ventral penile deviation. Arch Ital Urol Nefrol Androl 64:349–351

Ahmed M, Chilton CP, Munson KW et al (1998) The role of colour Doppler imaging in the management of Peyronie's disease. Br J Urol 81:604–606

Amin Z, Patel U, Friedman EP et al (1993) Colour Doppler and duplex ultrasound assessment of Peyronie's disease in impotent men. Br J Radiol 66:398–402

Andresen R, Wegner HE, Miller K, Banzer D (1998) Imaging modalities in Peyronie's disease. An intrapersonal comparison of ultrasound sonography, X-ray in mammography technique, computerized tomography, and nuclear magnetic resonance in 20 patients. Eur Urol 34:128–134; discussion 135

Bertolotto M, de Stefani S, Martinoli C et al (2002) Color Doppler appearance of penile cavernosal-spongiosal communications in patients with severe Peyronie's disease. Eur Radiol 12:2525–2531

Brant WO, Bella AJ, Garcia MM et al (2007) Isolated septal fibrosis or hematoma–atypical Peyronie's disease? J Urol 177:179–182; discussion 183

Carbone M, Rossi E, Iurassich S et al (1999) [Assessment of microvascularization around the plaques in Peyronie's disease with Doppler color ultrasonography, power Doppler and ultrasonography contrast media]. Radiol Med (Torino) 97:66–69

Chen TY, Zahran AR, Carrier S (2001) Penile curvature associated with scleroderma. Urology 58:282

Fornara P, Gerbershagen HP (2004) Ultrasound in patients affected with Peyronie's disease. World J Urol 22:365–367

Hakim LS (2002) Peyronie's disease: an update. The role of diagnostics. Int J Impot Res 14:321–323

Hauck EW, Hackstein N, Vosshenrich R et al (2003) Diagnostic value of magnetic resonance imaging in Peyronie's disease – a comparison both with palpation and ultrasound in the evaluation of plaque formation. Eur Urol 43:293–299; discussion 299–300

Jordan GH, Angermeier KW (1993) Preoperative evaluation of erectile function with dynamic infusion cavernosometry/cavernosography in patients undergoing surgery for Peyronie's disease: correlation with postoperative results. J Urol 150:1138–1142

Kadioglu A, Tefekli A, Erol H et al (2000) Color Doppler ultrasound assessment of penile vascular system in men with Peyronie's disease. Int J Impot Res 12:263–267

Lopez JA, Jarow JP (1993) Penile vascular evaluation of men with Peyronie's disease. J Urol 149:53–55

Montorsi F, Guazzoni G, Bergamaschi F et al (1994) Vascular abnormalities in Peyronie's disease: the role of color Doppler sonography. J Urol 151:373–375

Pretorius ES, Siegelman ES, Ramchandani P, Banner MP (2001) MR imaging of the penis. Radiographics 21 Spec No:S283-298; discussion S298-289

Ralph DJ, Hughes T, Lees WR, Pryor JP (1992) Pre-operative assessment of Peyronie's disease using colour Doppler sonography. Br J Urol 69:629–632

Sirikci A, Bayram M, Demirci M et al (1999) Penile epithelioid sarcoma: MR imaging findings. Eur Radiol 9:1593–1595

Usta MF, Adams DM, Zhang JW et al (2003) Penile epithelioid sarcoma and the case for a histopathological diagnosis in Peyronie's disease. BJU Int 91:519–521

Vosshenrich R, Schroeder-Printzen I, Weidner W et al (1995) Value of magnetic resonance imaging in patients with penile induration (Peyronie's disease). J Urol 153:1122–1125

Vossough A, Pretorius ES, Siegelman ES et al (2002) Magnetic resonance imaging of the penis. Abdom Imaging 27:640–659

Wegner HE, Andresen R, Knispel HH, Miller K (1997) Local interferon-alpha 2b is not an effective treatment in early-stage Peyronie's disease. Eur Urol 32:190–193

Weidner W, Schroeder-Printzen I, Weiske WH, Vosshenrich R (1997) Sexual dysfunction in Peyronie's disease: an analysis of 222 patients without previous local plaque therapy. J Urol 157:325–328

Wilkins CJ, Sriprasad S, Sidhu PS (2003) Colour Doppler ultrasound of the penis. Clin Radiol 58:514–523

Pathophysiology and Treatment of Priapism

Giovanni Liguori, Stefano Bucci, Sara Benvenuto, Carlo Trombetta, and Emanuele Belgrano

CONTENTS

9.1 Background 71
9.2 Incidence 71
9.3 Etiology and Pathophysiology of Priapism 72
9.4 Low-Flow Priapism 72
9.4.1 Etiology of Low-Flow Priapism 72
9.5 High-Flow Priapism 73
9.6 Recurrent or Stuttering Priapism 74
9.7 Diagnosis of Priapism 74
9.8 Treatment of Priapism 74
9.8.1 Treatment of Low-Flow Priapism 74
9.8.2 Treatment of High-Flow Priapism 76
9.9 Complications 76
9.10 Prognosis 76
References 76

9.1 Background

Priapism is defined as a persistent erection of the penis not accompanied by sexual desire or stimulation, usually lasting more than 6 h and typically involving only the corpora cavernosa and resulting in dorsal penile erection with the ventral penis and glans being flaccid (Keoghane et al. 2002). Rare exceptions with involvement of the corpus spongiosum and sparing of the cavernosal spaces have been reported (Tarry et al. 1987). This condition has many different causes and in some cases can be a urological emergency. The recently published American Urological Association Guideline on the management of priapism sheds further light on the management of this potentially emergent condition, but the guideline does not establish a fixed set of rules or define the legal standard of care for the treatment of priapism (Montague et al. 2003).

9.2 Incidence

In a population-based, retrospective cohort study, the incidence of priapism was found to be 1.5 per 100,000 person-years and 2.9 per 100,000 person-years for men aged 40 years and older (Eland et al. 2001). For men using intracorporal injections to treat erectile dysfunction, the incidence ranges from 1% for the patients who receive prostaglandin E1 to 17% for patients who receive papaverine (Linet and Ogrinc 1996). In children with sickle cell anemia, the incidence is reported to range from 6–27% (Tarry et al. 1987; Ewalt et al. 1996b). In adults, the incidence increases up to 42% (Emond et al. 1980). A different study in this population reports 89% of males with sickle cell anemia will have an episode of priapism by age 20. The mean period is 125 min per event (Mantadakis et al. 1999).

G. Liguori, MD; S. Bucci, MD; S. Benvenuto, MD;
C. Trombetta, MD, Associate Professor;
E. Belgrano, MD, Professor and Chairman
Department of Urology, University of Trieste, Ospedale di Cattinara, Strada di Fiume 447, Trieste, 34124, Italy

9.3
Etiology and Pathophysiology of Priapism

In broad terms, priapism may be regarded as an alteration of imbalance between arterial inflow and outflow. Burnett (2003) has recently reviewed the pathophysiology of priapism and suggested derangements in the diverse systems of regulatory control in erectile function. These dysregulatory functions include possible overactivity of the veno-occlusive mechanism, arterial inflow, or neurogenic processes that can affect inflow or outflow. Conversely, the problem may be secondary to malfunction of the normal contractile activities of cavernosal smooth muscle cells.

The etiology of priapism has been traditionally divided into primary or idiopathic and secondary to some other condition or disease process. However, in accordance with Pryor (2004), for the purposes of clinical management, it is appropriate to distinguish between high-flow, low-flow, and recurrent or stuttering priapism.

9.4
Low-Flow Priapism

The spectrum of clinical symptoms and signs of low-flow, ischemic or anoxic priapism is analogous to those found in other compartment syndromes. It is a prolongation of a normal painful erection and in the idiopathic form is frequently present on walking. During erection there is smooth muscle relaxation in the cavernous arteries and tissue, associated with increased arterial inflow and decreased venous outflow. The intracorporal pressure may rise above mean arterial pressure and the inflow of blood then ceases. The persistence of erection and failure of detumescence, the persistent relaxation and failure of contraction of cavernous smooth muscle, are associated with increasing anoxia, a rising pCO_2 and acidosis (Broderick and Harkaway 1994). The prolonged erection becomes painful after a variable length of time; therefore, patients are warned to seek urgent medical attention for an erection lasting more than 4 h. Early relief is associated with return of normal flaccidity, but more prolonged ischemia is associated with tissue edema.

Histological studies have shown a defined pattern of the pathology (Spycher and Hauri 1986). Interstitial edema and thickening are present up to 12 h. By 24 h, endothelial thrombocytic adherence is present, and by 48 h, necrosis of cavernosal smooth muscle cells and fibroblast proliferation has occurred, which may result in subsequent fibrosis and calcification.

In organ-bath preparations using isolated rabbit corpus cavernosum, Broderick et al. (1994) suggest that corporeal smooth muscle tone, spontaneous contractile activity and the response to α-agonists depends on the state of corporal oxygenation. These observations might be an explanation for the failure of locally administered α-antagonists to relieve ischemic priapism because of smooth muscle paralysis.

Daley et al. (1996a) documented a significant reduction in prostacyclin (PGI-2) production during hypoxia in rabbit corpus cavernosal cells, which was attributed to inhibition of the enzyme PG-2 synthase. In view of the role of PGI-2 as an inhibitor of platelet aggregation and white cell adhesion, these studies may provide some insight into the changes in corporeal hemostasis during ischemic priapism. Further studies have shown that re-oxygenation of these hypoxic rabbit cavernosal cells generates oxidative stress that interferes with the recovery of prostanoid production (Daley et al. 1996b).

The production of nitric oxide (NO) in the corpus cavernosum is altered by hypoxia because NO synthase activity is affected by changes in oxygen tension (Kim et al. 1993). During veno-occlusive ischemic priapism, the entrapped pool of blood that is initially at arterial oxygenation becomes progressively hypoxic. The combined reduction of PGI-2 and NO expected under hypoxic conditions would favor platelet aggregation and white cell adhesion, leading to thrombus formation and tissue damage.

The end result of muscle necrosis after priapism is fibrosis, which may be patchy in distribution, and it is thought that TGF-beta has an important role in this process

9.4.1
Etiology of Low-Flow Priapism

Nieminen and Tammala (1995) found that in 21% of cases the cause of priapism was intracavernosal injection of a vasoactive agents. Papaverine has been associated with a 5% risk at initial diagnostic testing, but with a much lower risk when used as therapy (JUNEMANN and ALKEN 1989); most cases of priapism were in patients with psychogenic or neurogenic impotence.

POHL et al. (1986) evaluated various etiologies for priapism in a study of 230 single case reports in the literature: idiopathic causes comprised one-third of the cases, whereas 21% were attributed to alcohol abuse or medications.

The incidence range of priapism following injection of prostaglandin E1 is around 1% (PORST 1996). The most likely cause of prolonged erection as a result of intracavernous injection therapy is overdose.

Sildenafil is an orally active agent for the treatment of erectile dysfunction, and in well-controlled trials the incidence of priapism appears extremely low, although it has been anecdotally reported in post-marketing surveillance studies.

Drug-induced priapism has been reported with a variety of medications, most commonly related to the antihypertensive drugs guanethidine, prazosin, hydralazine and the anticoagulants, including intravenous heparin, and the oral coumarins (ROUTLEDGE et al. 1998). Generally priapism occurred after cessation of anticoagulant therapy, thus resulting in a rebound hypercoagulable state. Priapism has been reported with a variety of centrally acting drugs including the phenothiazines, paroxetine, fluoxetine and trazodone and cocaine may have synergistic effects in promoting priapism (JIVA and ANWER 1994; BERTHOLON et al. 1996). Cocaine-induced priapism has been reported in association with topical application to enhance sexual performance and intranasal and intracavernous injections. Priapism has also been reported in association with the recreational drug ecstasy (DUBIN and RAZACK 2000).

Examples of neurologic etiologic factors include priapism in patients with degenerative stenosis of the lumbar canal, priapism secondary to cauda equine syndrome and herniated disk (BABA et al. 1995).

Trauma to the perineum, penis or groin, while usually resulting in high-flow priapism, can result in venous compression secondary to penile hematoma or edema.

Different solid tumors have been associated with priapism, including both bladder and prostate cancer (SCHROEDER-PRINTZEN et al. 1994). Malignant priapism has been reported as the initial presentation of metastatic renal cell cancer, metastatic tumors of the gastrointestinal tract and rarely from testis, lung, liver cancer, bone tumors and sarcomas as a result of invasion of both the corpora cavernosa and the corpus spongiosum. Besides infiltration of the corpora cavernosa, priapism may result from infiltration of the perineal veins producing venous drainage impairment (KRCO et al. 1984; CHAN et al. 1998).

Total parenteral nutrition, appendicitis, amyloid and rabies have all been reported as rare causes of priapism (DUTTA 1992; DUTTA 1994; FRIEDMAN 1998).

9.5
High-Flow Priapism

This situation is less common than low-flow priapism and can be classified as congenital due to arterial malformations, traumatic usually associated with penile, perineal or pelvic trauma, iatrogenic following revascularization procedures or idiopathic. The local blood gas tension in these patients is arterial, and therefore the penis is not at risk of ischemia and subsequent fibrosis.

The onset of a post-traumatic, high-flow priapism may occur up to 72 h after the injury. Pain is never as severe as in an ischemic priapism: the penis is often not maximally rigid and pulsation may be recognized.

A mechanism for the pathophysiology of high-flow priapism is described by BASTUBA et al. (1994). Unlike a traditional arteriovenous fistula, the condition is described as an arterial-lacunar fistula where the helicine arteries are bypassed, and the blood passes directly into the lacunar spaces. The high-flow in the lacunar space creates shear stress in adjacent areas, leading to increased nitric oxide release, activation of the cGMP pathway, smooth muscle relaxation and trabecular dilatation. These authors also postulate that the delay in onset of high-flow priapism may be secondary to a delay in the complete necrosis of the arterial wall after the initial trauma or secondary to clot formation at the site of injury followed by the normal lytic pathway, which progresses in a few days.

A rare condition associated with high-flow priapism is Fabry's disease, which may be caused by an unregulated high arterial inflow (FODA et al. 1996).

9.6
Recurrent or Stuttering Priapism

Priapism is associated with the hyper-viscosity syndrome, the most common of which is sickle-cell disease, which still ranks as the most frequent cause of priapism in children (MILLER et al. 1995). In boys with sickle cell disease the incidence of priapism is of 18–27% (EWALT et al. 1996a). This poorly understood condition is uncommon and not confined to men with sickle cell disease. The erection usually presents during sleep, and detumescence does not occur upon waking. These erections usually do not become painful for about an hour. SERJANT et al. (1985) described "stuttering" nocturnal attacks in 42% of Jamaican adults with homozygous sickle-cell disease. Recurrent episodes may result in a markedly enlarged penis with fibrotic corpora, which may later lead to erectile dysfunction.

Other hemoglobinopathies including the rare unstable haemoglobin Hb Olmsted, thrombophilia, leukemias and myeloma and erythropoietin therapy have also been associated with priapism (QUIGLEY and FAWCETT 1999).

9.7
Diagnosis of Priapism

A thorough history and physical examination are prerequisites to diagnostic accuracy. The fundamental aim of the initial phase of assessment is to distinguish arterial from ischemic priapism. The sexual and medical history should especially focus on medications, trauma and predisposing comorbidities. Presence or absence of pain is a fairly reliable predictor of low-flow versus high-flow priapism, respectively. Absence of pain in arterial priapism frequently results in less patient anxiety and discomfort as compared with veno-occlusive priapism. Consequently, patients with arterial priapism may present days or even weeks after the original injury (RICCIARDI et al. 1993).

Physical examination of the penis is critical and typically reveals firm corpora cavernosa and a soft glans, indicating sparing of the corpus spongiosum in low-flow priapism. Findings in high-flow states usually reveal a partial to full erection and sparing of the corpus spongiosum in most cases (BURNETT 2003).

General diagnostic tests include urine toxicology screening for psychoactive drugs and metabolites of cocaine. It has additionally suggested reticulocyte count, urinalysis, complete blood count, platelets and differential white blood cell count.

Urologic management of priapism requires assessment of corporal blood flow status with corporal aspirate, visual inspection by color and consistency or corporal blood, and blood gas analysis including pH, pO_2, and pCO_2. As described in Chapter 10, color Doppler ultrasonography is the imaging modality of choice (BERGER et al. 2001).

Low-flow priapism is suggested by finding low oxygen tension, high carbon dioxide and low pH in the blood gas analysis of the aspirate. When a high-flow state is suspected based on the bright red appearance or blood gas analysis of the corporal aspirate, color Doppler ultrasound is indicated to identify the arterial sinusoidal fistula.

In patients with low-flow states the degree of cavernosal blood acidosis can give an indication of the urgency of treatment. A pH less than 7.10 reflects the need for immediate treatment also with aggressive management options because the tissue is at risk for necrosis (LUE et al. 1986)

9.8
Treatment of Priapism

Therapeutic options for low-flow and high-flow priapism are essentially different, reflecting profound differences in etiology and pathophysiology. While ischemic priapism is a urological emergency that must be treated immediately, also using invasive procedures, patients with high-flow states are in general at low risk of developing irreversible erectile dysfunction and can be managed more conservatively.

9.8.1
Treatment of Low-Flow Priapism

Therapy is based on the underlying cause and will typically follow a pattern of least invasive to more invasive procedures. Any primary factors involved in the cause of the priapism should be addressed and treated. Pain and anxiety also require therapy, which includes the use of parenteral opioids and an anxiolytic if indicated. Ice and elevation are also components of the initial conservative therapy. A penile dorsal nerve block utilizing local anesthesia, circumferential penile block, subcutaneous local penile shaft block and oral conscious sedation for pediatric patients may be of benefit to control pain (Vilke et al. 2004).

For patients with low-flow priapism of relatively short duration (approximately 4 h) penile aspiration and irrigation with saline remain the standard first line management strategies.

Oral terbutaline, a β-adrenoreceptor agonist, in a dose of 5–10 mg has been advocated for treatment of patients with prostaglandin-induced priapism with a response rate of 36% (Lowe and Jarow 1993). Terbutaline can also be given subcutaneously in doses of 0.25–0.5 mg and can be repeated in 15–20 min. Oral pseudoephedrine, an α-adrenoreceptor agonist, in a dose of 60–120 mg has been used to treat priapism due to intracavernosal injected agents, but efficacy is not well studied.

Treatment with injections into the corpus cavernosum of alpha adrenergic receptor agonists after aspiration would be the next therapy after terbutaline. Phenylephrine, 10 cc, which corresponds to a dose of 200 µg, is injected into the penis after aspiration. Frequent blood pressure measurements and preferably ECG monitoring are required throughout, and failure to respond may require a second injection of 200 µg and a final dose of 500 µg. Alternatively, epinephrine can be injected in 1–3-cc boluses up to 10 cc (O'Brien et al. 1989). Methylene blue has been shown to be useful as an alternative to alpha agonists, with a mechanism felt to be related to inhibition of cyclic GMP, which in turn inhibits smooth muscle relaxation (Steers and Selby 1991). Intracavernosal injection with 50 mg of methylene blue is followed by aspiration and penile compression for 5 min. Transient penile burning and blue discoloration lasting for about 3 days were the reported side effects (Martinez Portillo et al. 2001).

If these relatively simple measures fail, surgical intervention is required. A variety of techniques has been described, including the Winter procedure (Fig. 9.1) using a Trucut needle (Winter 1978), the Ebbehoj method using a pointed scalpel blade to create a shunt between the glans and corpora cavernosa (Ebbehoj 1974), and the more radical El-Ghorab procedure that involves excision of a small disk of tunica albuginea (Ercole et al. 1981). These techniques fail in about a third of patients (Carter et al. 1976).

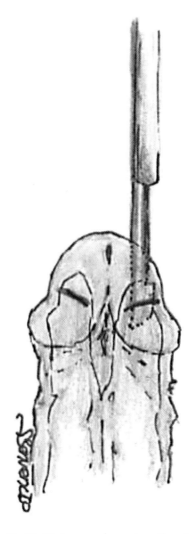

Fig. 9.1. Winter procedure using a Trucut

Use of intracavernosal thrombolytic medications, including tissue plasminogen activator, has been recently described, although the efficacy is uncertain and long-term prognosis is lacking (Rutchik et al. 2001).

The treatment of sickle cell priapism requires more disease-specific treatment, including oxygenation, hydration, alkalinization, exercise, analgesia and exchange transfusion. Anecdotal evidence supports the use of oral therapy with hydroxyurea and hydralazine (Al Jam'a and Al Dabbous 1998). Etilefrine is an oral α-adrenoreceptor agonist that in the form of maintenance therapy may help prevent further attacks, with little effect on systemic blood pressure (Virag et al. 1996). Surgical spinal decompression has been recommended to alleviate priapism associated with lumbar spinal stenosis.

9.8.2
Treatment of High-Flow Priapism

The clinical history and initial investigation, coupled with selective angiography, should confirm the diagnosis. The initial treatment should be observation. This approach is based on the finding that expectant management results in spontaneous resolution in 62% of the report cases. The others cases are best managed by an interventional radiological procedure to embolize the responsible vessels of the cavernous fistula using different embolizing materials such as autologous blood clots, coils, Geolfoam sponge, polyvinyl alcohol particles or N-butylcyanocyalate. Sometimes more than one procedure may be necessary to achieve a complete result (Bastuba et al. 1994).

Open surgical ligation of the responsible vessels using intraoperative ultrasonographic guidance may be used when conservative and minimally invasive methods have failed.

9.9
Complications

Early complications typically result from injection of α-adrenergic agents and include headache, palpitation, hypertension and cardiac arrhythmias. Vital signs should be monitored during this phase of therapy. Additional adverse events include urethral injury and urethrocutaneous or urethrocavernosal fistula from aggressive needle decompression, bleeding and infection (De Stefani et al. 2001). Rare cases of gangrene of the penis after corporospongiosal shunt have been reported.

9.10
Prognosis

Impotence rates between 35–60% have been reported when priapism persists for 5–10 days, respectively (Mulhall and Honig 1996). When the priapism has been ongoing for over 24 h, treatment with aspiration alone is often unsuccessful and will usually require irrigation and often injection. Treatment should be initiated within 12 h of the onset of symptoms to avoid long-term erectile dysfunction and irreversible infarction, with the corollary being the earlier the resolution of symptoms, the better the long-term prognosis.

References

Al Jam'a AH, Al Dabbous IA (1998) Hydroxyurea in the treatment of sickle cell associated priapism. J Urol 159:1642

Baba H, Maezawa Y, Furusawa N, et al. (1995) Lumbar spinal stenosis causing intermittent priapism. Paraplegia 33:338–345

Bastuba MD, Saenz de Tejada I, Dinlenc CZ et al (1994) Arterial priapism: diagnosis, treatment and long-term followup. J Urol 151:1231–1237

Berger R, Billups K, Brock G et al (2001) Report of the American Foundation for Urologic Disease (AFUD) Thought Leader Panel for evaluation and treatment of priapism. Int J Impot Res 13 [Suppl 5]:S39–43

Bertholon F, Krajewski Y, el Allali A (1996) [Adverse effects: priapism caused by paroxetine]. Ann Med Psychol (Paris) 154:145–146; discussion 146–147

Broderick GA, Gordon D, Hypolite J, Levin RM (1994) Anoxia and corporal smooth muscle dysfunction: a model for ischemic priapism. J Urol 151:259–262

Broderick GA, Harkaway R (1994) Pharmacologic erection: time-dependent changes in the corporal environment. Int J Impot Res 6:9–16

Burnett AL (2003) Pathophysiology of priapism: dysregulatory erection physiology thesis. J Urol 170:26–34

Carter RG, Thomas CE, Tomskey GC (1976) Cavernospongiosum shunts in treatment of priapism. Urology 7:292–295

Chan PT, Begin LR, Arnold D et al (1998) Priapism secondary to penile metastasis: a report of two cases and a review of the literature. J Surg Oncol 68:51–59

Daley JT, Brown ML, Watkins T et al (1996a) Prostanoid production in rabbit corpus cavernosum: I. regulation by oxygen tension. J Urol 155:1482–1487

Daley JT, Watkins MT, Brown ML et al (1996b) Prostanoid production in rabbit corpus cavernosum. II. Inhibition by oxidative stress. J Urol 156:1169–1173

De Stefani S, Savoca G, Ciampalini S et al (2001) Urethrocutaneous fistula as a severe complication of treatment for priapism. BJU Int 88:642–643

Dubin NN, Razack AH (2000) Priapism: ecstasy related? Urology 56:1057

Dutta JK (1992) Priapism in rabies. J Assoc Physicians India 40:555

Dutta JK (1994) Rabies presenting with priapism. J Assoc Physicians India 42:430

Ebbehoj J (1974) A new operation for priapism. Scand J Plast Reconst Surg 8:241–245

Eland IA, van der Lei J, Stricker BH, Sturkenboom MJ (2001) Incidence of priapism in the general population. Urology 57:970–972

Emond AM, Holman R, Hayes RJ, Serjeant GR (1980) Priapism and impotence in homozygous sickle cell disease. Arch Intern Med 140:1434–1437

Ercole CJ, Pontes JE, Pierce JM Jr (1981) Changing surgical concepts in the treatment of priapism. J Urol 125:210–211

Ewalt D, Cavender J, Buchanan G, Rogers Z (1996a) Characterization and incidence of priapism in boys with sickle cell anaemia. Paediatrics 88:643

Ewalt D, Cavender J, Buchanan G, Rogers Z (1996b) Leuprolide therapy prevents recurrent priapism in teenage boys with sickle cell anaemia. Paediatrics 88:610

Foda MM, Mahmood K, Rasuli P et al (1996) High-flow priapism associated with Fabry's disease in a child: a case report and review of the literature. Urology 48:949–952

Friedman J (1998) Priapism: an unusual presentation of appendicitis. Pediatr Emerg Care 14:143–144

Jiva T, Anwer S (1994) Priapism associated with chronic cocaine abuse. Arch Intern Med 154:1770

Junemann K, Alken P (1989) Pharmacotherapy of erectile function: a review. Int J Impot Res 1:71–93

Keoghane SR, Sullivan ME, Miller MA (2002) The aetiology, pathogenesis and management of priapism. BJU Int 90:149–154

Kim N, Vardi Y, Padma-Nathan H et al (1993) Oxygen tension regulates the nitric oxide pathway. Physiological role in penile erection. J Clin Invest 91:437–442

Krco MJ, Jacobs SC, Lawson RK (1984) Priapism due to solid malignancy. Urology 23:264–266

Linet OI, Ogrinc FG (1996) Efficacy and safety of intracavernosal alprostadil in men with erectile dysfunction. The Alprostadil Study Group. N Engl J Med 334:873–877

Lowe FC, Jarow JP (1993) Placebo-controlled study of oral terbutaline and pseudoephedrine in management of prostaglandin E1-induced prolonged erections. Urology 42:51–53; discussion 53–54

Lue TF, Hellstrom WJ, McAninch JW, Tanagho EA (1986) Priapism: a refined approach to diagnosis and treatment. J Urol 136:104–108

Mantadakis E, Cavender JD, Rogers ZR et al (1999) Prevalence of priapism in children and adolescents with sickle cell anemia. J Pediatr Hematol Oncol 21:518–522

Martinez Portillo F, Hoang-Boehm J, Weiss J et al (2001) Methylene blue as a successful treatment alternative for pharmacologically induced priapism. Eur Urol 39:20–23

Miller ST, Rao SP, Dunn EK, Glassberg KI (1995) Priapism in children with sickle cell disease. J Urol 154:844–847

Montague DK, Jarow J, Broderick GA et al (2003) American Urological Association guideline on the management of priapism. J Urol 170:1318–1324

Mulhall JP, Honig SC (1996) Priapism: etiology and management. Acad Emerg Med 3:810–816

Nieminen P, Tammala T (1995) Aetiology of priapism in 207 patients. Eur Urol 28:241–245

O'Brien WM, O'Connor KP, Lynch JH (1989) Priapism: current concepts. Ann Emerg Med 18:980–983

Pohl J, Pott B, Kleinhans G (1986) Priapism: a three-phase concept of management according to aetiology and prognosis. Br J Urol 58:113–118

Porst H (1996) The rationale for prostaglandin E1 in erectile failure: a survey of worldwide experience. J Urol 155:802–815

Pryor J, Akkus E, Alter G et al (2004) Priapism. J Sex Med 1:116–120

Quigley M, Fawcett DP (1999) Thrombophilia and priapism. BJU Int 83:155

Ricciardi R, Jr., Bhatt GM, Cynamon J et al (1993) Delayed high flow priapism: pathophysiology and management. J Urol 149:119–121

Routledge PA, Shetty HG, White JP, Collins P (1998) Case studies in therapeutics: warfarin resistance and inefficacy in a man with recurrent thromboembolism, and anticoagulant-associated priapism. Br J Clin Pharmacol 46:343–346

Rutchik S, Sorbera T, Rayford RW, Sullivan J (2001) Successful treatment of recalcitrant priapism using intercorporeal injection of tissue plasminogen activator. J Urol 166:628

Schroeder-Printzen I, Vosshenrich R, Weidner W, Ringert RH (1994) Malignant priapism in a patient with metastatic prostate adenocarcinoma. Urol Int 52:52–54

Serjeant GR, de Ceulaer K, Maude GH (1985) Stilboestrol and stuttering priapism in homozygous sickle-cell disease. Lancet 2:1274–1276

Spycher MA, Hauri D (1986) The ultrastructure of the erectile tissue in priapism. J Urol 135:142–147

Steers WD, Selby JB, Jr (1991) Use of methylene blue and selective embolization of the pudendal artery for high flow priapism refractory to medical and surgical treatments. J Urol 146:1361–1363

Tarry WF, Duckett JW Jr, Snyder HM 3rd (1987) Urological complications of sickle cell disease in a pediatric population. J Urol 138:592–594

Vilke GM, Harrigan RA, Ufberg JW, Chan TC (2004) Emergency evaluation and treatment of priapism. J Emerg Med 26:325–329

Virag R, Bachir D, Lee K, Galacteros F (1996) Preventive treatment of priapism in sickle cell disease with oral and self-administered intracavernous injection of etilefrine. Urology 47:777–781; discussion 781

Winter CC (1978) Priapism cured by creation of fistulas between glans penis and corpora cavernosa. J Urol 119:227–228

Imaging Priapism:
The Diagnostic Role of Color Doppler US

Michele Bertolotto, Fabio Pozzi Mucelli, Giovanni Liguori, and Daniela Sanabor

CONTENTS

10.1 Background 79

10.2 Post-Traumatic Priapism 80
10.2.1 Grey-Scale Ultrasonography 80
10.2.2 Color and Duplex Doppler Ultrasonography 80
10.2.3 Identification of Feeding Vessels 81
10.2.4 Evaluation of Treatment Outcome 82

10.3 Ischemic Priapism 84
10.3.1 Grey-Scale Ultrasonography 84
10.3.2 Color and Duplex Doppler Ultrasonography 85

10.4 Metastatic Priapism 86

10.5 Diagnostic Role of Other Imaging Modalities 86

References 87

10.1
Background

As described in Chapter 9, priapism is an uncommon medical condition defined as persistent tumescence or erection not associated with sexual desire or stimulation (Pautler and Brock 2001). Different pathophysiologies have been described. Low-flow or ischemic priapism is characterized by complete painful erection secondary to inadequate venous outflow leading to hypoxia, acidosis and pain (Lue et al. 1986; Pautler and Brock 2001). High-flow priapism is usually associated with penile or perineal blunt trauma and cavernosal artery tear (Pautler and Brock 2001). Patients with high-flow priapism usually develop a painless partial erection and are able to increase rigidity with sexual stimulation. Venous outflow can be relatively compromised (Bertolotto et al. 2003), but usually is maintained, preventing complete erection, stasis and tissue hypoxia.

Recently, recurrent or stuttering priapism has been described as a poorly understood condition that may present clinically with low-flow or, more frequently, with high-flow episodes, alternatively (Pautler and Brock 2001; Pryor et al. 2004).

Malignant priapism (Pautler and Brock 2001) is a rare complication of hematologic malignancies, with pathogenesis being ascribed to the sludging effect of leukemic cells within the corpora cavernosa of the penis (Winter and McDowell 1988). Also other causes such as disturbance of the central or peripheral nervous system have been advocated (Vadakan and Ortega 1972; Winter and McDowell 1988). Metastatic priapism (Pautler and Brock 2001) is related to secondary penile tumor involvement presenting clinically with painful penile stiffness.

Priapism is a rare manifestation of aortocaval fistula that should be considered in elderly patients with large aortic aneurysms (Abela et al. 2003; Gordon et al. 2004). Similar to posttraumatic priapism, the corpus spongiosum is usually turgid, and blood gas analysis reveals nonischemic blood. Other signs suggestive for the presence of an aortocaval fistula are associated frank hematuria and renal failure. The high-pressure congestion within the venous compartments distal to the fistula is the cause of both penile turgescence and hematuria, lower limb pain and edema, and arterial pulsation in the leg veins. Renal insufficiency is probably caused by decreased renal perfusion, as a result of preferential shunting of blood flow through the fistula, possibly complicated by increased renal vein pressure.

Although diagnosis of priapism and differentiations between the non-ischemic and the ischemic sub-

M. Bertolotto, MD; F. Pozzi Mucelli, MD; D. Sanabor, MD
Department of Radiology, University of Trieste, Ospedale di Cattinara, Strada di Fiume 447, Trieste, 34124, Italy
G. Liguori, MD
Department of Urology, University of Trieste, Ospedale di Cattinara, Strada di Fiume 447, Trieste, 34124, Italy

types can be accomplished based on history, clinics and aspiration of blood from the corpora cavernosa, grey-scale and color Doppler ultrasonography provide clinically useful information that are essential for the management of the patient (HAKIM et al. 1996).

10.2
Post-Traumatic Priapism

Color Doppler ultrasonography is currently considered the imaging modality of choice for the diagnosis of high-flow priapism since it is sensitive, noninvasive and widely available (HAKIM et al. 1996; BERTOLOTTO et al. 2003). No cavernosal injection of vasoactive drugs is required.

10.2.1
Grey-Scale Ultrasonography

At ultrasound, an irregular hypoechoic region within the echogenic cavernous tissue is usually identified, consistent with cavernosal tissue laceration, extravasation of blood from the torn arterial vessel and distension of the lacunar spaces (Fig. 10.1). Distinguishing between these factors is difficult, if not impossible, at US (BERTOLOTTO et al. 2003; BERTOLOTTO et al. 2005a).

Grey-scale ultrasound appearance of the corpora cavernosa can be different in longstanding disease. In fact, patients with high-flow priapism occasionally undergo evaluation several days, or even months or years after the onset of symptoms. In longstanding priapism it is conceivable that the area encompassing the arterial-lacunar wound is covered with endothelium, mimicking a pseudoaneurysm that appears at grey-scale US more regular and circumscribed than previously described (BERTOLOTTO et al. 2003).

10.2.2
Color and Duplex Doppler Ultrasonography

Direct identification of the arterial-lacunar fistula is obtained with Doppler techniques. Color Doppler ultrasonography allows identification of the lesion in virtually all patients; only one case has been reported in which the fistula was not detected both at color Doppler and at angiography, but became evident only after empiric selective embolization of the contralateral internal pudendal artery (ANKEM et al. 2001).

Unilateral or bilateral cavernosal artery tear can be demonstrated. This information has a profound

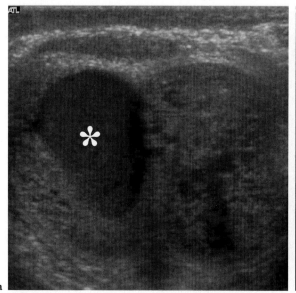
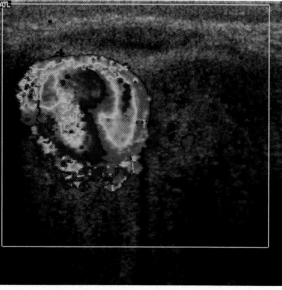

Fig. 10.1a,b. Postraumatic high-flow priapism. Axial scans of the penis. **a** Grey-scale ultrasonography showing an hypoechoic region within the right corpus cavernosum (*). **b** Color Doppler interrogation showing characteristic color blush that is consistent with extravasation of blood from the lacerated cavernosal artery [reprinted with permission from: Bertolotto M, Calderan L, Cova MA (2005) Imaging of penile traumas-therapeutic implications. Eur Radiol 15:2475–2482]

effect in the choice of the treatment. In particular, color Doppler ultrasonography demonstrates extravasation of blood from the lacerated cavernosal artery presenting with a characteristic color blush extending into the erectile tissue (Fig. 10.1).

A careful Doppler technique allows a better evaluation of all vascular structures involved (Bertolotto et al. 2003). Optimization of the color Doppler parameters to detect slow velocity flows allows evaluation of the penile vessels and eases identification of the color blush from the torn artery. However, visualization of high velocity flows is not correct, and aliasing hampers visualization of the exact site of the cavernosal tear. When color Doppler velocity scale is increased, depiction of lower velocity flows is reduced, and the cavernosal tear is immediately recognized as a circumscribed color spot displaying aliasing. Duplex Doppler interrogation of the arterial-lacunar fistula displays characteristically high velocity, turbulent flows (Fig. 10.2).

10.2.3
Identification of Feeding Vessels

Besides identification of the arterial-lacunar fistula, color Doppler ultrasonography allows evaluation of the penile vasculature to identify hemodynamically significant feeding vessels that present with high velocity flow. Both unilateral and bilateral feeding

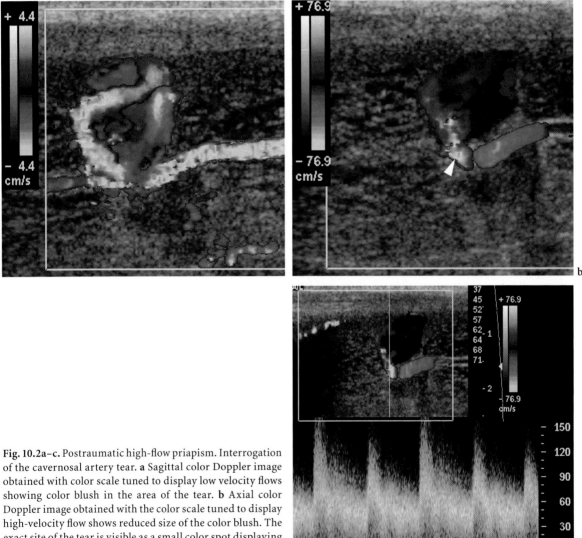

Fig. 10.2a–c. Postraumatic high-flow priapism. Interrogation of the cavernosal artery tear. **a** Sagittal color Doppler image obtained with color scale tuned to display low velocity flows showing color blush in the area of the tear. **b** Axial color Doppler image obtained with the color scale tuned to display high-velocity flow shows reduced size of the color blush. The exact site of the tear is visible as a small color spot displaying aliasing (*arrowhead*). **c** Duplex Doppler interrogation of the fistula shows high velocity, turbulent flow

vessels can be identified, providing useful information in patients undergoing embolization to plan the angiographic approach from the left or from the right side (BERTOLOTTO et al. 2003). Usually the main feeding vessel is a cavernosal artery; however, a variety of collateral vessels can be associated. In particular, dorsal to cavernosal artery communications represent large vascular pathways that are able to feed the fistula and may be responsible for treatment failure after embolization of the torn cavernosal artery. Also intercavernosal arterial communications can connect the proximal portion of the torn artery with the controlateral cavernosal artery and can be responsible for treatment failure. Cavernosal-spongiosal communications and other small collaterals can feed the fistula as well.

In patients with high-flow priapism Doppler interrogation shows flows with increased velocity in both cavernosal arteries also in patients with unilateral tear. In fact, large communications exist between the corpora cavernosa, and nitric oxide released at the level of the fistula diffuses freely in the contralateral side. Cavernosal diastolic flow is variable, depending on blood pressure within the partially erected penis. The firmer the erection is, the lower the diastolic pressure. In general, lower resistances are observed at the site of the fistula, with progressively higher diastolic flows while approaching the lesion. Although in general patients with high-flow priapism have painless incomplete erection, nearly complete painful erection can occasionally be detected (BERTOLOTTO et al. 2003). Immediate embolization of the fistula is recommended in these patients to avoid irreversible cavernosal tissue damage.

10.2.4
Evaluation of Treatment Outcome

High-flow priapism can occasionally undergo spontaneous resolution (ARANGO et al. 1999). Superselective embolization of the torn artery, however, is currently considered the treatment of choice (BASTUBA et al. 1994; CIAMPALINI et al. 2002; SAVOCA et al. 2004). After embolization, closure of the torn artery can be observed at grey-scale ultrasonography by the presence of embolizing material within the vessel. If the arterial tear is large, embolizing material can pour into the hypoechoic lacuna within the cavernosal tissue. When the fistula is successfully embolized, a cavernosal hematoma is left in the lacuna, which usually appears hypoechoic and then organizes presenting with complex echogenic areas, anechoic regions and septations. The hematoma progressively reduces in size resulting in complete restoration of the normal ultrasound appearance of the injured cavernosal tissue or, more often, in tissue scar (Fig. 10.3).

Color Doppler ultrasonography allows evaluation of penile blood flow changes after embolization of the diseased vessel. This evaluation is useful in the clinical practice because in many cases erection does not subside immediately after embolization, but might require several days. As a consequence, it is usually not possible to evaluate the success of therapy basing on clinics alone.

Different ultrasound findings can be appreciated after embolization (BERTOLOTTO et al. 2003). In about 33% of patients the fistula closes completely. However, in about 44% of patients the fistula is still patent despite arteriographic evidence of occlusion (Fig. 10.4). The fistula is usually markedly reduced in size, fed by small homolateral and contralateral vessels that usually are not detected before embolization because of non-significant flows, but widen when the main feeding pathways are obliterated.

In our experience, the type of vessels that are involved in refilling the fistula is of concern for the outcome of the patients. In fact, previous studies have shown that if the size of the fistula reduces after embolization, penile turgidity reduces as well, and the fistula is likely to heal spontaneously. After incomplete embolization the fistula can be fed by non-obliterated collaterals such as accessory pudendal arteries, recurrent cavernosal branches, communications with the contralateral cavernosal artery or with the dorsal artery, and cavernosal-spongiosal communications with inverted flow (BERTOLOTTO et al. 2003). In our experience, if penile turgidity reduces after embolization, the fistula is likely to heal spontaneously in a few days due to reduced hyperoxygenation and endothelial shear stress. In general, this condition occurs when the fistula is supplied by small feeding vessels with limited blood flow, such as cavernosal-spongiosal communications. Watchful observation is recommended in these patients. Conversely, when a more significant blood supply is demonstrated at color Doppler ultrasound or penile turgidity remains unchanged, repeat angiography should be considered.

In about 23% of patients with high-flow priapism and apparently successful embolization of the lacer-

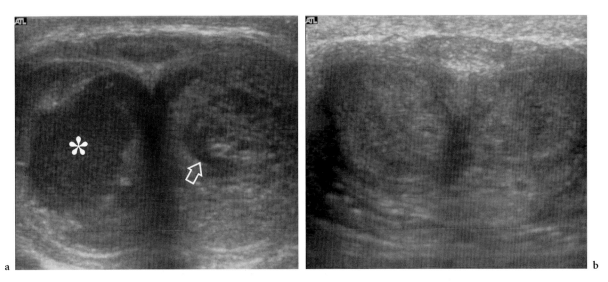

Fig. 10.3a,b. Grey-scale appearance of the penile shaft after successful angiographic embolization of a right cavernosal artery tear. **a** Axial scan obtained 1 h after embolization shows a cavernous hematoma (*) in the site of the embolized fistula within the right corpus cavernosum. A smaller hematoma (*open arrow*) not associated to cavernosal artery injury is recognized within the left corpus cavernosum as well. **b** Axial scan obtained 6 months later shows that the echotexture of the corpora cavernosa in the site of the previously embolized fistula is inhomogeneous due to fibrous changes. The patient, however, reported normal erections

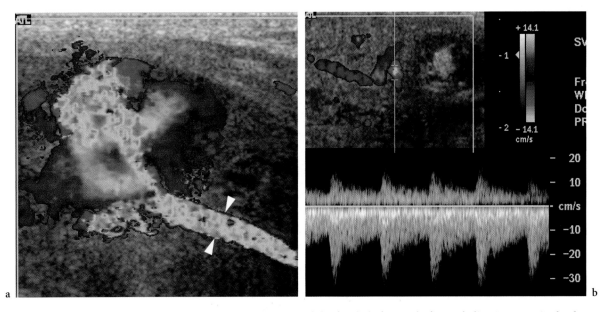

Fig. 10.4a,b. High-flow priapism. Color Doppler appearance of the fistula before and after embolization. **a** Sagittal color Doppler image of the right crus shows extravasation of blood from the cavernosal artery (*arrowheads*). **b** Duplex Doppler ultrasound image obtained soon after angiography shows that the fistula is still patent, but reduced in size. The fistula closed spontaneously within 5 days

ated artery, color Doppler ultrasonography demonstrates early recanalization of the embolized artery and the need for repeated treatment.

During the follow-up of patients with high-flow priapism, we recommend color Doppler ultrasound 1–2 months after embolization to confirm the absence of recurrent fistula. Recanalization of the embolized cavernosal artery can be observed also when non-reabsorbable embolization material has been used (Savoca et al. 2004). In patients with erectile dysfunction, the study should be performed after intracavernosal prostaglandin injection to determine whether the functional impairment is caused by insufficient penile blood flow or not.

10.3
Ischemic Priapism

Imaging is usually not required before the operation in patients with ischemic priapism, because this condition is considered a urological emergency, and history and examination are often sufficient to make the diagnosis. It is commonly accepted that prompt treatment is mandatory in all patients with low-flow priapism because recovery of function becomes increasingly unlikely over time (Winter and McDowell 1988).

However, there is increasing evidence that the degree of venous outflow obstruction and ischemia varies from person to person. In fact, some degree of blood circulation is maintained in many cases and several patients regain potency even after days of priapism. On the contrary, other patients lose potency in a much shorter period of time (Lue et al. 1986).

In patients with low-flow priapism grey-scale and color Doppler ultrasonography provide useful information on the vascular status of the penis that can be of prognostic value and may influence the clinical or surgical management.

10.3.1
Grey-Scale Ultrasonography

At ultrasound the corpora cavernosa initially present with the same echogenicity and echotexture that is observed in patients with normal erection. When the patient is left supine for a few minutes without manipulating the penis, the corpuscolate component of the blood into the corpora cavernosa tends to sediment downwards forming a fluid-fluid level; this situation documents blood stasis within the corpora cavernosa (Fig. 10.5). In more advanced situations the corpora cavernosa present with increased echogenicity, probably associated with tissue edema. Occasionally echogenic material obliterates the cavernosal arteries (Fig. 10.6). Initially, the glans is turgid, while it is usually flaccid later. In long-standing ischemic priapism, wide echo-texture alterations of the corpora cavernosa are recognized, consistent with fibrotic changes.

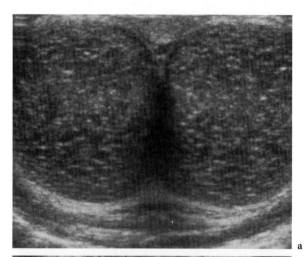

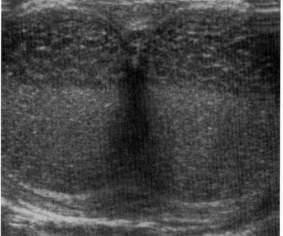

Fig. 10.5a,b. Cocaine-induced priapism lasting for 10 h. a Grey-scale axial image showing normal echogenicity of the corporal bodies. b Grey-scale axial image of the same patient left supine for few minutes without manipulating the penis. The corpuscolate component of blood sedimented downwards forming a fluid-fluid level consistent with stasis. The patient underwent corporal blood aspiration and medical treatment injecting alpha-adrenoreceptor drugs and recovered normal erectile function

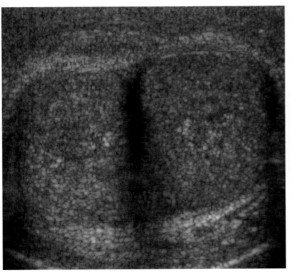 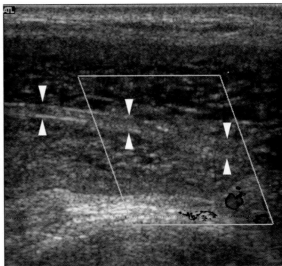

Fig. 10.6a,b. Idiopatic ischemic priapism lasting since 25 h. a Grey-scale axial image showing increased echogenicity of the corporal bodies, consistent with tissue edema. b Longitudinal color Doppler image of the same patient showing obliteration of the cavernosal arteries (*arrowheads*). The patient underwent surgical shunting, but developed irreversible erectile dysfunction

10.3.2
Color and Duplex Doppler Ultrasonography

In patients with low-flow priapism, color Doppler interrogation of the cavernosal arteries shows flows of different characteristics from person to person. Early on, flow with high peak systolic velocity and holodiastolic flow reversal can be appreciable. As venous occlusion progresses and cavernosal blood pressure approaches systolic blood pressure, the systolic envelope sharpens with progressive reduction of the peak systolic velocity. These flow characteristics are indistinguishable from flows that are recognized in subjects with normal rigid erection. Termination of cavernosal artery flow indicates that the intracorporeal pressure rose above mean arterial pressure causing intracavernous stasis, ischemia and progressive cavernous tissue damage.

In our clinical experience in patients presenting with cavernosal artery flows, priapism usually relieves injecting an alpha-adrenoreceptor after blood aspiration from the corpora cavernosa. In general, these patients are able to achieve an erection sufficient for penetration within a few weeks. In patients presenting with no cavernosal artery flows shunt surgery is often required, and the incidence of irreversible erectile dysfunction is high. Patients presenting with echogenic material obliterating the cavernosal arteries usually develop irreversible erectile dysfunction.

It has been recently suggested that priapism induced by intracavernous injection of papaverine/phentolamine could be successfully predicted with color Doppler ultrasonography (Metawea et al. 2005). Cavernosal artery flows with peak systolic velocity greater than 66 cm/s and end diastolic velocity of 0 to 1 cm/s should be accurate predictors of persistent erection requiring intervention. In our experience, however, when prostaglandin E1 is used, cavernosal artery flows with peak systolic velocity of 66 cm/s or greater are often recognized in young patients who reach full erection that undergo detumescence within 2–3 h without requiring intervention.

In patients with priapism and clinical signs and symptoms suggestive of the presence of an aortocaval fistula, abdominal color Doppler ultrasonography can be used to confirm the diagnosis revealing the presence of an aortic aneurysm. High velocity, pulsatile flows in the inferior vena cava confirm the diagnosis. Renal hypoperfusion is often recognized. Diagnosis, however, may be difficult in obese patients, and direct visualization of the fistula can be problematic using conventional Doppler techniques. We found no description of the ultrasound appearance of the penis in these patients; it is conceivable, however, that grey-scale and color Doppler ultrasound findings would be similar to those observed in operated patients with deep dorsal vein arterialization (Bertolotto et al. 2005c).

10.4
Metastatic Priapism

Invasion of the corpora cavernosa by a malignant neoplasm can present with penile stiffness and pain simulating low-flow priapism. In these patients greyscale ultrasonography can show circumscribed tumor nodules within the corpora cavernosa or diffuse infiltration of the shaft (BERTOLOTTO et al. 2005b). Doppler interrogation of the cavernosal arteries usually shows hypervascular cavernosal bodies due to tumor lesion vascularity; cavernosal artery flows are variable. Venous stasis can be associated, resulting from infiltrations of the normal venous leakage pathways.

10.5
Diagnostic Role of Other Imaging Modalities

Internal pudendal angiography followed by superselective embolization of the torn artery with autologous blood clots or reabsorbable synthetic substances is usually considered a satisfactory therapy for high-flow priapism (BASTUBA et al. 1994; CIAMPALINI et al. 2002; SAVOCA et al. 2004). Other operators perform obliteration of the shunt with coils (HARMON and NEHRA 1997). In order to reduce the rate of recurrent priapism, however, non-reabsorbable embolizing material can be used (BERTOLOTTO et al. 2003). In our department embolization is usually done using polyvinyl alcohol particles of variable size between 350–500 microns (Fig. 10.7). We observed early recanalization of the embolized artery in 3/16 patients. Despite the use of non-reabsorbable embolizing material, both cavernosal arteries were patent within 2 months in 60% of the patients who had undergone complete embolization. All but one patient recovered normal erectile function. The remaining patient had nearly complete, painful erection. Repeated embolization and surgical ligation of a large accessory artery were needed.

Besides color Doppler ultrasonography and angiography other imaging modalities are rarely needed in evaluating patients with priapism. Retrograde urethrography and micturition cystourethrography can be considered in patients with suspected associated urethral injury, which can rarely occur especially after iatrogenic maneuvers.

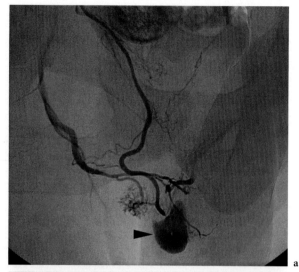
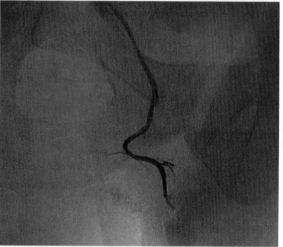

Figure 10.7a,b. Postraumatic high-flow priapism. **a** Angiogram showing extravasation of contrast material (*arrowhead*) from a tear of the right cavernosal artery. **b** After embolization using polyvinyl alcohol particles the angiogram shows occlusion of the fistula. Penile tumescence decreased markedly within a few hours [reprinted with permission from: Bertolotto M, Calderan L, Cova MA (2005) Imaging of penile traumas-therapeutic implications. Eur Radiol 15:2475–2482]

Dynamic infusion cavernosometry and cavernosography have been used to document the absence of cavernosal venous outflow in patients with ischemic low-flow priapism (GOTO et al. 1999) and to identify postischemic fibrotic cavernosal tissue changes (VELCEK and EVANS 1982; VAN DER HORST et al. 2003). Clinical evaluation and ultrasound, however, provide enough useful information to manage the patients.

In patients with high-flow priapism and complex traumas undergoing contrast-enhanced CT with state-of-the-art multiple detector-row systems, the arterial-sinusoidal fistula can be identified (Fig. 10.8). This examination, however, cannot replace angiography, because interventional maneuvers cannot be performed. In malignant priapism contrast-enhanced CT is indicated to evaluate the perineal and pelvic extent of the disease. In patients with priapism secondary to aortocaval fistula contrast-enhanced CT reveals the communication between the aorta and the inferior vena cava and congestion of the pelvic vessels (ABELA et al. 2003; GORDON et al. 2004). Poor enhancement of the kidneys reveals renal hypoperfusion.

Magnetic resonance imaging findings in patients with priapism have been described in a limited number of cases. In patients with high-flow priapism this technique is able to identify the site of the fistula (ENGIN et al. 1999). In patients with ischemic and metastatic priapism, the presence of corporeal thrombosis (PTAK et al. 1994; VOSSOUGH et al. 2002) and tumor infiltration of the corpora cavernosa (VOSSOUGH et al. 2002) can be recognized.

During the follow-up of ischemic priapism this examination allows evaluation of circumscribed (PARK et al. 2001) or diffuse fibrous changes of the cavernous tissue as heterogeneous areas of low signal intensity on both T1- and T2 weighted sequences.

During the follow-up of high-flow priapism, magnetic resonance imaging is able to document persistent closure or recanalization of the embolized cavernosal artery (PARK et al. 2001). Color Doppler ultrasonography, however, usually provides enough clinically useful information in these patients.

References

Abela R, Khan S, Wells A (2003) Priapism at age 94. J R Soc Med 96:407–408

Ankem MK, Gazi MA, Ferlise VJ et al (2001) High-flow priapism: a novel way of lateralizing the lesion in radiologically inapparent cases. Urology 57:800

Arango O, Castro R, Dominguez J, Gelabert A (1999) Complete resolution of post-traumatic high-flow priapism with conservative treatment. Int J Impot Res 11:115–117

Bastuba MD, Saenz de Tejada I, Dinlenc CZ et al (1994) Arterial priapism: diagnosis, treatment and long-term follow-up. J Urol 151:1231–1237

Bertolotto M, Calderan L, Cova MA (2005a) Imaging of penile traumas–therapeutic implications. Eur Radiol 15:2475–2482

Bertolotto M, Quaia E, Mucelli FP et al (2003) Color Doppler imaging of posttraumatic priapism before and after selective embolization. Radiographics 23:495–503

Bertolotto M, Serafini G, Dogliotti L et al (2005b) Primary and secondary malignancies of the penis: ultrasound features. Abdom Imaging 30:108–112

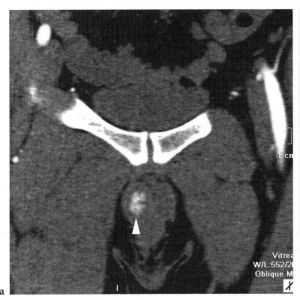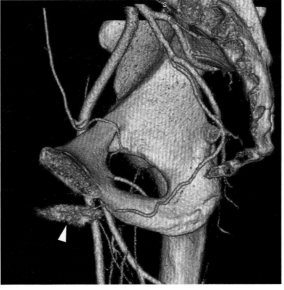

Fig. 10.8a,b. Postraumatic high-flow priapism. Imaging features with multidetector-row CT angiography. **a** Coronal image showing iodinated contrast extravasation within the right corpus cavernosum (*arrowhead*). **b** 3D reconstruction of the vascular supply to the penis on the right side, from the pudendal artery to the cavernosal artery tear (*arrowhead*)

Bertolotto M, Serafini G, Savoca G et al (2005c) Color Doppler US of the postoperative penis: anatomy and surgical complications. Radiographics 25:731-748

Ciampalini S, Savoca G, Buttazzi L et al (2002) High-flow priapism: treatment and long-term follow-up. Urology 59:110-113

Engin G, Tunaci M, Acunas B (1999) High-flow priapism due to cavernous artery pseudoaneurysm: color Doppler sonography and magnetic resonance imaging findings. Eur Radiol 9:1698-1699

Gordon S, Marsh P, Day A, Chappell B (2004) Priapism as the presenting symptom of an aortocaval fistula. Emerg Med J 21:265

Goto T, Yagi S, Matsushita S et al (1999) Diagnosis and treatment of priapism: experience with five cases. Urology 53:1019-1023

Hakim LS, Kulaksizoglu H, Mulligan R et al (1996) Evolving concepts in the diagnosis and treatment of arterial high flow priapism. J Urol 155:541-548

Harmon WJ, Nehra A (1997) Priapism: diagnosis and management. Mayo Clin Proc 72:350-355

Lue TF, Hellstrom WJ, McAninch JW, Tanagho EA (1986) Priapism: a refined approach to diagnosis and treatment. J Urol 136:104-108

Metawea B, El-Nashar AR, Gad-Allah A et al (2005) Intracavernous papaverine/phentolamine-induced priapism can be accurately predicted with color Doppler ultrasonography. Urology 66:858-860

Park JK, Jeong YB, Han YM (2001) Recanalization of embolized cavernosal artery: restoring potency in the patient with high flow priapism. J Urol 165:2002-2003

Pautler SE, Brock GB (2001) Priapism. From Priapus to the present time. Urol Clin North Am 28:391-403

Pryor J, Akkus E, Alter G et al (2004) Priapism. J Sex Med 1:116-120

Ptak T, Larsen CR, Beckmann CF, Boyle DE Jr (1994) Idiopathic segmental thrombosis of the corpus cavernosum as a cause of partial priapism. Abdom Imaging 19:564-566

Savoca G, Pietropaolo F, Scieri F et al (2004) Sexual function after highly selective embolization of cavernous artery in patients with high flow priapism: long-term follow-up. J Urol 172:644-647

Vadakan VV, Ortega J (1972) Priapism in acute lymphoblastic leukemia. Cancer 30:373-375

Van der Horst C, Stuebinger H, Seif C et al (2003) Priapism-etiology, pathophysiology and management. Int Braz J Urol 29:391-400

Velcek D, Evans JA (1982) Cavernosography. Radiology 144:781-785

Vossough A, Pretorius ES, Siegelman ES et al (2002) Magnetic resonance imaging of the penis. Abdom Imaging 27:640-659

Winter CC, McDowell G (1988) Experience with 105 patients with priapism: update review of all aspects. J Urol 140:980-983

Penile Injuries:
Mechanism, Presentation and Management

Gianfranco Savoca

CONTENTS

11.1 Presentation and Diagnosis 89

11.2 Management 91
11.2.1 Injury to the Suspensory Ligament 91
11.2.2 Blunt Trauma to the Flaccid Penis 91
11.2.3 Penile Fracture 91
11.2.4 Anterior Urethral Injuries 91
11.2.5 Posterior Urethral Injuries 92
11.2.6 Penile Amputation 92

References 93

11.1
Presentation and Diagnosis

From the clinical point of view, the first important distinction in patients presenting with penile traumas is between penetrating and non-penetrating lesions.

Penetrating injuries usually occur while flaccid, and severity is variable depending of whether the skin, the urethra or the erectile tissues are involved (Selikowitz 1977). The most common penetrating injuries to the penis are iatrogenic, following cavernosal injection of vasoactive drugs and inappropriate circumcision maneuvers, or result from farm and war accidents, gunshot wounds, animal or human bites. Zipper injuries are rare and often not significant. Most of the penetrating traumas are self inflicted in mentally deranged patients or inflicted by a second party.

G. Savoca, MD
Department of Urology, Ospedale Fondazione San Raffaele Giglio, Contrada Pietrapollastra, Cefalù, 90015, Italy

The most common cause of non-penetrating injury is sexual intercourse with the compression of the shaft against the symphysis or with the sudden bending of the shaft (Nicolaisen et al. 1983). This condition is due to an excessive force applied to the long axis of the penis in the erect status (Coogan and Levine 1998; Shaeer 2006). Fracture of the penis may also occur by rolling over in bed during a deep sleep or during penile manipulation (Mellinger 1993; Chung et al. 2006). Blunt perineal trauma of the flaccid penis is generally due to bicycle or motorcycle accidents with the compression of the corpora cavernosa and the urethra against the ischial rami.

In patients with penile injury another clinically important distinction is between trauma with associated urethral rupture and without urethral rupture. Albugineal rupture is associated with urethral injury in approximately 15% of cases (Webster 1989).

The rupture of the suspensory ligament can occur from sudden ventral displacing of the penis in the erect status, during masturbation or placing the erect penis into underpants. The patient typically hears a cracking sound followed by pain at the basis of the shaft. If the snatch involves only the suspensor ligament, a slight hematoma of the soft tissue at the basis of shaft can appear, and the rigidity of the penis remains unchanged (Sagalowsky and Peters 1998). Afterwards the patient will note an abnormal angle during erection. During an accurate physical examination a gap between the pubis and the base of the penile shaft can be noted. In this case imaging is not required, but ultrasonography can be helpful to exclude more significant lesions or hematomas.

In case of fracture of the corpora cavernosa, a significant hematoma can occur. The fascial layers of the genitalia will determine the distribution and the extent of blood extravasion. If the Buck's fascia is involved, the extravasated blood will be contained within the limits of the Colles' fascia with a resulting perineal hematoma in a typical "butterfly" distribution (Fig. 11.1). If the Buck's fascia remains intact, blood extravasion will direct along the shaft of the penis with a typical "eggplant" distribution (Fig. 11.2).

Moreover, in case of rupture of the corpora cavernosa, the typical snap sound is followed by severe pain, rapid detumescence, penile swelling and deformity (Jack et al. 2004).

For many years cavernosography has been considered the standard diagnostic procedure to identify the tear of the tunica albuginea (Jack et al. 2004). This procedure, however, is invasive and at risk for contrast reaction and fibrosis of the corpora cavernosa (Tsang and Demby 1992).

We advocate ultrasound as the first-choice imaging modality in these patients because it is easily performed and non-invasive. Immediate ultrasonography enables to determine the entity of hematoma and allows detection of the site and the length of the tear of the tunica albuginea (Bertolotto and Pozzi Mucelli 2004). Moreover, ultrasonography permits to exclude the concomitant presence of cavernosal artery rupture with formation of an arteriallacunar fistula.

Other imaging modalities besides ultrasonography, such as magnetic resonance imaging, are rarely needed in the clinical practice to evaluate patients with penile traumas and to plan the proper therapy (Coogan and Levine 1998; Bertolotto et al. 2005).

Patients with penile fracture may present with associated injury to the corpus spongiosum and to the anterior urethra. The severity of the lesions can be variable, ranging from urethral contusion to partial or complete rupture.

Posterior urethra can be injured in patients with pelvic traumas. Precise definition of pelvic fracture location may enable prediction of which subjects are at risk for posterior urethral injury (Basta et al. 2007).

Diagnosis of associated urethral injury can be problematic. The patient can report a difficulty voiding, or present with blood at the meatus. In this case diagnostic catheterization must be avoided because it may convert a minimal tear into a complete tear of the urethra. The diagnosis is confirmed by a retrograde urethrography with extravasation of contrast material at the site of the disruption.

Penile amputation is due to self-mutilation, assaults and accidents. About 200 cases have been reported in the literature. In penile amputation both the corpora cavernosa and corpus spongiosum with the urethra are involved (Aboseif et al. 1993), and the neurovascular dorsal bundle is dissected. Diagnosis is straightforward because the distal portion of the penile shaft is partially or totally dismembered from the proximal part and important hemorrhage is evident. Diagnostic imaging procedures are not necessary.

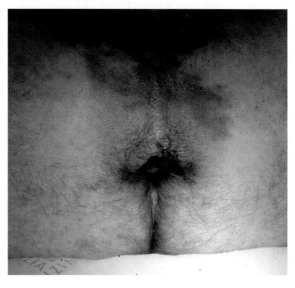

Fig. 11.1. Penile fracture with rupture of the Buck's fascia. The hematoma spreads to the attachment of the Colles' fascia involving the penis, scrotum and perineum with typical "butterfly" configuration

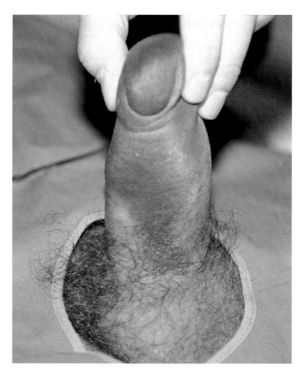

Fig. 11.2. Penile fracture with intact Buck's fascia. The hematoma is confined to the shaft

11.2
Management

A variety of surgical of conservative procedures can be used for treatment of the different penile traumas depending of the type and severity of injuries.

11.2.1
Injury to the Suspensory Ligament

Rupture of the suspensory ligament does not cause loss of penile rigidity, and the erectile function is unchanged. However, the patients can complain of an abnormal angle during erection. In this case a simple suture of the ligament through a suprapubic access can be easily performed.

11.2.2
Blunt Trauma to the Flaccid Penis

Most traumas to the flaccid penis result in hematoma without lesion of the tunica albuginea. Immediate treatment consists in catheterization, ice packs and anti-inflammatory agents.

It is mandatory to exclude an arterial priapism by ultrasonography. If an arterial-lacunar fistula is demonstrated, the immediate treatment is conservative and consists of prolonged compression of the site of the fistula. Primary delayed treatment consists in percutaneous embolization of the fistula or microsurgical repair. Highly selective embolization of the cavernous artery seems to be the best option in order to prevent erectile dysfunction at long term (Savoca et al. 2004).

11.2.3
Penile Fracture

When a defect of the tunica albuginea is demonstrated by ultrasonography and/or cavernosography, early repair of the tunica albuginea is recommended by most of the authors (Ozen et al. 1986; Orvis and McAninch 1989; Jack et al. 2004; Kulovac et al. 2007)

Several approaches have been proposed. In case of a single, evident defect of one corpus cavernosum, some authors suggest direct incision over the lesion with minimal dissection (Ozen et al. 1986).

In our experience we prefer a circumcising type of incision with complete degloving of the skin of the penile shaft. Buck's fascia is opened longitudinally and laterally in order to avoid accidental lesion of the dorsal neurovascular bundle.

This approach permits an excellent exposure of both corpora cavernosa and urethra, and it is very helpful in case of bilateral rupture with or without associated urethral injury. Actually surgical management can be confusing and time consuming due to the concealment of the tear in organized blood and edematous tissue. In these cases a minimal dose of methylene blue can be injected into the corpora cavernosa to point out the tear (Shaeer 2006).

After the removal of the hematoma, the tunical defect is repaired by running or interrupted absorbable 3–0 polydioxanone or vicryl suture. Then the Buck's fascia is reconstructed to perform compression and hemostasis. If a urethral injury is present, treatment depends on the site and extent of the injury.

Posttraumatic scarring of the tunica albuginea and fibrosis of the corpora cavernosa are common sequelae of penile trauma with or without immediate surgical repair. Fibrotic changes are generally localized in the site of the tunical tear and can cause a curvature on the same side. In these cases a delayed second operation is often required to straighten the penis. If the entity of the curvature is inferior to 60 degrees and penile shortening is not significant, we prefer a Nesbit or Yachia procedure to correct the curvature and preserve the erectile function. In case of significant curvature and penile shortening, the use of saphenous vein or eterologous grafts can be considered.

11.2.4
Anterior Urethral Injuries

Lesions of the anterior urethra are more frequent than those of the posterior urethra. Complications of anterior urethral injuries include infections and strictures. Most of the urethral strictures will necessitate surgical treatment also many months later. Moreover, extravasion of urine could cause fibrosis of the corpus spongiosum. Incontinence and impotence are uncommon complications.

The management of anterior urethral injury is variable depending on several factors such as etiology, site and the extent. Urethral contusion due to external trauma can be managed by the placement of a Foley catheter for a few days. In case of partial urethral disruption a conservative approach can be chosen. Some authors propose the placement of a suprapubic catheter without urethral catheterization with delayed cistourethrography at 3–4 weeks after the trauma. This approach has a potential for stricture-free healing providing the surviving portion of the urethral lumen is not further traumatized by strumentation. Then, if a short stricture is evident at urethrography, endoscopic treatment can be performed.

Immediate repair of urethral transection is performed only if urethral injury is concomitant to penile fracture. In this case the injury is generally due to more severe external trauma with significant extravasation of blood and urine that necessitates immediate drainage. If the injury involves the bulbar urethra or the proximal penile urethra, a perineal approach is suggested. In case of lesion of the distal part of anterior urethra, circumcision with degloving of the penile shaft is generally preferred. After surgical exploration evacuation of the hematoma is performed, and necrotic tissue is debrided. Direct repair of the lesion is performed over a 16-F Foley catheter. The urethral stumps are spatulated and approximated by end-to-end two layer anastomosis. For the mucosa approximation, we suggest a 4–0 or 5–0 Monocryl uninterrupted suture followed by a second layer with absorbable interrupted suture for the tunica spongiosa.

In most cases primary repair is not possible because hematoma and urine extravasation at the site of urethral defect cause infection, inflammation and stuffing of the tissues. In these cases, suprapubic placement of the catheter is necessary, and the repair of the urethra is delayed 3 weeks later.

11.2.5
Posterior Urethral Injuries

The major percentages of injuries of the posterior urethra are caused by blunt traumas of the bony pelvis. Approximately 10% of patients with pelvic fractures have an associated urethral injury. In these traumas the involvement of the penis is very rare. However, the first symptom is the presence of blood at the meatus associated with difficult voiding. The disruption of the urethra may be partial or complete. Immediate diagnosis is made by retrograde urethrography and urography or CT urography, which are necessary to evaluate the upper urinary tract and the bladder. The presence of contrast into the bladder during retrograde urethrography suggests partial disruption. Immediate urethral realignment is not generally suggested because the risk to create a morbidity during exploration is too high. The complications of injuries of the posterior urethra include incontinence, impotence and strictures. The incidence of impotence and incontinence decreases significantly in patients treated with delayed repair. In fact, iatrogenic injury to the sphincter or neurovascular bundle can occur more frequently at the time of immediate surgical realignment (WEBSTER 1989), which therefore can be considered mostly when early abdominal exploration is necessary because of associated rectal, vascular or bladder neck injury (WEBSTER 1989).

In case of minimal disruption, immediate urethral catheterization can be tried by gentle maneuver. If the catheter placement is not simple, it is better to avoid further handling. Suprapubic catheter placement is performed, and the lesion is then repaired within 15 days from the injury. This delayed primary repair seems to be the best choice because it avoids the risk of immediate abdominal exploration. The urethra can be repaired by endoscopic realignment or by surgical tension-free anastomosis via a perineal approach using one of a variety of techniques.

11.2.6
Penile Amputation

Immediate treatment begins by placement of a tourniquet around the proximal shaft of the penis to avoid important hemorrhage. Then clots are removed, and the different structures are identified. Microsurgical approach is required for vascular and neural structures (HEYMANN et al. 1977; CARROLL et al. 1985). The urethra is reapproximated, and end-to-end spatulated anastomosis is performed using a 4–0 Monocryl suture for the mucosa followed by a second layer suture of the spongiosa.

The tunica albuginea is reapproximated with 3–0 Polydioxanone suture. Finally, the Buck's fascia, dartos and skin are sutured. The urethral catheter is left in place for 2–3 weeks. Postoperative complications include erectile dysfunction, strictures of the urethra and necrosis of distal portions of the shaft or glans.

When reimplantation is not possible, the patient may undergo neo-phallic reconstruction using the Chang radial forearm flap (CHANG and HWANG 1984) or pedicled pubic phalloplasty (BETTOCCHI et al. 2005).

References

Aboseif S, Gomez R, McAninch JW (1993) Genital self-mutilation. J Urol 150:1143–1146

Basta AM, Blackmore CC, Wessells H (2007) Predicting urethral injury from pelvic fracture patterns in male patients with blunt trauma. J Urol 177:571–575

Bertolotto M, Calderan L, Cova MA (2005) Imaging of penile traumas–therapeutic implications. Eur Radiol 15:2475–2482

Bertolotto M, Pozzi Mucelli R (2004) Nonpenetrating penile traumas: sonographic and Doppler features. AJR Am J Roentgenol 183:1085–1089

Bettocchi C, Ralph DJ, Pryor JP (2005) Pedicled pubic phalloplasty in females with gender dysphoria. BJU Int 95:120–124

Carroll PR, Lue TF, Schmidt RA et al (1985) Penile replantation: current concepts. J Urol 133:281–285

Chang TS, Hwang WY (1984) Forearm flap in one-stage reconstruction of the penis. Plast Reconstr Surg 74:251–258

Chung CH, Szeto YK, Lai KK (2006) Fracture' of the penis: a case series. Hong Kong Med J 12:197–200

Coogan C, Levine L (1998) Injuries to the external genitalia In: Whitfield H, Hendry W, Kirby R, Duckett J (eds) Textbook of genitourinary surgery, vol 2. Blackwell Science Inc, London, pp 1044–1054

Heymann AD, Bell-Thompson J, Rathod DM, Heller LE (1977) Successful reimplantation of the penis using microvascular techniques. J Urol 118:879–880

Jack GS, Garraway I, Reznichek R, Rajfer J (2004) Current treatment options for penile fractures. Rev Urol 6:114–120

Kulovac B, Aganovic D, Junuzovic D et al (2007) Surgical treatment and complications of penile fractures. Bosn J Basic Med Sci 7:37–39

Mellinger B (1993) Blunt traumatic injuries of the penis. In: Hashmat A, Das S (eds) The penis. Lea and Febiger, Philadelphia, pp 105–113

Nicolaisen GS, Melamud A, Williams RD, McAninch JW (1983) Rupture of the corpus cavernosum: surgical management. J Urol 130:917–919

Orvis BR, McAninch JW (1989) Penile rupture. Urol Clin North Am 16:369–375

Ozen HA, Erkan I, Alkibay T et al (1986) Fracture of the penis and long-term results of surgical treatment. Br J Urol 58:551–552

Sagalowsky A, Peters P (1998) Genitourinary trauma. In: Walsh P, Retik A, Vaughan EJ, Wein A (eds) Campbell's urology. Saunders, Philadelphia, pp 3085–3100

Savoca G, Pietropaolo F, Scieri F et al (2004) Sexual function after highly selective embolization of cavernous artery in patients with high flow priapism: long-term follow-up. J Urol 172:644–647

Selikowitz SM (1977) Penetrating high-velocity genitourinary injuries. Part I. Statistics, mechanisms, and renal wounds. Urology 9:371–376

Shaeer O (2006) Methylene blue-guided repair of fractured penis. J Sex Med 3:349–354

Tsang T, Demby AM (1992) Penile fracture with urethral injury. J Urol 147:466–468

Webster GD (1989) Perineal repair of membranous urethral stricture. Urol Clin North Am 16:303–312

US Evaluation of Patients with Penile Traumas

Michele Bertolotto, Carmelo Privitera, and Ciro Acampora

CONTENTS

12.1 Background 95
12.2 Penetrating Penile Traumas 95
12.3 Non-Penetrating Penile Traumas 98
12.3.1 Extra-Albugineal and Cavernosal Hematoma 98
12.3.2 Acute Intracavernosal Hemorrhage 99
12.3.3 Rupture of the Dorsal Penile Vessels 99
12.3.4 Rupture of the Suspensory Ligament 99
12.3.5 Penile Fracture 100
12.3.6 Isolated Urethral Trauma and High Flow Priapism 102
12.3.7 Isolated Septal Hematoma 102
12.4 Postraumatic Erectile Dysfunction 103
12.5 Diagnostic Role of Other Imaging Modalities 104
References 105

12.1 Background

Since the penis is mobile and largely protected by its position, it is much less frequently injured than other parts of the body. As mentioned in Chapter 11, however, it can be wounded as a result of various accidents, and in the erect state it is more prone to trauma in the form of penile fracture. Distinction between penetrating and non-penetrating penile

M. Bertolotto, MD
Department of Radiology, University of Trieste, Ospedale di Cattinara, Strada di Fiume 447, Trieste, 34124, Italy
C. Privitera, MD
Servizio di Radiologia Ospedale Vittorio Emanuele, azienda Ospedaliera-Universitaria V. Emanuele, Ferrarotto, S.Bambino, Via Plebiscito 628, Catania, 95100, Italy
C. Acampora, MD
Azienda Ospedaliera A. Cardarelli, Via Cardarelli 9, Napoli, 80131, Italy

trauma is important because the management of the patient is different, and as regards non-penetrating traumas, the erectile state of the penis during the traumatic event must be recognized as well.

In the presence of typical history and physical findings, imaging studies are not usually required in patients with penile trauma to establish the diagnosis, and actually many urologists think that with the exception of post-traumatic priapism, imaging plays little or no role in the management of the patient (Morey et al. 2004). Ultrasonography and other imaging techniques, however, provide clinically useful information in selected cases.

12.2 Penetrating Penile Traumas

The different types of penetrating injuries to the penis have been described in Chapter 11. The most common lesions are iatrogenic, following cavernosal injection of vasoactive drugs that may be accidentally done outside the corpora cavernosa or may be occasionally complicated with small hemorrhage, granulomata and cavernosal artery tear. While the former complications are relatively common, the latter is extremely rare. Gunshot wounds to the genitalia are not frequent; however, they need to be immediately investigated to assess the extension of the lesion to reproductive organs and prevent complications, such as bleeding, infection, penile curvature, erectile dysfunction and urethral stenosis.

Diagnosis of penetrating traumas of the penis is usually straightforward, and imaging is rarely required, but in the more complex situations that need careful preoperative assessment, in particular, grey-scale and color Doppler ultrasonography can be useful to identify cavernosal or albugineal hematoma and to assess integrity of the tunica albuginea and of the cavernosal arteries. Although retrograde uretrography is considered the imaging modality of choice to evaluate the integrity of the urethra, when injury to the penile portion of the urethra is suspected, sonourethrography can be considered as well.

Grey-scale and color Doppler ultrasonography are the imaging modalities of choice to evaluate complications of cavernosal injection (Fig. 12.1). In particular, when injection is accidentally done outside the corpora cavernosa, a small fluid collection is usually recognized in the injection site (BERTOLOTTO et al. 2005). Postinjection acute hemorrhage within the corpora cavernosa is uncommon and usually recognized, in our experience, in patients with cavernosal fibrotic changes. In these patients hemorrhage usually appears as relatively echogenic spots along the insertion of the niddle, mimicking air bubbles.

Post-injection granulomata are painful and usually present at ultrasound as circumscribed nodules with variable echogenicity. Ultrasound is indicated also during the follow-up to prove tissue restoration or development of fibrotic nodules that present as heterogeneously echogenic lesions (BERTOLOTTO et al. 2005). Among the rare complications of cavernosal injection, intracorporeal needle breakage has been reported (GREENSTEIN et al. 1997; IACONO and BARRA 1998; SHAMLOUL and KAMEL 2005). Grey scale ultrasonography is indicated to localize the needle, which presents with the typical appearance of metallic objects, to identify associated cavernosal fibrotic changes and to guide retrieval (SHAMLOUL and KAMEL 2005).

Rarely, needle insertion can produce cavernosal artery tear resulting in high flow priapism (WITT et al. 1990; BASTUBA et al. 1994).

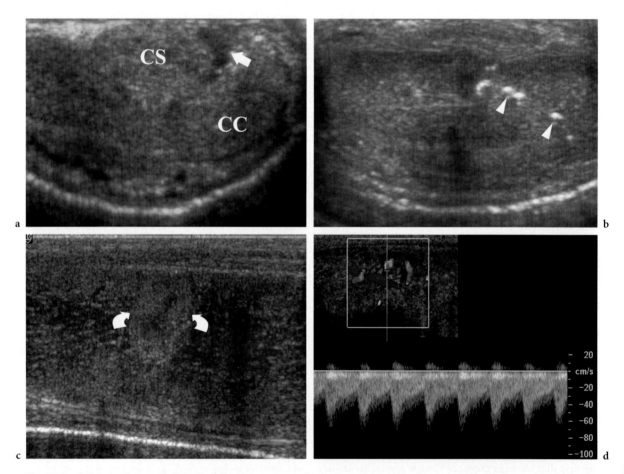

Fig. 12.1a–d. Penetrating penile injuries following cavernosal injection of vasoactive drugs. a Injection (*arrow*) accidentally done outside the corpora cavernosa, between the corpus spongiosum (*CS*) and the left corpus cavernosum (*CC*). b Post-injection acute hemorrhage in a patient with cavernosal fibrotic changes presenting as echogenic spots along the insertion of the niddle. c Post-injection granuloma presenting as a slightly echogenic, painful nodule (*curved arrows*). d Postinjection cavernosal artery injury demonstrated by the presence of high velocity, turbulent flows causing high flow priapism

In patients with gunshot wounds to the genitalia, ultrasonography can have a role to identify hematomas, localize bullets and other foreign bodies retained within the penis (Fig. 12.2) and guide retrieval (FICARRA et al. 1999; CAVALCANTI et al. 2006). Visualization of injured tissues, however, may be hampered by air. The appearance of associated penile hematomas varies with the age of the lesion. Acutely, they appear relatively echogenic; with time they become hypoechoic and then organize and present with complex, echogenic areas, cystic components and septations. Cavernosal hematomas can evolve with complete tissue restoration or with a fibrotic scar (BERTOLOTTO and NEUMAIER 1999).

In patients with genital gunshot wounds, the exact location of bullets or other foreign bodies, such as cloth fragments, does not only allow for easier extraction, but also avoids unnecessary manipulation of the cavernous tissue, which can further affect the erectile condition of the patient. Color Doppler interrogation of cavernosal arteries allows the evaluation of associated vascular injuries (GIAMMUSSO et al. 2006). Also, associated cavernositis and abscess formation can be evaluated. Although retrograde urethrography is commonly considered the imaging modality of choice to identify associated urethral lesions (MOREY et al. 2004), also sonourethrography can help identify interruption of the urethral wall (BHATT et al. 2005).

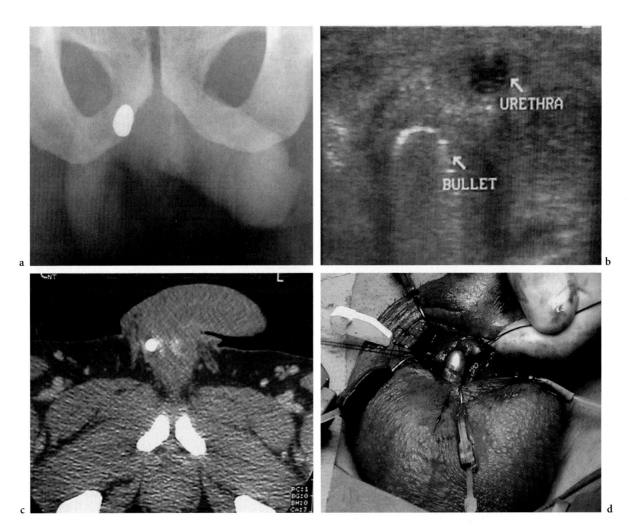

Fig. 12.2a–d. Gunshot penile injury. a X-ray demonstrates the bullet projecting on the right ischiatic bone. b,c Grey-scale ultrasonography (b) and CT (c) show that the bullet is located within the right corpus cavernosum. d Surgical removal of the bullet

12.3
Non-Penetrating Penile Traumas

Ultrasound findings in non-penetrating injuries to the flaccid and to the erect penis are essentially different. A variety of lesions may result from injury to the erect penis including extra-albugineal and intracavernosal hematoma, acute intracavernosal hemorrhage, rupture of the dorsal penile vessels with intact albuginea, rupture of the suspensory ligament, isolated injury to the urethra and to the corpus spongiosum, and rupture of the tunica albuginea and of the cavernosal bodies, which may be associated with urethral and vascular injury. Non-penetrating trauma to the flaccid penis usually follows blunt perineal injury and involves the crura, where the corpora cavernosa are anchored and can be crushed against the pelvic bones. Extra-albugineal or intracavernous hematoma may result, or cavernosal artery rupture followed by high-flow priapism. Color Doppler ultrasonography can accurately delineate the nature and extent of these lesions, though false-negative results have been occasionally reported. The most challenging differential diagnosis is differentiating lesions that require surgery or interventional maneuvers from lesions that may be treated conservatively.

12.3.1
Extra-Albugineal and Cavernosal Hematoma

Direct traumas to the genitalia may result in blood extravasation within the subepithelial connective tissue or in the space between the Colles' and the Buck's fascia. Location of the penile hematomas can be evaluated with ultrasonography (Fig. 12.3). In fact, as illustrated in Chapter 11, penile hematomas present clinically with a different appearance when they are restricted below the Buck's fascia or when they spread in the more superficial layers. Ultrasonography, however, allows evaluation of the relationships between the penile envelops and the

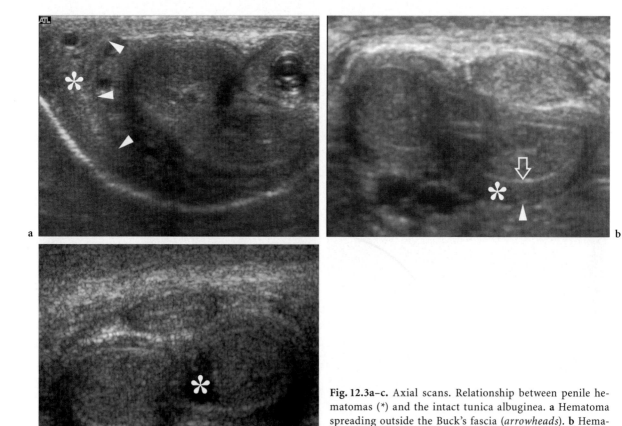

Fig. 12.3a–c. Axial scans. Relationship between penile hematomas (*) and the intact tunica albuginea. **a** Hematoma spreading outside the Buck's fascia (*arrowheads*). **b** Hematoma between the tunica albuginea (*open arrow*) and the Buck's fascia (*arrowhead*). **c** Hematoma within the left corpus cavernosum

hematoma and, in particular, provides differential diagnosis between injuries that can be managed conservatively when the tunica albuginea is intact and injuries associated with albugineal rupture that required surgical repair.

12.3.2
Acute Intracavernosal Hemorrhage

Vigorous intercourse can occasionally result in injury to the subtunical venous plexus or to the smooth muscle trabeculae below the tunica albuginea producing intracavernosal hemorrhage (BHATT et al. 2005). Greyscale ultrasonography reveals a hyperechoic area with an ill-defined margin in the site of the trauma that usually disappears rapidly during the follow-up.

12.3.3
Rupture of the Dorsal Penile Vessels

A variety of injuries to extraalbugineal vessels can occur during intercourse mimicking penile fracture (NEHRU-BABU et al. 1999; ARMENAKAS et al. 2001). Deformation and immediate penile detumescence, however, do not occur following isolated vascular injury to the penis because the tunica albuginea is intact. When identified, these lesions can be treated conservatively.

Rupture of small venous collaterals is more common than injury of the main venous branches, and rupture of the dorsal artery is rare. Ultrasound is useful to confirm diagnosis when an intact tunica albuginea is identified (BERTOLOTTO and POZZI MUCELLI 2004). In patients with rupture of the deep dorsal vessels, the hematoma is confined to the penile shaft if the Buck's fascia is intact. If on the contrary the Buck's fascia is injured, or after avulsion of the superficial dorsal vein, the hematoma spreads involving the pubis, the scrotum and the perineum. In general, torn veins collapse and are not visible directly with ultrasonography, but occasionally may undergo posttraumatic thrombosis (Fig. 12.4) and present at ultrasonography as non-compressible vessels with echogenic content (BHATT et al. 2005). If an arterial injury is associated, a posttraumatic arteriovenous fistula may result, with increased venous pressure and dilatation of the injured vein. Doppler interrogation of the lesion reveals high velocity, low resistance arterial flows and high velocity, turbulent venous flows (BERTOLOTTO and POZZI MUCELLI 2004).

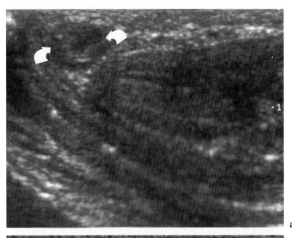
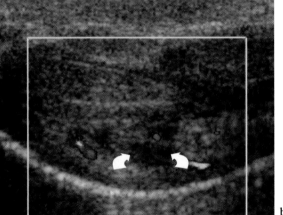

Fig. 12.4a,b. Rupture of the deep dorsal vein (*curved arrows*) following vigorous intercourse. **a** The torn vessel presents with posttraumatic thrombosis identified by presence of echogenic material within the lumen. **b** Color Doppler interrogation shows absence of color signal within the obliterated vessel

12.3.4
Rupture of the Suspensory Ligament

This lesion can occur when the erect penis is forcibly displaced towards the feet (PRYOR and HILL 1979). Diagnosis of rupture of the suspensory ligament is made by history and by palpation of a gap between the base of the shaft of the penis and the symphysis pubis. An abnormal angle is noted during erection. Ultrasonography is able to document the gap between the pubis and the penile shaft and associated hematomas of the soft tissues (Fig. 12.5), but usually does not provide additional useful information (BERTOLOTTO and POZZI MUCELLI 2004).

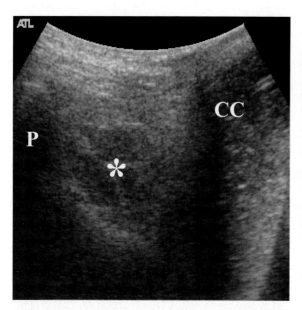 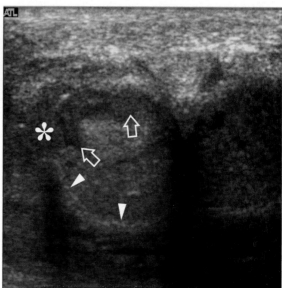

Fig. 12.5. Rupture of the suspensory ligament. The patient experienced pain after his partner's fall during standing intercourse. Longitudinal scan showing a small hematoma (*) in the gap between the corpora cavernosa (CC) and pubis (P)

Fig. 12.6. Penile fracture. Axial scan showing a large albugineal tear (*open arrows*) as interruption of the thin echogenic line of the tunica albuginea (*arrowheads*) of the right corpus cavernosum. Associated extraalbugineal hematoma (*) is also recognized

12.3.5
Penile Fracture

This pathological condition is characterized by monolateral or bilateral rupture of the tunica albuginea of the corpora cavernosa, associated with injury to the urethra and to the corpus spongiosum in 10 to 20% of cases (EL-BAHNASAWY and GOMHA 2000). Diagnosis is usually made from a characteristic history of sharp pain and hearing a cracking or popping sound during the acute bending of the erect penis followed by rapid detumescence, penile swelling and deformity. Rare conditions exist, however, in which albugineal disruption does not produce immediate penile detumescence because of a very small tear or in patients with complete penile corporeal septation presenting with monolateral albuginea disruption. Identification of the albugineal tear is the most important factor in determining the necessity for surgical intervention (EL-BAHNASAWY and GOMHA 2000).

In patients with penile fracture, imaging is used to confirm the diagnosis when clinical presentation is atypical, or when severe local pain and swelling prohibit a thorough physical examination. Ultrasonography is able to detect the exact site of the tear as an interruption of the thin echogenic line of the tunica albuginea (Fig. 12.6), determine whether cavernosal tissue protrudes through the defect and examine for associated hematoma (BERTOLOTTO and POZZI MUCELLI 2004; BHATT et al. 2005). As described before, penile hematoma is confined to the shaft when the Buck's fascia is intact; otherwise, it spreads to the attachment of the Colles' fascia involving the pubis, the scrotum and the perineum.

Small albugineal ruptures may be identified with color Doppler ultrasonography by squeezing the penile shaft and demonstrating a blood flush from the cavernosal bodies through the lesion (BERTOLOTTO and NEUMAIER 1999). Identification of the albugineal tear at ultrasound largely depends on operator skill and available equipment. In fact, false-negative cases have been reported (KOGA et al. 1993; PÉREZ 1997). Increasing clinical evidence exists, however, showing that ultrasound should be currently considered the imaging modality of choice to evaluate patients with suspicious penile fracture (EL-BAHNASAWY and GOMHA 2000). When performed by a dedicated sonologist, indeed, the sensitivity of ultrasonography in detecting albugineal disruption has recently increased due to improved spatial and contrast resolution provided by the latest generation of equipment (PAVLICA 1998; BERTOLOTTO and POZZI MUCELLI 2004; BERTOLOTTO et al. 2005; BHATT et al. 2005). False-negative studies may occur only in the presence of very small tears having minimal or no blood extravasation. In our experience, conservative management of these patients could be considered even though the tear has been identified at ultrasound or with other imaging modalities, with low risk of complications such as penile angulation or other disturbances.

In patients with penile fracture, injury can occasionally involve the cavernosal tissue deeply, and associated cavernosal artery tear can be detected at color Doppler ultrasound (Fig. 12.7). High-flow priapism, however, does not develop in these patients, probably because of blood leakage from the albugineal tear. In our experience no attempt should be made during the operation to repair the arterial tear in these patients because of the high risk of corporeal fibrosis following surgical ligation of the cavernosal arteries within the corpora cavernosa. In fact, the injured cavernosal artery usually heals spontaneously.

While albugineal disruption can be identified at ultrasound in almost all surgical cases, associated urethral injuries can be difficult to detect with ultrasound techniques (Fig. 12.8). Sonourethrography can help identifying interruption of the urethral wall, but retrograde urethrography could be needed. In the absence of external penetrating traumas, an indirect sign of urethral injury is the presence of air (Fig. 12.9) in the cavernosal bodies (BERTOLOTTO and POZZI MUCELLI 2004).

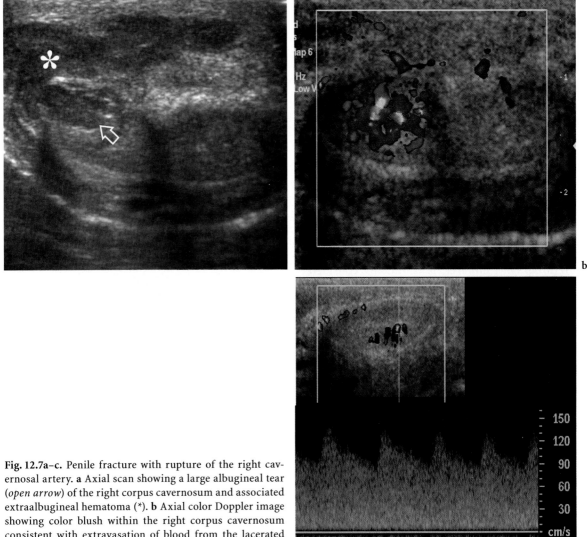

Fig. 12.7a–c. Penile fracture with rupture of the right cavernosal artery. a Axial scan showing a large albugineal tear (*open arrow*) of the right corpus cavernosum and associated extraalbugineal hematoma (*). b Axial color Doppler image showing color blush within the right corpus cavernosum consistent with extravasation of blood from the lacerated cavernosal artery. c Duplex Doppler interrogation of the torn cavernosal artery shows high-velocity turbulent flows

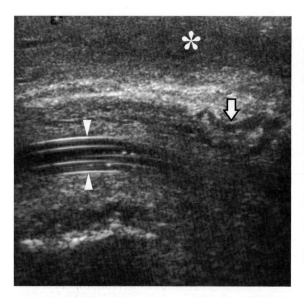

Fig. 12.8. Rupture of the corpus spongiosum. Longitudinal scan showing interruption of the echogenic line of the spongiosal albuginea (*arrow*) and associated soft-tissue hematoma (*). A catheter (*arrowheads*) is placed in the urethra

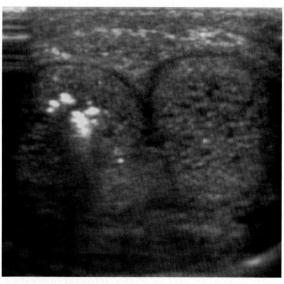

Fig. 12.9. Small rupture of the tunica albuginea with associated urethral injury identified by presence of air within the right corpus cavernosum

12.3.6
Isolated Urethral Trauma and High Flow Priapism

While about 20% of penile fractures are associated with injury to the corpus spongiosum and urethra, isolated urethal traumas are uncommon. Evaluation of the urethra with sonourethrography can help identify interruption of the urethral wall; retrograde urethrography, however, is commonly considered the imaging modality of choice. High-flow priapism is usually secondary to penile or perineal trauma causing cavernosal artery laceration with an intact tunica albuginea.

The ultrasound appearance of urethral injuries, grey-scale and Doppler features in patients with high flow priapism are illustrated in Chapters 10 and 19.

12.3.7
Isolated Septal Hematoma

Recently it has been reported that injury to the erect penis may produce isolated disruption of the penile septum. Ultrasound evaluation allows early identification of the resulting hematoma (Fig. 12.10), which can be recognized as a well-defined cystic-like area in the septal region (Brant et al. 2007). Hematoma aspiration under ultrasound guidance is recommended in these patients to prevent circumscribed septal fibrosis and its associated symptoms, such as penile shortening or focal lack of rigidity.

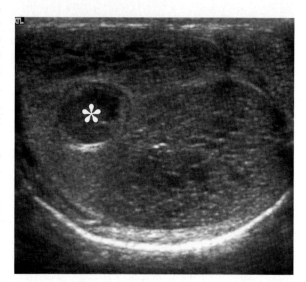

Fig. 12.10. Isolated septal hematoma. Patient presenting with a lump in the mid shaft 1 month after severe bending of the erect penis during intercourse associated with pain and a snapping sensation. Axial scan showing a well-defined cystic-like area in the septal region (*) consistent with postraumatic hematoma

12.4 Postraumatic Erectile Dysfunction

Patients with vertebral, pelvic or perineal injuries and patients undergoing extensive pelvic surgery can present with posttraumatic erectile dysfunction (Machtens et al. 2001).

Trauma-related neurogenic impotence can result from isolated spinal cord injury and isolated damage to the penile nerves. Doppler ultrasound findings may be normal in these patients or may show exaggerated response to vasoactive agents (Kim and Kim 2006). In fact, a sustained erection can often be obtained after intracavernosal injection of 5 µg prostaglandin E1 indicating intact cavernosal smooth muscle function and vascular supply (Machtens et al. 2001). However, impaired response to the vasoactive agent is sometimes encountered and may be due to combined vascular injury. Also, duration of erectile dysfunction is important. In fact, experimental and clinical evidence exists showing that denervation causes progressive cavernous fibrosis and consequent venous occlusive dysfunction, often refractory to symptomatic therapy (Leungwattanakij et al. 2003; Iacono et al. 2005).

Postraumatic penile arterial obstruction characteristically involves the proximal portion of the dorsal penile and cavernosal arteries and the distal internal pudendal artery at the level of the urogenital diaphragm. The integrity of arterial vascular supply to the penis can be assessed by Doppler interrogation of the cavernosal arteries. A peak systolic velocity of 25 cm/s or less after prostaglandin E1 intracavernosal injection reflects arterial insufficiency (Fig. 12.11).

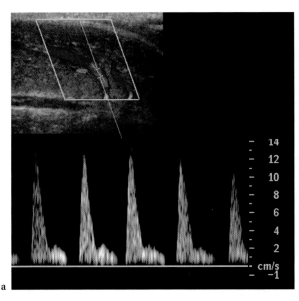
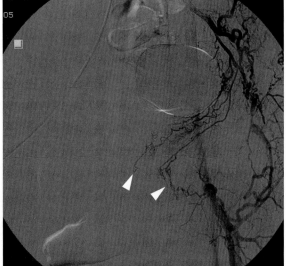
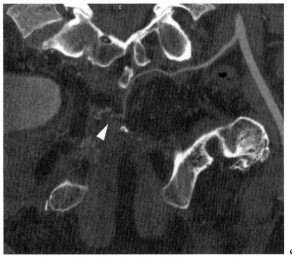

Fig. 12.11a–c. Postraumatic erectile dysfunction. A 32-year-old patient who received pelvic bone fractures during a traffic accident. **a** Doppler interrogation of the cavernosal arteries shows low velocity flows of 12 cm/s, consistent with postraumatic arterial insufficiency. **b** Left internal pudendal arteriogram shows interruption of the vascular supply to the penis with no opacification of the cavernosal artery. **c** MDCT angiography demonstrates the same vascular features noninvasively

12.5 Diagnostic Role of Other Imaging Modalities

In patients with penetrating penile traumas X-ray allows identification of bullets, needle fragments and other radiopaque foreign bodies (Fig. 12.2). Cavernosography has been used to assess corporal and tunical rupture, with extravasation from the corpora considered to be diagnostic (PLISKOW and OHME 1979; MYDLO et al. 1998). This procedure, however, is invasive and is not currently recommended. Potential risks include infection, priapism, contrast reaction and cavernosal fibrosis from extravasated contrast medium. Moreover, false-negative results may occur in the presence of small tears presenting with minimal or no extravasation, and false-positive results may occur if the corpora are underfilled or when filling of the contralateral normal cavernosal body is misinterpreted as extravasation (MOREY et al. 2004). In fact, when performed by a skilled operator, the diagnostic accuracy of ultrasound approaches that of cavernosography without the potential hazard and radiation.

Retrograde urethrography is commonly considered the imaging modality of choice to evaluate urethral injury. The sensitivity of this technique, however, is controversial. While some authors assess that virtually all urethral injury can be identified (KOIFMAN et al. 2003), in other published series a lower efficiency has been demonstrated (MYDLO et al. 1998).

For most patients with widespread acute trauma, CT scanning is performed as an initial diagnostic tool. In penetrating perineal and penile traumas, the presence and location of foreign bodies can be fully evaluated. In non-penetrating traumas injury to the pelvic and perineal organs can be investigated. In patients undergoing CT for complex pelvic injuries urethral disruption can be identified (ALI et al. 2003). In patients with post-traumatic erectile dysfunction high-resolution CT angiography allows evaluation of the arterial vascular supply to the penis (Fig. 12.11). Although small terminal branches and collaterals usually cannot be identified, even when the blood supply to the penis is maximized with pharmacologically induced erection, when state-of-the-art multiple detector-row CT equipment is used, CT angiography allows replacing diagnostic conventional angiography to evaluate the blood supply to the penis in the pelvis and in the perineum.

Magnetic resonance imaging (MRI) is an excellent modality for evaluating patients with acute penile trauma, and it has been suggested to be more sensitive in detecting cavernosal tissue injury compared to ultrasound and cavernosography (FEDEL et al. 1996). Due to limited availability, however, MRI is not often performed in the acute setting, but may be useful in selected cases to confirm that a penile fracture is absent and that a non-operative approach is appropriate. Disruption of the tunica appears on T1- and T2-weighted images as loss of continuity of the low signal intensity tunica with or without associated high signal intensity penile hematoma. Although T1-weighted gadolinium-enhanced images may easily show the hematoma and the tunical tear, non-contrast imaging is sufficient in almost all cases to reach diagnosis. Associated injury to the corpus spongiosum and urethra can be identified. Due to excellent visualization of the intact tunica albuginea, isolated extracorporal or intracorporal hematomas without tunical rupture can be diagnosed (Fig. 12.12), suggesting a conservative management of the patient (CHOI et al. 2000). Extravasation of urine from the injured urethra appears as a high signal intensity collection on T2-weighted images. Post-traumatic periurethral and corporal fibrosis is depicted as low signal intensity tissue on both T1- and T2-weighted images.

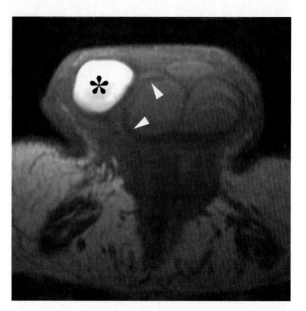

Fig. 12.12. Extraalbugineal hematoma. T1-weighted MR image showing a high signal intensity lesion (*) outside the intact tunica albuginea of the right corpus cavernosum, which is recognized as a low signal intensity linear structure (*arrowheads*). (Courtesy of P. Pavlica, Bologna, Italy)

In patients with complex pelvic traumas MRI can accurately depict pelvic anatomy and provide useful preoperative information that cannot be obtained with other imaging modalities. In this regard, it has been shown helpful in changing the clinically planned surgical approach in a significant percentage of traumatized patients (Narumi et al. 1993). In particular, MRI provides information regarding the degree and direction of prostate dislocation and determines accurately the length of associated urethral disruption. MRI can demonstrate associated fractures of the pelvic bones, avulsion of the corpora cavernosa from the ischium and the presence of pelvic hematomas.

In patients with post-traumatic erectile dysfunction, dynamic gadolinium-enhanced MR angiography can be used to evaluate the aorta, internal iliac arteries and internal pudendal arteries (John et al. 1999). While the proximal iliac and pudendal arteries are reliably delineated, however, evaluation of the more distal portions of these vessels is often limited by the presence of artifacts. A major disadvantage of MR angiography compared to conventional digital angiography is non-specific image presentation. In fact, both arteries and veins are often represented in the images and distal penile arteries are usually obscured by the cavernosal venous plexus. Since anatomical variations in the distal portions of penile arteries cannot be investigated, the indication for revascularization procedures cannot be based on MR angiography alone, and other imaging modalities are needed, such as color Doppler ultrasonography.

References

Ali M, Safriel Y, Sclafani SJ, Schulze R (2003) CT signs of urethral injury. Radiographics 23:951–963; discussion 963–956

Armenakas NA, Hochberg DA, Fracchia JA (2001) Traumatic avulsion of the dorsal penile artery mimicking a penile fracture. J Urol 166:619

Bastuba MD, Saenz de Tejada I, Dinlenc CZ et al (1994) Arterial priapism: diagnosis, treatment and long-term follow-up. J Urol 151:1231–1237

Bertolotto M, Calderan L, Cova MA (2005) Imaging of penile traumas–therapeutic implications. Eur Radiol 15:2475–2482

Bertolotto M, Neumaier CE (1999) Penile sonography. Eur Radiol 9 [Suppl 3]:S407–412

Bertolotto M, Pozzi Mucelli R (2004) Nonpenetrating penile traumas: sonographic and Doppler features. AJR Am J Roentgenol 183:1085–1089

Bhatt S, Kocakoc E, Rubens DJ et al (2005) Sonographic evaluation of penile trauma. J Ultrasound Med 24:993–1000; quiz 1001

Brant WO, Bella AJ, Garcia MM et al (2007) Isolated septal fibrosis or hematoma–atypical Peyronie's disease? J Urol 177:179–182; discussion 183

Cavalcanti AG, Krambeck R, Araujo A et al (2006) Penile lesion from gunshot wound: a 43-case experience. Int Braz J Urol 32:56–60; discussion 60–53

Choi MH, Kim B, Ryu JA et al (2000) MR imaging of acute penile fracture. Radiographics 20:1397–1405

El-Bahnasawy MS, Gomha MA (2000) Penile fractures: the successful outcome of immediate surgical intervention. Int J Impot Res 12:273–277

Fedel M, Venz S, Andreessen R et al (1996) The value of magnetic resonance imaging in the diagnosis of suspected penile fracture with atypical clinical findings. J Urol 155:1924–1927

Ficarra V, Caleffi G, Mofferdin A et al (1999) Penetrating trauma to the scrotum and the corpora cavernosa caused by gunshot. Urol Int 62:192–194

Giammusso B, Pomara G, Giannarini G, Motta M (2006) Ninth commandment: 'Thou shalt not covet thy neighbor's wife!' Penetrating trauma to the corpora cavernosa caused by gunshot. Int J Impot Res 18:566–567

Greenstein A, Sofer M, Chen J (1997) Delayed retrieval of fragment after needle breakage during intracavernous self-injection. J Urol 157:953

Iacono F, Barra S (1998) Intracorporeal needle breakage as an unusual complication of intracavernous self-injection. Tech Urol 4:54–55

Iacono F, Giannella R, Somma P et al (2005) Histological alterations in cavernous tissue after radical prostatectomy. J Urol 173:1673–1676

John H, Kacl GM, Lehmann K et al (1999) Clinical value of pelvic and penile magnetic resonance angiography in preoperative evaluation of penile revascularization. Int J Impot Res 11:83–86

Kim SH, Kim SH (2006) Post-traumatic erectile dysfunction: Doppler US findings. Abdom Imaging 31:598–609

Koga S, Saito Y, Arakaki Y et al (1993) Sonography in fracture of the penis. Br J Urol 72:228–229

Koifman L, Cavalcanti AG, Manes CH et al (2003) Penile fracture–experience in 56 cases. Int Braz J Urol 29:35–39

Leungwattanakij S, Bivalacqua TJ, Usta MF et al (2003) Cavernous neurotomy causes hypoxia and fibrosis in rat corpus cavernosum. J Androl 24:239–245

Machtens S, Gansslen A, Pohlemann T, Stief CG (2001) Erectile dysfunction in relation to traumatic pelvic injuries or pelvic fractures. BJU Int 87:441–448

Morey AF, Metro MJ, Carney KJ et al (2004) Consensus on genitourinary trauma: external genitalia. BJU Int 94:507–515

Mydlo JH, Hayyeri M, Macchia RJ (1998) Urethrography and cavernosography imaging in a small series of penile fractures: a comparison with surgical findings. Urology 51:616–619

Narumi Y, Hricak H, Armenakas NA et al (1993) MR imaging of traumatic posterior urethral injury. Radiology 188:439–443

Nehru-Babu M, Hendry D, Ai-Saffar N (1999) Rupture of the dorsal vein mimicking fracture of the penis. BJU Int 84:179–180

Pavlica PB (1998) Ultrasound of penile tumors and trauma. Ultrasound Q 14:95–109

Pérez EE, Arbej JAP, Gimeno MAN, Mayor VC, Orgaz RE (1997) Fractura de pene: dos nuevos casos. Revision de literatura. Utilidad de la ecografia. Arch Esp Urol 50:1.099–091.102

Pliskow RJ, Ohme RK (1979) Corpus cavernosography in acute "fracture" of the penis. AJR Am J Roentgenol 133:331–332

Pryor JP, Hill JT (1979) Abnormalities of the suspensory ligament of the penis as a cause for erectile dysfunction. Br J Urol 51:402–403

Shamloul R, Kamel I (2005) A broken intracavernous needle: successful ultrasound-guided removal. J Sex Med 2:147–148

Witt MA, Goldstein I, Saenz de Tejada I, et al (1990) Traumatic laceration of intracavernosal arteries: the pathophysiology of nonischemic, high flow, arterial priapism. J Urol 143:129–132

Penile Tumors: Classification, Clinics and Current Therapeutic Approach

Mariela Pow-Sang and Víctor Destéfano

CONTENTS

13.1 Incidence 107
13.2 Epidemiology 107
13.3 Pathology 107
13.4 Clinical Presentation 108
13.5 Staging 109
13.6 Treatment of the Primary Lesion 110
13.7 Treatment of Regional Lymph Nodes 110
13.8 Lymphoscintigraphy and Sentinel Node Biopsy 111
13.9 Chemotherapy 111
13.10 Prognostic Factors and Survival 112
13.11 Conclusions 112
References 112

13.1 Incidence

Penile cancer is an uncommon malignancy in developed countries. In the United States, 1,530 cases occur per year. Higher incidence rates (Narayana et al. 1982) are seen in Africa and Asia (10% to 20%), and in areas of Brazil penile cancer accounts for 17% of all malignancies in men (Ornellas et al. 1994). Penile cancer most commonly affects men between 50 and 70 years of age (Hoppmann and Fraley 1978). Younger individuals are also affected; approximately 22% of patients are less than 40 years of age.

M. Pow-Sang, MD; V. Destéfano, MD
Instituto Nacional de Enfermedades Neoplasicas "Dr. Eduardo Caceres Graziani", Av. Angamos 2520, Lima 34 (Surquillo), Peru

13.2 Epidemiology

The most important etiologic factor of penile cancer is the presence of an intact foreskin. Penile cancer is rarely seen in circumcised individuals (Daling et al. 2005). A history of phimosis (i.e., narrowness of the opening of the prepuce) is found in approximately 25% of penile cancer patients. Phimosis (Fig. 13.1) is strongly associated with invasive carcinoma of the penis (Tsen et al. 2001). Precancerous lesions are found in an additional 15% to 20% of patients (Maiche 1992).

The protective effect of circumcision is likely due to the lack of accumulation of smegma, which forms from desquamated epithelial cells. To date, the precise carcinogenic substance in smegma is not known. The protective effect of circumcision is diminished when performed later in life as evidenced by the higher incidence of penile carcinoma in Muslims as compared to Jews. Poor hygiene also contributes to the development of penile carcinoma through accumulation of smegma and other irritants. In populations that practice good hygiene but are uncircumcised, the incidence of penile carcinoma approaches that of circumcised populations.

Many studies have shown the association of human papillomavirus (HPV) types 16 and 18 with penile carcinoma in as many as 50% of cases, as well as with penile carcinoma in situ (CIS) and basaloid and warty verrucous varieties in more than 90% of cases (Guerrero et al. 2000; Daling et al. 2005; Pascual et al. 2007).

13.3 Pathology

Malignancies of the penis are divided into primary malignancies, those that originate either from the

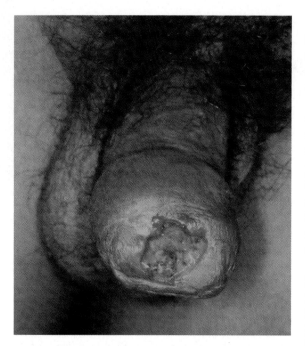

Fig. 13.1. Patient with phimosis and an exofitic lesion on the glans penis

Many penile lesions have been identified as premalignant to the development of invasive squamous cell carcinoma, including leukoplakia, balanitis xerotica obliterans, Bowen's disease, erythroplasia of Queyrat, and giant condyloma accuminatum.

Balanitis xerotica obliterans is typically benign with 12 cases of squamous cell carcinoma association reported in the past 30 years. Erythroplasia of Queyrat describes CIS involving the glans penis, prepuce, or shaft, whereas Bowen's disease describes CIS involving the remainder of the genitalia or perineal region. Bowen's disease and erythroplasia of Queyrat have been noted to degenerate into invasive carcinoma in 5 to 10% and 10% to 33% of cases, respectively (SCHELLHAMMER et al. 1992).

The histopathologic grading is based upon the Broder's Classification System (I–IV) (LUCIA and MILLER 1992): grade I – cells well differentiated with keratinization, prominent intercellular bridges, and keratin pearls; grade II to III – greater nuclear atypia, increased mitotic activity, and decreased keratin pearls; grade IV – marked nuclear pleomorphism, nuclear mitoses, necrosis, lymphatic and perineural invasion, no keratin pearls, and deeply invasive.

soft tissues, urethral mucosa, or covering epithelium, and secondary malignancies, those that represent metastatic disease and often affect the corpus cavernosum. The first step in histologic diagnosing malignancy is the confirmation of the diagnosis and assessment of depth of invasion by microscopic examination of a biopsy specimen.

Squamous cell carcinoma (SCC) represents 95% of malignant disease of the penis. Sarcomas are the most frequent non-squamous penile cancers, followed by melanomas, basal cell carcinomas, and lymphomas. Kaposi's sarcoma presents as a well-marginated red nodule, often isolated to the glans, and represents the initial site of presentation in 3% of patients (KATONA et al. 2006).

Secondary malignancies (metastatic tumors) should be suspected in patients with a known diagnosis of cancer and present with new-onset priapism (involvement of the corpora cavernosa) or an unusual penile lesion. Metastatic lesions are often multiple, palpable, painless nodules that may mimic syphilitic chancres. The primary malignancy is most often bladder, prostate, rectosigmoid areas, and the kidney, in 32, 30, 13, and 8%, respectively, and it is spread most commonly by retrograde venous dissemination (HIZLI and BERKMEN 2006).

13.4
Clinical Presentation

The clinical presentation of an invasive penile carcinoma is varied and may range from an area of induration or erythema to a non-healing ulcer or a warty exophytic growth. Phimosis may obscure the tumor, and not until there is a bloody or foul smelling discharge is the tumor diagnosed.

All penile lesions, particularly those under a non-retractile foreskin, require a high index of suspicion for neoplasia. A penile lesion that does not respond after a short period of 2–3 weeks of careful observation and skin care requires biopsy.

Presentation is on the glans in 48% of cases (Fig. 13.2), the prepuce in 21%, glans and prepuce in 9%, coronal sulcus in 6%, and shaft in less than 2% of cases (BURGERS et al. 1992).

The physical examination is key to the clinical evaluation of the patient with penile cancer. The assessment of the primary tumor should include the size, location, fixation, and involvement of the corporal bodies. The penile base and scrotum should be inspected to exclude neoplastic extension.

13.5
Staging

There are two staging systems employed in penile carcinoma (Tables 13.1 and 13.2); the Jackson classification and the TNM classification (JACKSON 1966; SOBIN and WITTEKIND 2002).

Table 13.1. Jackson classification for carcinoma of the penis

Stage	Description
I	Confined to glans of prepuce
II	Invasion into shaft or corpora
III	Operable inguinal lymph node metastasis
IV	Tumor invades adjacent structures; inoperable inguinal lymph node metastasis

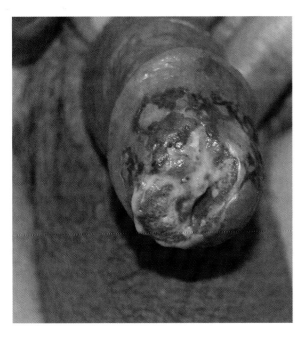

Fig. 13.2. Penile tumor originating on the glans

Table 13.2. TNM classification for carcinoma of the penis

Stage	Description
Tumor (T)	
TX	Primary tumor cannot be assessed
T0	No evidence of primary tumor
TIS	Carcinoma in situ (Bowen's disease, erythroplasia of Queyrat)
T1	Tumor invades usbepithelial connective tissue
T2	Tumor invades corpus spongiosum or cavernosum
T3	Tumor invades urethra or prostate
T4	Tumor invades other organs
Node (N)	
NX	Regional lymph nodes cannot be assessed
N0	No evidence of regional node involvement
N1	Metastasis in a single, superficial, inguinal lymph node
N2	Metastasis in multiple or bilateral superficial inguinal lymph nodes
N3	Metastasis in deep inguinal or pelvis lymph node(s) unilateral or bilateral
Metastasis (M)	
MX	Distant metastasis cannot be assessed
M0	No evidence of distant metastasis
M1	Distant metastasis present

Careful palpation of the inguinal regions should be done since palpable inguinal lymphadenopathy is present at diagnosis in 58% of patients (range 20%–96%). Of these patients, 45% will ultimately be diagnosed with metastatic carcinoma. The remainder will have inflammatory lymphadenopathy, which resolves following resection of the primary tumor and a 4–6 week course of oral antibiotics. In patients with nonpalpable inguinal lymph nodes at the time of resection of the primary tumor, 20% will ultimately be found to have metastatic disease in the superficial groin nodes. Late in the course of the disease, metastasis to retroperitoneal nodes, liver, lung, and brain can occur.

As illustrated in Chapter 14, diagnostic imaging, gray scale ultrasound and color Doppler ultrasound can assist in identifying the depth of tumor invasion, particularly with regard to corpora cavernosa infiltration (LONT et al. 2003a; BERTOLOTTO et al. 2005). An assessment of distant metastasis should only be performed in patients with proven positive nodes. Pelvis/abdominal CT scanning is used in the identification of pelvic and/or retroperitoneal nodes in patients with inguinal metastases. A chest radiograph should be performed on patients with positive lymph nodes (HORENBLAS et al. 1991; BURGERS et al. 1992; HORENBLAS et al. 1993).

13.6
Treatment of the Primary Lesion

Small tumors limited to the foreskin can be treated by circumcision with a 2-cm margin of clearance. Circumcision alone, especially with tumors in the proximal foreskin, may be associated with recurrence rates of 32%. These high recurrence rates underscore the need for careful follow-up of patients treated by circumcision alone.

Other treatment options are Mohs' micrographic surgery (Mohs et al. 1992), laser ablation using a neodnium-yitrium-aluminum garnet (Nd:YAG) or carbon dioxide (CO_2) laser for the treatment of selected patients with small, superficial penile cancers (Lont et al. 2006), and radiation therapy (Crook et al. 2002; Kharchenko et al. 2006).

Carcinomas of the penis involving the glans and the distal shaft are best managed by partial penectomy excising 1.5 to 2 cm of normal tissue proximal to the margin of the tumor. This should leave a 2.5- to 3-cm stump of the penis to allow directable micturition in a standing posture, with some coital function as well. Recently, several studies have concluded that a 10-mm clearance is adequate for grade 1 and 2 lesions, leaving a more acceptable penile stump (Agrawal et al. 2000; Minhas et al. 2005).

For bulky T3 or T4 proximal tumors involving the base of the penis, total penectomy with perineal urethrostomy is done. Often these proximal tumors are advanced and associated with regional metastatic disease.

13.7
Treatment of Regional Lymph Nodes

The presence of palpable inguinal lymph nodes at the time of diagnosis may be due to inflammatory reaction or metastatic disease. Only 50% of patients presenting with palpable lymphadenopathy actually have metastatic disease, the remainder having lymph node enlargement secondary to inflammation. After 4 to 6 weeks of oral antibiotics following treatment of the primary lesion, the patient is reevaluated for the presence of palpable regional lymphadenopathy. The development of new adenopathy during follow-up is more likely due to tumor in 70% of the cases (Ornellas et al. 1994).

The issue of the timing of a lymph node dissection is important, especially in those patients who present with no clinical sign of metastatic disease. Solsona proposed three risk groups: low, intermediate, and high, for occult lymph node metastasis in patients with penile carcinoma and clinically negative lymph nodes.

Low-risk group were patients with stage T1-grade 1 tumors. None of these patients developed lymph node metastasis on follow-up. Intermediate risk group were patients with stage T1-grades 2–3 tumors or stages T2–3-grade 1 tumors. These patients had a 36.4% incidence of positive lymph nodes on follow-up. High-risk groups were patients with stages T2–3-grades 2–3 tumors with an 80% incidence of lymph node involvement on follow-up (Solsona et al. 2001). Similar data are reported by Hungerhuber (Hungerhuber et al. 2006).

In patients in the low-risk group of lymph node metastasis, a surveillance program is advised. If patients are considered unreliable for follow-up, a modified inguinal lymphadenectomy is an optional recommendation. In patients in the intermediate risk group, a modified lymphadenectomy is recommended. The current high reliability of dynamic sentinel node biopsy demonstrated in recent reports (Lont et al. 2003b) can replace the use of a predictive factor in indicating the need for modified lymphadenectomy in this risk group. In patients at high risk of nodal involvement, a modified or radical inguinal lymphadenectomy should be performed.

In patients who present with positive palpable nodes, a bilateral radical inguinal lymphadenectomy is recommended. Pelvic lymphadenectomy is recommended in cases where two or more positive inguinal lymph nodes or extracapsular invasion is found upon inguinal lymphadenectomy. In these cases the probability of pelvic lymph nodes is 23% when two to three inguinal nodes are involved and 56% when more than three nodes are involved (Ornellas et al. 1994).

In patients with unilateral nodal recurrence during the follow-up, bilateral lymph node dissection should be done. In these cases, the probability of occult contralateral involvement is 60%–79% of cases due to crossover lymphatics at the base of the penis (Horenblas et al. 1993).

Metastasis to the pelvic nodes in the absence of inguinal node metastasis is an extremely rare event and has not been observed in many modern series (Fraley et al. 1989). In the setting of negative superficial and deep inguinal lymphadenectomies and a negative pelvic CT scan, pelvic lymphadenectomy is not required.

A modification of the standard inguinal lymphadenectomy has been developed by CATALONA (1988) as another option for patients with clinically negative inguinal lymph nodes. In patients with histological negative inguinal nodes, pelvic lymphadenectomy is not performed. In patients with positive lymph nodes on frozen section, a bilateral iliac lymphadenectomy also is performed. The technique has been associated with less morbidity than the standard lymphadenectomy.

13.8
Lymphoscintigraphy and Sentinel Node Biopsy

Sentinel node biopsy, which has been extensively validated in breast cancer and melanoma, is being used increasingly in the evaluation of penile cancer. The concept of the sentinel node, the first lymph node to contain metastatic cancer within a tumor's lymphatic basin, was introduced by CABANAS in 1977 (CABANAS 1977). Anatomically, the sentinel lymph node was discovered to be part of the lymphatic system around the superficial inferior epigastric vein, and theoretically, skip metastases beyond this node were suppose to be a very rare event. Cabanas recommended bilateral sentinel node biopsy followed by inguino-femoral dissection only when biopsy of the sentinel node was positive. When the sentinel node is negative for metastatic disease, no further surgical treatment was recommended. The reliability of Cabana's approach was limited by its relatively poor localization technique, and therefore failed to gain widespread acceptance.

By combining preoperative lymphatic mapping with intra-operative gamma probe detection, this nuclear medicine procedure is used to identify sentinel nodes. Horenblas et al. reported on a series of 55 patients with clinically node-negative disease, T2 or greater penile cancer that underwent lymphoscintigraphy with ^{99m}Technetium nanocolloid injected intradermally around the tumor (HORENBLAS et al. 2000). Sentinel nodes were found intraoperatively using patent Blue dye injected intradermally around the tumor and a gamma detection probe. Regional node dissections were limited to patients with tumor-positive sentinel nodes. A total of 108 sentinel nodes were removed, and 11 patients underwent a regional node dissection secondary to a sentinel node positive for metastatic disease. A median follow-up of 22 months showed one patient having nodal metastasis despite prior excision of a tumor-free sentinel node. Lymphocintigraphy offers a valid, well-tolerated method for lymphatic mapping and sentinel node identification (KROON et al. 2005; PERDONA et al. 2006).

13.9
Chemotherapy

For patients with inguinal masses (Fig. 13.3) or clinically positive pelvic lymph nodes, induction courses of chemotherapy can provide partial or complete clinical responses. Some response has been observed with a combination of cisplatin, bleomycin and methotrexate (CBM). PIZZOCARO evaluated neoadjuvant chemotherapy with combined vincristine, bleomycin and methotrexate in 16 patients with fixed inguinal nodes (PIZZOCARO et al. 1996). Nine of the 16 patients (56%) underwent successful surgical resection, and 5 (31%) achieved 5-year disease-free survival. The Southwest Oncology Group evaluated combination chemotherapy with CBM in patients with metastatic disease. Forty patients were evaluated for response. There were five complete and eight partial responses for a 32.5% response rate. The therapy was associated with excessive toxicity; five treatment-related deaths

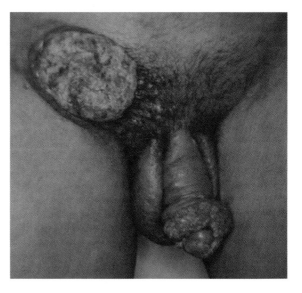

Fig. 13.3. Penile lesion with involvement of inguinal lymph nodes at diagnosis

occurred, and 6 of the 36 remaining patients evaluable for toxicity had one or more life-threatening toxic episodes. Recently, Hakenberg evaluated the efficacy and toxicity of chemotherapy with CMB in the adjuvant and palliative setting, and its effect on survival in 13 patients with locally advanced or metastatic penile carcinoma (Hakenberg et al. 2006). Three of the eight patients with adjuvant treatment showed no evidence of disease, while four in this group died from disease progression after a mean of 11 (5–20) months, and one died from treatment-related toxicity. All five patients with metastatic disease died from disease progression after they had shown temporary signs of regression. They conclude that chemotherapy with CMB had little effect on metastatic penile cancer, and responses were transient. However, patients with minimal disease after radical local and lymphatic resection seemed to benefit from adjuvant therapy.

13.10
Prognostic Factors and Survival

The pathologic variables with known prognostic value are the presence of lymph node metastasis, tumor thickness, stage, grade, and lymphatic and venous embolization, pattern of invasion and vertical growth (Lopes et al. 2002; Ficarra et al. 2005; Guimaraes et al. 2006).

An overall 5-year survival rate of 52% has been reported. This ranges from 66% in patients with negative lymph nodes to 27% in patients with positive nodes (Horenblas and van Tinteren 1994; Ornellas et al. 1994) and 0–38% in patients with pelvic node involvement (Horenblas and van Tinteren 1994; Ornellas et al. 1994; Lopes et al. 2000).

13.11
Conclusions

Penile cancer, though a rare disease, poses many diagnostic, staging and treatment challenges. Accurate treatment and staging of the primary lesion are important to aid in predicting the status of the regional lymph nodes. Modified groin lymph node dissection has decreased morbidity, and the recent description of sentinel node localization offers the possibility of less extensive surgery in a significant number of patients. For patients with inguinal masses or clinically positive pelvic lymph nodes, induction courses of CMB can provide partial or complete clinical responses.

References

Agrawal A, Pai D, Ananthakrishnan N et al (2000) The histological extent of the local spread of carcinoma of the penis and its therapeutic implications. BJU Int 85:299–301

Bertolotto M, Serafini G, Dogliotti L et al (2005) Primary and secondary malignancies of the penis: ultrasound features. Abdom Imaging 30:108–112

Burgers JK, Badalament RA, Drago JR (1992) Penile cancer. Clinical presentation, diagnosis, and staging. Urol Clin North Am 19:247–256

Cabanas RM (1977) An approach for the treatment of penile carcinoma. Cancer 39:456–466

Catalona WJ (1988) Modified inguinal lymphadenectomy for carcinoma of the penis with preservation of saphenous veins: technique and preliminary results. J Urol 140:306–310

Crook J, Grimard L, Tsihlias J et al (2002) Interstitial brachytherapy for penile cancer: an alternative to amputation. J Urol 167:506–511

Daling JR, Madeleine MM, Johnson LG et al (2005) Penile cancer: importance of circumcision, human papillomavirus and smoking in in situ and invasive disease. Int J Cancer 116:606–616

Ficarra V, Zattoni F, Cunico SC et al (2005) Lymphatic and vascular embolizations are independent predictive variables of inguinal lymph node involvement in patients with squamous cell carcinoma of the penis: Gruppo Uro-Oncologico del Nord Est (Northeast Uro-Oncological Group) Penile Cancer data base data. Cancer 103:2507–2516

Fraley EE, Zhang G, Manivel C, Niehans GA (1989) The role of ilioinguinal lymphadenectomy and significance of histological differentiation in treatment of carcinoma of the penis. J Urol 142:1478–1482

Guerrero I, Pow-Sang M, Pow-Sang J et al (2000) Improved DNA extraction from paraffin-embedded tissue for human papillomavirus detection in penile cancer by polymerase chain reaction. Urologia Panamericana 12:20–21

Guimaraes GC, Lopes A, Campos RS et al (2006) Front pattern of invasion in squamous cell carcinoma of the penis: new prognostic factor for predicting risk of lymph node metastases. Urology 68:148–153

Hakenberg OW, Nippgen JB, Froehner M et al (2006) Cisplatin, methotrexate and bleomycin for treating advanced penile carcinoma. BJU Int 98:1225–1227

Hizli F, Berkmen F (2006) Penile metastasis from other malignancies. A study of ten cases and review of the literature. Urol Int 76:118–121

Hoppmann HJ, Fraley EE (1978) Squamous cell carcinoma of the penis. J Urol 120:393–398

Horenblas S, Jansen L, Meinhardt W et al (2000) Detection of occult metastasis in squamous cell carcinoma of the penis using a dynamic sentinel node procedure. J Urol 163:100–104

Horenblas S, van Tinteren H (1994) Squamous cell carcinoma of the penis. IV. Prognostic factors of survival: analysis of tumor, nodes and metastasis classification system. J Urol 151:1239–1243

Horenblas S, Van Tinteren H, Delemarre JF et al (1991) Squamous cell carcinoma of the penis: accuracy of tumor, nodes and metastasis classification system, and role of lymphangiography, computerized tomography scan and fine needle aspiration cytology. J Urol 146:1279–1283

Horenblas S, van Tinteren H, Delemarre JF et al (1993) Squamous cell carcinoma of the penis. III. Treatment of regional lymph nodes. J Urol 149:492–497

Hungerhuber E, Schlenker B, Karl A et al (2006) Risk stratification in penile carcinoma: 25-year experience with surgical inguinal lymph node staging. Urology 68:621–625

Jackson SM (1966) The treatment of carcinoma of the penis. Br J Surg 53:33–35

Katona TM, Lopez-Beltran A, MacLennan GT et al (2006) Soft tissue tumors of the penis: a review. Anal Quant Cytol Histol 28:193–206

Kharchenko VP, Kaprin AD, Timova VA et al (2006) [Radiation assisted diagnosis and complex treatment of penile carcinoma]. Vopr Onkol 52:315–321

Kroon BK, Valdes Olmos RA, van Tinteren H et al (2005) Reproducibility of lymphoscintigraphy for lymphatic mapping in patients with penile carcinoma. J Urol 174:2214–2217

Lont AP, Besnard AP, Gallee MP et al (2003a) A comparison of physical examination and imaging in determining the extent of primary penile carcinoma. BJU Int 91:493–495

Lont AP, Gallee MP, Meinhardt W et al (2006) Penis conserving treatment for T1 and T2 penile carcinoma: clinical implications of a local recurrence. J Urol 176:575–580; discussion 580

Lont AP, Horenblas S, Tanis PJ et al (2003b) Management of clinically node negative penile carcinoma: improved survival after the introduction of dynamic sentinel node biopsy. J Urol 170:783–786

Lopes A, Bezerra AL, Pinto CA et al (2002) p53 as a new prognostic factor for lymph node metastasis in penile carcinoma: analysis of 82 patients treated with amputation and bilateral lymphadenectomy. J Urol 168:81–86

Lopes A, Bezerra AL, Serrano SV, Hidalgo GS (2000) Iliac nodal metastases from carcinoma of the penis treated surgically. BJU Int 86:690–693

Lucia MS, Miller GJ (1992) Histopathology of malignant lesions of the penis. Urol Clin North Am 19:227–246

Maiche AG (1992) Epidemiological aspects of cancer of the penis in Finland. Eur J Cancer Prev 1:153–158

Minhas S, Kayes O, Hegarty P et al (2005) What surgical resection margins are required to achieve oncological control in men with primary penile cancer? BJU Int 96:1040–1043

Mohs FE, Snow SN, Larson PO (1992) Mohs micrographic surgery for penile tumors. Urol Clin North Am 19:291–304

Narayana AS, Olney LE, Loening SA et al (1982) Carcinoma of the penis: analysis of 219 cases. Cancer 49:2185–2191

Ornellas AA, Seixas AL, Marota A et al (1994) Surgical treatment of invasive squamous cell carcinoma of the penis: retrospective analysis of 350 cases. J Urol 151:1244–1249

Pascual A, Pariente M, Godinez JM et al (2007) High prevalence of human papillomavirus 16 in penile carcinoma. Histol Histopathol 22:177–183

Perdona S, Autorino R, Gallo L et al (2006) Role of dynamic sentinel node biopsy in penile cancer: our experience. J Surg Oncol 93:181–185

Pizzocaro G, Piva L, Nicolai N (1996) [Treatment of lymphatic metastasis of squamous cell carcinoma of the penis: experience at the National Tumor Institute of Milan]. Arch Ital Urol Androl 68:169–172

Schellhammer PF, Jordan GH, Robey EL, Spaulding JT (1992) Premalignant lesions and nonsquamous malignancy of the penis and carcinoma of the scrotum. Urol Clin North Am 19:131–142

Sobin L, Wittekind C (2002) TNM classification of malignant tumors. Wiley, New York

Solsona E, Iborra I, Rubio J et al (2001) Prospective validation of the association of local tumor stage and grade as a predictive factor for occult lymph node micrometastasis in patients with penile carcinoma and clinically negative inguinal lymph nodes. J Urol 165:1506–1509

Tsen HF, Morgenstern H, Mack T, Peters RK (2001) Risk factors for penile cancer: results of a population-based case-control study in Los Angeles County (United States). Cancer Causes Control 12:267–277

Penile Tumors: US Features

Giovanni Serafini, Michele Bertolotto, Luca Scofienza, Francesca Lacelli, and Nicoletta Gandolfo

CONTENTS

14.1	Background	115
14.2	Staging Primary Penile Malignancies	116
14.3	Ultrasound Features of Squamous Cell Carcinoma	116
14.3.1	Examination Technique	116
14.3.2	Tumor Appearance	116
14.3.3	Local Staging	116
14.4	Ultrasound Features of Other Penile Primary Tumors	118
14.4.1	Hemangioma	118
14.4.2	Neurilemmoma	118
14.4.3	Epithelioid Sarcoma	118
14.4.4	Kaposi's Sarcoma	118
14.4.5	Lymphoma	119
14.5	Secondary Penile Malignancies	119
14.6	Ultrasound Features of Penile Metastases	120
14.7	Diagnostic Role of Other Imaging Modalities	120
14.7.1	Cavernosography	120
14.7.2	CT	120
14.7.3	Magnetic Resonance Imaging	121
14.7.3.1	Examination Technique	121
14.7.3.2	Appearance of Squamous Cell Carcinoma	122
14.7.3.3	Appearance of Other Penile Primary Tumors	122
14.7.3.4	Appearance of Secondary Tumors	123
	References	124

G. Serafini, MD; L. Scofienza, MD; F. Lacelli, MD; N. Gandolfo, MD
U.O. Radiologia, Ospedale S. Corona, Via XXV Aprile, Pietra Ligure, 17027, Italy
M. Bertolotto, MD
Department of Radiology, University of Trieste, Ospedale di Cattinara, Strada di Fiume 447, Trieste, 34124, Italy

14.1 Background

Penile tumor is uncommon in developed countries. As illustrated in Chapter 13, however, in some developing countries it accounts for as many as 10% to 20% of all malignancies in men (Algaba et al. 2002; Pow-Sang et al. 2002).

Worldwide differences of prevalence must be referred to the different social and economic situations in developed and in developing countries, to lack of personal hygiene and preputial phimosis. The prevalence of penile malignancies is very low in circumcised men (Burgers et al. 1992).

The role of tobacco has been emphasized recently. Smoking seems to be an independent risk factor. There is evidence that penile malignancies are associated with human papilloma virus infection (HPV), particularly with types 16 and 18, even though it is not possible to say on a scientific basis that cancer of the penis is a sexually transmitted disease (Bezerra et al. 2001).

Most penile tumors are squamous cell carcinomas. Non-squamous cell primary tumors are very uncommon and include benign lesions, such as hemangiomas (Kim et al. 1991), neurilemmomas (Kousseff and Hoover 1999; Jung et al. 2006) and leiomyomas (Stehr et al. 2000; Bartoletti et al. 2002; Liu et al. 2007), and malignant lesions such as epithelioid sarcoma (Sirikci et al. 1999), Kaposi's sarcoma (Hermida Gutierrez et al. 1995), lymphoma (El-Sharkawi and Murphy 1996; Lo et al. 2003; Wei et al. 2006) and melanoma (Sanchez-Ortiz et al. 2005). Other penile tumors are extremely rare.

A typical tumor involving the penis of AIDS patients is Kaposi's sarcoma (Hermida Gutierrez et al. 1995), but also frequency of squamous cell carcinoma increases. In patients with AIDS a highly aggressive progression of the disease has been reported, possibly as a consequence of interaction between HIV-1 and HPV (Theodore et al. 2002).

14.2
Staging Primary Penile Malignancies

As illustrated in Chapter 13, there are two staging systems employed in penile carcinoma: the Jackson classification and the TNM classification. Staging criteria include tumor size, depth, localization, histological type, grade of differentiation and involvement of the erectile bodies. Neoplastic embolization of lymphatic and venous vessels is predictive for positive groin lymph nodes (Sanz Mayayo et al. 2004).

14.3
Ultrasound Features of Squamous Cell Carcinoma

Penile cancer is usually visible at physical examination, and diagnosis is confirmed with biopsy. Imaging, however, is indicated for staging purposes. Ultrasonography is more accurate than clinical examination for measuring the extent of tumor (Agrawal et al. 2000; Lont et al. 2003). In particular, pathologic nodes and involvement of the corpora cavernosa are better recognized.

14.3.1
Examination Technique

Local staging of penile cancer requires intracavernosal PGE1 injection. In fact, with artificial erection, the penile shaft enlarges, the tunica albuginea is distended, and the boundary between the corpora cavernosa and the surrounding structures are better evaluated (Kayes et al. 2007).

Unfortunately, many patients with penile cancer are old men with preexisting erectile dysfunction in whom artificial erection cannot be obtained even following intracavernosal injection of large quantities of vasoactive drugs. Failure to obtain artificial erection could produce inaccuracy in demonstrating the boundaries between the different penile compartments, resulting in staging errors. Moreover, the tunica albuginea is not distended, and focal thickening or subtle alteration of the echotexture cannot be evaluated. Pharmacologically induced erection can be very difficult to obtain, also in patients with very large tumors, because it could be difficult to identify a suitable injection site in a normal portion of the corpus cavernosum and because extensive corporeal infiltration prevents blood entrapment within the erectile bodies and cavernosal pressure increase.

14.3.2
Tumor Appearance

At ultrasound, squamous cell carcinoma of the penis usually presents as an hypoechoic lesion with poor vascularization at Doppler interrogation. Gas bubbles entrapped in ulcerations present as hyperechogenic spots (Horenblas et al. 1994; Agrawal et al. 2000; Bertolotto et al. 2005). Tumor inflammation is common in large ulcerated tumors, especially in diabetic patients. Ultrasound can show increased vascularity of the inflamed tumor and of the surrounding tissues and abscess formation (Fig. 14.1).

14.3.3 Local Staging

Frank infiltration of the corpora cavernosa (Fig. 14.2) is identified at ultrasound as an interruption of the echogenic interface of the tunica albuginea (Horenblas et al. 1994; Agrawal et al. 2000; Bertolotto et al. 2005).

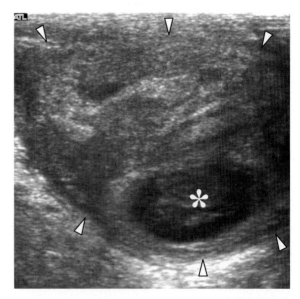

Fig. 14.1. An 84-year-old diabetic patient with penile cancer and inflammation. Axial scan showing a large tumor (*arrowheads*) involving the entire glans. A fluid collection is appreciable within the lesion (*) with thickened echogenic wall and internal debris consistent with abscess formation

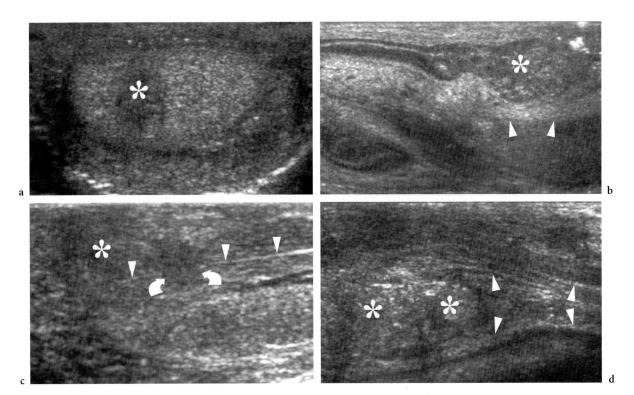

Fig. 14.2a–d. Squamous cell carcinoma of the penis. Local staging. a Axial scan showing a small tumor (*) confined to the glans. b Longitudinal scan showing a tumor (*) confined to the subepithelial connective tissue. The tunica albuginea of the corpora cavernosa (*arrowheads*) is intact. c Larger tumor (*) with focal infiltration (*curved arrows*) of the tunica albuginea (*arrowheads*). d Large penile cancer (*) with widespread infiltration of the corpora cavernosa. The tunica albuginea (*arrowheads*) cannot be identified at the tip of the corpora where the cavernosal tissue is replaced by tumor tissue

In patients with initial infiltration the tunica albuginea may be not interrupted; ultrasonography, however, shows that the tumor is not cleaved from the corpora and that the tunica albuginea in contact with the lesion is thickened and less echogenic than in the remaining portions (Fig. 14.3). Identification of these subtle changes requires an adequate penile turgescence and high resolution wideband probes. Local staging of large tumors extending to the pelvis cannot be obtained with ultrasound. Evaluation of these rare lesions requires other imaging modalities, in particular, magnetic resonance imaging.

Previous studies have shown that the diagnostic accuracy of ultrasound in evaluating infiltration of the tunica albuginea is limited, especially in the presence of microscopic tumor invasion (Horenblas et al. 1994; Agrawal et al. 2000). These studies, however, are more than 10 years old, or have been performed with inadequate equipment, and artificial erection was not obtained. Ultrasound technology progressed significantly in the last years. Using recent apparatuses and an appropriate imaging technique, tumors circumscribed in the subepithelial tissue can be effectively distinguished from those spreading to the erectile bodies (Bertolotto et al. 2005). Large studies, however, are needed to substantiate these findings.

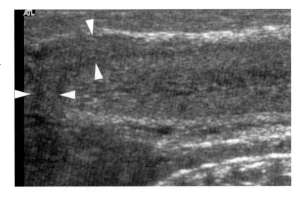

Fig. 14.3. Squamous cell carcinoma of the penis. Local staging. Longitudinal scan showing thickening and reduced echogenicity of the tunica albuginea at the tip of the corpus cavernosum (*arrowheads*) consistent with tumor infiltration. The tunica albuginea is not interrupted

14.4
Ultrasound Features of Other Penile Primary Tumors

Ultrasound appearance of benign and malignant penile tumors different from squamous cell carcinoma is usually non specific. Diagnosis is based on history, clinics and biopsy. Echographic characteristics, however, can help in characterization of some tumors and, as occurs for squamous cell carcinomas, imaging may be required for staging purpose.

14.4.1
Hemangioma

This lesion represents the more frequent benign tumor of the penis and typically presents as a superficial reddish spot in the glans barely visible at ultrasound or not visible at all. Occasionally, however, giant cavernous hemangiomas may involve the entire glans and a variable portion of the corpora cavernosa. In these patients the lesion typically appears as a heterogeneously echogenic mass with multiple hypoechoic lacunae (KIM et al. 1991). As occurs for venous hemangiomas elsewhere in the body, no vascularization is appreciable at color Doppler ultrasonography. Involvement of the corpora cavernosa is recognized by disappearance of the normal echotexture of the sinusoidal spaces at the tip of the corpora cavernosa (Fig. 14.4).

14.4.2
Neurilemmoma

This extremely rare benign tumor, usually capsulated, arises from the nerve sheaths of peripheral nerves. It presents at ultrasound as a well-defined, hypoechoic rounded mass hypervascularized at color Doppler interrogation (KOUSSEFF and HOOVER 1999; JUNG et al. 2006).

14.4.3
Epithelioid Sarcoma

This rare, slowly growing mesenchymal neoplasm may mimic benign pathologies such as granuloma and Peyronie's disease (SIRIKCI et al. 1999; USTA et al. 2003) and should be considered in the differential diagnosis of growing plaques. Ultrasonography reveals a solid mass with multiple focal calcifications infiltrating the corpora cavenosa (SIRIKCI et al. 1999).

14.4.4
Kaposi's Sarcoma

Kaposi's sarcoma is a rare neoplasm of vascular origin. Four variants with different clinical manifestations are recognized (RESTREPO et al. 2006): classic (sporadic or Mediterranean), endemic (African), iat-

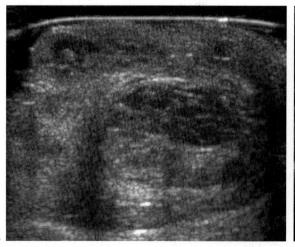
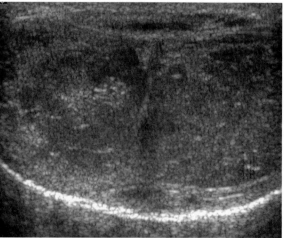

Fig. 14.4a,b. Giant hemangioma of the penis. **a** Axial scan of the glans showing inhomogeneous echotexture by presence of multiple hypoechoic lacunae. **b** Axial scan on the tip of the corpora cavernosa showing a coarse echotexture of the sinusoidal spaces consistent with extension of the lesion into the corpora

rogenic (organ transplant related) and AIDS related (epidemic). Kaposi's sarcoma is the most common neoplasm in AIDS patients.

The exact nature of the disease is not clear, but current data support a tight link to human herpes virus 8 (HHV-8) infection (Iscovich et al. 2000).

Kaposi's sarcoma is usually multifocal and affects primarily the skin, but can cause disseminated disease in a variety of organs (Restrepo et al. 2006). It usually presents with hyperpigmented maculopapular, plaque-like lesions, or multiple nodules often prevalent on the lower limbs (Kagu et al. 2006). Nodal involvement is frequent.

While penile involvement of disseminated Kaposi's sarcoma is relatively common, Kaposi's sarcoma limited to the penis is rare. Occasionally it can also affect HIV-seronegative patients (Guy et al. 1994; Koyuncuoglu et al. 1996; Mir et al. 1998; Micali et al. 2003). The lesion can present with diffuse penile swelling or with reddish maculo-papules and penile deformation. Excision of the penile lesion and local irradiation is currently considered the treatment of choice.

Ultrasound appearance of penile Kaposi's sarcoma is not specific. The lesion usually presents as a heterogeneously hypoechoic vascularized mass with ill-defined margins.

14.4.5
Lymphoma

Penile lymphoma is a rare neoplasm, generally due to a direct invasion of neighboring organs or to a retrograde lymphatic or hematogenic spread (secondary lymphoma). The real existence of a primary lymphomatous affection of the penis is a much debated question; some authors suppose that penile lymphoma is just an early symptom of an unknown lymphonodal disease (Bunesch Villalba et al. 2001; Lo et al. 2003; Wei et al. 2006).

Clinically the lesion appears with diffuse penile swelling or like a mass, a plaque or an ulcer in the penile skin. Contrary to squamous cell carcinoma, lymphoma usually presents in the penile shaft rather than in the glans and prepuce. At color Doppler ultrasonography penile lymphoma presents as an isoechoic or relatively hypoechoic hypervascularized lesion (Fig. 14.5). Infiltration of the corpora cavernosa is often present.

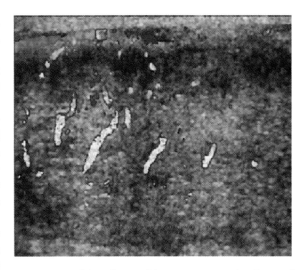

Fig. 14.5. B-cell lymphoma of the penis. Longitudinal scan of the penile shaft demonstrates a slightly heterogeneous, well-vascularized mass infiltrating the corpora cavernosa

14.5
Secondary Penile Malignancies

The first case report about a secondary penile malignancy was written in 1870 by Eberth, who described penile metastases originating from an adenocarcinoma of the rectum (Eberth 1870). Two years later, Roberts described a secondary penile malignancy from a genitourinary primary tumor (Roberts 1872).

Most penile metastases originate from the genital apparatus or from the lower urinary tract (Belville and Cohen 1992). In the past, bladder tumor was considered the major source responsible for penile metastases, but a relatively recent revision of the literature pointed out that most secondary penile tumors originate from prostate cancer (Perez et al. 1992). Tumors from different organs, however, can be involved, such as renal, testicle, bowel and rectum, lung, skin and bone malignancies. The reason why penile metastases are rare despite rich penile vascularization remains unexplained.

Several mechanisms can account for penile metastatic deposits (Cherian et al. 2006). Retrograde venous spread is perhaps the most common way. An easy transportation of malignant cells is provided by the rich anastomotic connections between the dorsal venous system of the penis and the venous plexuses draining the pelvic viscera. This is the reason why most secondary penile tumors arise from the bladder, the prostate and the recto-sigmoid.

Retrograde lymphatic spread occurs in a similar way. The posterior portion of the prostate, the bladder base and the penis have the same lymphatic drainage into the external iliac nodes. This route of spread primarily brings metastases to the penile skin, rather than to the corpora or the glans. Arterial dissemination is uncommon. It can occur by direct tumor infiltration of arterial vessels, or by secondary tumor emboli originating from lung metastases.

Contact extension is possible from highly invasive primary tumors in organs with close anatomical relationship with the penis, like the bladder and prostate. Tumor cell dissemination from an aggressive rectal carcinoma can occur along the ischiorectal fossa until the base of the penis. Implantation secondary to instrumentation has been described, but appears highly unlikely.

Clinically penile metastases present with penile masses or diffuse induration of the penis. Priapism is reported with varying frequency. Obstructive voiding symptoms and hematuria are rarely reported. Pain is not a prominent symptom in most patients and when present is localized partly to the penis and partly to the perineum.

The diagnosis of penile metastases is based on history and clinical appearance. Biopsy can be useful to confirm diagnosis and to distinguish metastases from primary malignancies. Imaging has a role in confirming the diagnosis and to rule out other causes of penile induration.

The prognosis of secondary malignancies of the penis is generally poor, having in those patients a widespread metastatic disease. Usually therapy has only a palliative purpose.

14.6
Ultrasound Features of Penile Metastases

As told before, hematogenous or lymphatic metastases from distant organs usually present with cavernosal and spongiosal nodules of variable echogenicity and vascularization. Metastatic involvement from adjacent organs can present with multiple nodules and with diffuse infiltration on the penile shaft (Fig. 14.6). Direct infiltration of the tunica albuginea from the primary tumor can be identified as a tunical interruption at the base of the penis. Focal infiltration of the tunica albuginea along the shaft can be detected as well as localized interruptions of the echogenic interface surrounding the corpora (BERTOLOTTO et al. 2005).

In patients with diffuse secondary involvement of the shaft or with isoechoic metastases, the lesions may be barely visible, except for mild alteration of the penile echotexture, diffuse or focal interruption of the tunica albuginea or irregular bulking of the shaft. In these cases, the use of ultrasonographic contrast media can help identify alteration of the penile vascular supply to the penis (BERTOLOTTO et al. 2005).

14.7
Diagnostic Role of Other Imaging Modalities

With the exception of magnetic resonance imaging, which actually represents the gold standard imaging modality for staging, if the sonologist is confident with ultrasound penile anatomy and its changes in pathological conditions, other imaging techniques are rarely needed to evaluate patients with penile tumors.

14.7.1
Cavernosography

This technique has been used in the past for evaluation of penile tumors that appear as filling defects within the erectile bodies (ESCRIBANO et al. 1987; HADDAD 1989). It is an invasive procedure, however, that may cause severe complications and currently is not indicated.

14.7.2
CT

This technique has a limited role in local staging of patients with penile tumors. In fact, while CT and magnetic resonance imaging are equally effective to identify pathological nodes, the relationships of the tumor with adjacent structures are better evaluated with magnetic resonance imaging because of higher contrast resolution. In advanced penile cancers TC has a role in identification of distant metastatic deposits. CT is also indicated in patients with lymphoma apparently localized to the penis to check for the presence of other localizations of the disease.

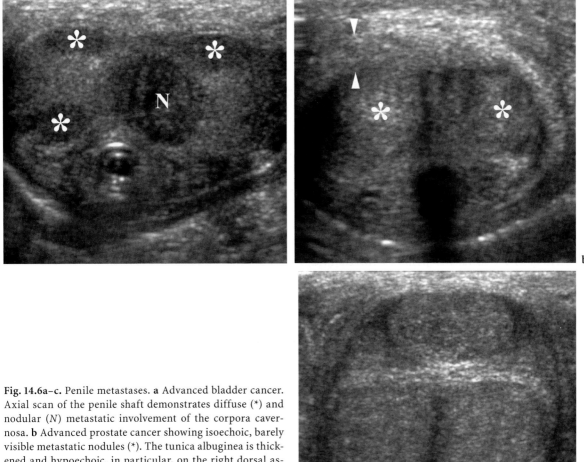

Fig. 14.6a–c. Penile metastases. a Advanced bladder cancer. Axial scan of the penile shaft demonstrates diffuse (*) and nodular (N) metastatic involvement of the corpora cavernosa. b Advanced prostate cancer showing isoechoic, barely visible metastatic nodules (*). The tunica albuginea is thickened and hypoechoic, in particular, on the right dorsal aspect (arrowheads), and boundaries with the right cavernosal body are ill defined, consistent with tumor infiltration. c Biopsy proved diffuse infiltration of the shaft from recurrent bladder cancer. No distinct nodules are appreciable. The tunica albuginea is thickened, but no interruption is visible

14.7.3
Magnetic Resonance Imaging

This technique represents the gold standard imaging modality for staging primary penile malignancies. Since it provides better contrast resolution than ultrasound, the margins between the mass and the erectile bodies are more clearly visualized, and better tumor staging is obtained (Fig. 14.7). A recent study on a large series of 55 tumors shows a sensitivity of 89%, 75% and 88% and a specificity of 83%, 89% and 98% in staging correctly T1, T2 and T3 tumors, respectively (Kayes et al. 2007).

14.7.3.1
Examination Technique

As occurs for ultrasound, intracavernosal PGE1 injection is required (Kayes et al. 2007) because with artificial erection the penile shaft enlarges, and the boundary between the tumor and the surrounding structures is better evaluated. Failure to obtain erection can lead to staging errors.

Different imaging protocols can be used. In general, when the tumor is small, superficial coils are preferred to obtain a better spatial resolution. At least an axial T1-weighted and axial, sagittal and coronal

T2-weighted sequences should be produced. If gadolinium is administered, fat-saturated T1-weighted images should be obtained on the three planes before and after contrast administration. Axial T1-weighted images of the pelvis are obtained using a pelvic coil to look for inguinal or obturator lymphadenopathy. In patients with large (T3–T4) tumors the pelvic coil is used to obtain information on invasion of adjacent organs producing images of the entire pelvis along different planes on both T1-weighted and T2-weighted images and after contrast administration.

14.7.3.2
Appearance of Squamous Cell Carcinoma

At magnetic resonance imaging, squamous cell carcinomas are usually hypointense or isointense relative to the corpora on T1-weighted images and hypointense on T2-weighted images (Pretorius et al. 2001; Vossough et al. 2002). Compared with the corpora poor enhancement is usually observed (Pretorius et al. 2001; Vossough et al. 2002). As a consequence, local staging of the disease is best accomplished on T2-weighted images.

14.7.3.3
Appearance of Other Penile Primary Tumors

Penile tumors different from squamous cell carcinoma usually present non-specific features. Urethral carcinoma and sarcomas are usually hypointense or isointense relative to the corpora on T1-weighted images and hypointense or heterogeneous on T2-weighted images (Pretorius et al. 2001; Vossough et al. 2002). They enhance less than the normal corpora. Large lesions present with inhomogeneous signal intensity and enhancement characteristics (Antunes et al. 2005).

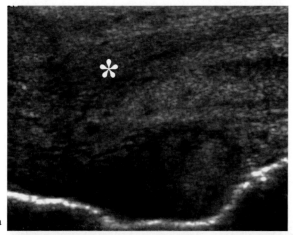

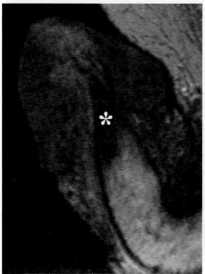

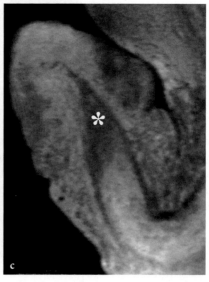

Fig. 14.7a–c. Comparison between ultrasound and magnetic resonance imaging in local staging of penile cancer. **a** Longitudinal ultrasound scan showing tumor infiltration of the right corpus cavernosum (*). **b,c** Tumor infiltration (*) is better depicted with sagittal T2-weighted images (**b**) and with sagittal T1-weighted images (**c**) after gadolinium administration

Penile hemangiomas present at magnetic resonance imaging with high signal intensity on T2-weighted images. This technique is indicated especially in large hemangiomas to assess the extent of the lesion and evaluate the involvement of the corpora cavernosa (KIM et al. 1991).

Neurilemmoma of the glans penis presents with high signal intensity on T2-weighted images and strong enhancement on contrast-enhanced T1-weighted images (JUNG et al. 2006).

Compared with signal intensity of the corpora cavernosa, epithelioid sarcoma is homogeneously isointense on T1-weighted images and inhomogeneously isointense (SIRIKCI et al. 1999) or hypointense (OTO and MEYER 1999) on T2-weighted images. Homogeneous or heterogeneous enhancement is observed after contrast agent injection. Kaposi's sarcoma is characterized by relatively strong tumoral enhancement after contrast material administration (RESTREPO et al. 2006).

Penile lymphomas are usually hypointense on T1-weighted images and hyperintense on T2-weighted images. After gadolinium administration the lesions show variable, usually prominent enhancement. Infiltration of the corporeal bodies can be recognized (KENDI et al. 2006). Primary melanoma of the penis is often hyperintense on both T1- and T2-weighted images and enhances strongly (VOSSOUGH et al. 2002).

14.7.3.4
Appearance of Secondary Tumors

Penile metastases present with variable features at magnetic resonance imaging. In most cases, single or multiple discrete enhancing nodules are identified, which usually display low signal intensity on both T1- and T2-weighted images and variable enhancement after gadolinium administration (KENDI et al. 2006). In case of diffuse infiltration of the shaft from adjacent cancer, invasion of the proximal portion of the tunica albuginea is recognized, and the cavernosal tissue is progressively replaced by enhancing tumor tissue (Fig. 14.8).

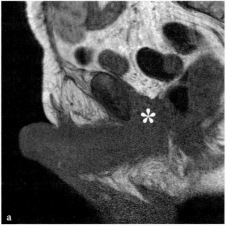
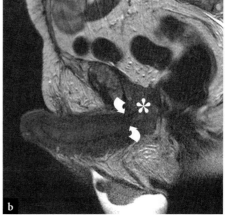
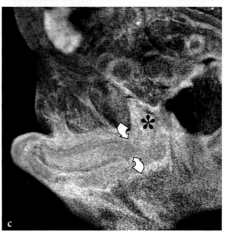

Fig. 14.8a–c. Diffuse metastatic involvement of the penis in a patient who had undergone cystectomy and prostatectomy 5 years before for bladder cancer. The patient presented with painless penile induration of 1-month duration and blood discharge from the urethral stump. Sagittal magnetic resonance scans. **a** T1-weighted image showing a relatively hypointense soft-tissue mass (*) between the rectum and the pubic bone consistent with tumor recurrence. Tissue of the same signal intensity fills up the corporeal bodies and the corpus spongiosum. **b** T2-weighted image confirming the presence of a recurrent tumor (*). The normally hyperdense cavernosal and spongiosal tissue is replaced by tissue with the same signal intensity of the recurrent tumor. The tunica albuginea is interrupted at the base of the penis (*curved arrow*), but is still visible along the shaft despite widespread corporeal infiltration. **c** T1-weighted image obtained after gadolinium administration showing diffuse homogeneous enhancement of the recurrent tumor mass involving the penile shaft

References

Agrawal A, Pai D, Ananthakrishnan N et al (2000) Clinical and sonographic findings in carcinoma of the penis. J Clin Ultrasound 28:399–406

Algaba F, Horenblas S, Pizzocaro-Luigi Piva G et al (2002) EAU guidelines on penile cancer. Eur Urol 42:199–203

Antunes AA, Nesrallah LJ, Goncalves PD et al (2005) Deep-seated sarcomas of the penis. Int Braz J Urol 31:245–250

Bartoletti R, Gacci M, Nesi G et al (2002) Leiomyoma of the corona glans penis. Urology 59:445

Belville WD, Cohen JA (1992) Secondary penile malignancies: the spectrum of presentation. J Surg Oncol 51:134–137

Bertolotto M, Serafini G, Dogliotti L et al (2005) Primary and secondary malignancies of the penis: ultrasound features. Abdom Imaging 30:108–112

Bezerra AL, Lopes A, Santiago GH et al (2001) Human papillomavirus as a prognostic factor in carcinoma of the penis: analysis of 82 patients treated with amputation and bilateral lymphadenectomy. Cancer 91:2315–2321

Bunesch Villalba L, Bargallo Castello X, Vilana Puig R et al (2001) Lymphoma of the penis: sonographic findings. J Ultrasound Med 20:929–931

Burgers JK, Badalament RA, Drago JR (1992) Penile cancer. Clinical presentation, diagnosis, and staging. Urol Clin North Am 19:247–256

Cherian J, Rajan S, Thwaini A et al (2006) Secondary penile tumours revisited. Int Semin Surg Oncol 3:33

Eberth C (1870) Krehsmetastasen des Corpus Cavernosum Penis. Virch Arch 51:145–146

el-Sharkawi A, Murphy J (1996) Primary penile lymphoma: the case for combined modality therapy. Clin Oncol (R Coll Radiol) 8:334–335

Escribano G, Allona A, Burgos FJ et al (1987) Cavernosography in diagnosis of metastatic tumors of the penis: five new cases and a review of the literature. J Urol 138:1174–1177

Guy M, Singer D, Barzilai N, Eisenkraft S (1994) Primary classic Kaposi's sarcoma of glans penis–appearance on magnetic resonance imaging. Br J Urol 74:521–522

Haddad FS (1989) Re: Cavernosography in diagnosis of metastatic tumors of the penis: 5 new cases and a review of the literature. J Urol 141:959–960

Hermida Gutierrez JF, Gomez Vegas A, Silmi Moyano A et al (1995) [Kaposi's sarcoma of the penis: our experience and review of the literature]. Arch Esp Urol 48:153–158

Horenblas S, Kroger R, Gallee MP et al (1994) Ultrasound in squamous cell carcinoma of the penis; a useful addition to clinical staging? A comparison of ultrasound with histopathology. Urology 43:702–707

Iscovich J, Boffetta P, Franceschi S et al (2000) Classic Kaposi's sarcoma: epidemiology and risk factors. Cancer 88:500–517

Jung DC, Hwang SI, Jung SI et al (2006) Neurilemmoma of the glans penis: ultrasonography and magnetic resonance imaging findings. J Comput Assist Tomogr 30:68–69

Kagu MB, Nggada HA, Garandawa HI et al (2006) AIDS-associated Kaposi's sarcoma in Northeastern Nigeria. Singapore Med J 47:1069–1074

Kayes O, Minhas S, Allen C et al (2007) The role of magnetic resonance imaging in the local staging of penile cancer. Eur Urol 51:1313–1318; discussion 1318–1319

Kendi T, Batislam E, Basar MM et al (2006) Magnetic resonance imaging (MRI) in penile metastases of extragenitourinary cancers. Int Urol Nephrol 38:105–109

Kim SH, Lee SE, Han MC (1991) Penile hemangioma: US and MR imaging demonstration. Urol Radiol 13:126–128

Kousseff BG, Hoover DL (1999) Penile neurofibromas. Am J Med Genet 87:1–5

Koyuncuoglu M, Yalcin N, Ozkan S, Kirkali Z (1996) Primary Kaposi's sarcoma of the glans penis. Br J Urol 77:614–615

Liu SP, Shun CT, Chang SJ et al (2007) Leiomyoma of the corpus cavernosum of the penis. Int J Urol 14:257–258

Lo HC, Yu DS, Lee CT et al (2003) Primary B cell lymphoma of the penis: successful treatment with organ preservation. Arch Androl 49:467–470

Lont AP, Besnard AP, Gallee MP et al (2003) A comparison of physical examination and imaging in determining the extent of primary penile carcinoma. BJU Int 91:493–495

Micali G, Nasca MR, De Pasquale R, Innocenzi D (2003) Primary classic Kaposi's sarcoma of the penis: report of a case and review. J Eur Acad Dermatol Venereol 17:320–323

Mir K, Buckley JF, Karanjavala JD, Elem B (1998) Penile Kaposi's sarcoma. Int Urol Nephrol 30:327–329

Oto A, Meyer J (1999) MR appearance of penile epithelioid sarcoma. AJR Am J Roentgenol 172:555–556

Perez LM, Shumway RA, Carson CC, 3rd et al (1992) Penile metastasis secondary to supraglottic squamous cell carcinoma: review of the literature. J Urol 147:157–160

Pow-Sang MR, Benavente V, Pow-Sang JE et al (2002) Cancer of the penis. Cancer Control 9:305–314

Pretorius ES, Siegelman ES, Ramchandani P, Banner MP (2001) MR imaging of the penis. Radiographics 21 Spec No:S283–298; discussion S298–289

Restrepo CS, Martinez S, Lemos JA et al (2006) Imaging manifestations of Kaposi sarcoma. Radiographics 26:1169–1185

Roberts W (1872) A practical treatise on urinary and renal disease. Smith, Elder and Co, London

Sanchez-Ortiz R, Huang SF, Tamboli P et al (2005) Melanoma of the penis, scrotum and male urethra: a 40-year single institution experience. J Urol 173:1958–1965

Sanz Mayayo E, Burgos Revilla FJ, Gomez Garcia I et al (2004) [Penile metastasis of a prostatic adenocarcinoma]. Arch Esp Urol 57:841–844

Sirikci A, Bayram M, Demirci M et al (1999) Penile epithelioid sarcoma: MR imaging findings. Eur Radiol 9:1593–1595

Stehr M, Rohrbach H, Schuster T, Dietz HG (2000) [Leiomyoma of the glans penis]. Urologe A 39:171–173

Theodore C, Androulakis N, Spatz A et al (2002) An explosive course of squamous cell penile cancer in an AIDS patient. Ann Oncol 13:475–479

Usta MF, Adams DM, Zhang JW et al (2003) Penile epithelioid sarcoma and the case for a histopathological diagnosis in Peyronie's disease. BJU Int 91:519–521

Vossough A, Pretorius ES, Siegelman ES et al (2002) Magnetic resonance imaging of the penis. Abdom Imaging 27:640–659

Wei CC, Peng CT, Chiang IP, Wu KH (2006) Primary B cell non-hodgkin lymphoma of the penis in a child. J Pediatr Hematol Oncol 28:479–480

Surgical Treatment of Penile Disease: Current Indications

Giovanni Liguori, Giuseppe Ocello, Stefano Bucci, Carlo Trombetta, and Emanuele Belgrano

CONTENTS

15.1 Background 125
15.2 Penile Cancer 125
15.3 Erectile Dysfunction 126
15.3.1 Penile Prosthesis Implantation 126
15.3.2 Penile Revascularization Surgery 126
15.3.3 Penile Venous Surgery 126
15.4 Reconstructive Phallic Surgery 127
15.5 Sex Reassignment Surgery Male-to-Female 128
15.6 Congenital and Acquired Deformity 129
15.6.1 Shortening Procedures 129
15.6.2 Lengthening Procedures 129

References 131

15.1 Background

A variety of surgical procedures have been described to treat various penile diseases. Nowadays the purpose of all surgical techniques in penile surgery is not only the correct treatment of the primary condition, but also to preserve sexual function and to maintain cosmesis of the penis.

G. Liguori, MD; G. Ocello, MD; S. Bucci, MD; C. Trombetta, MD
Department of Urology, University of Trieste, Ospedale di Cattinara, Strada di Fiume 447, Trieste, 34124, Italy
E. Belgrano, MD
Professor and Chairman, Department of Urology, University of Trieste, Ospedale di Cattinara, Strada di Fiume 447, Trieste, 34124, Italy

15.2 Penile Cancer

Penile cancer is a rare tumour in Europe with an incidence of 1 per 100,000 men per year (Busby and Pettaway 2005). As illustrated in Chapter 13, it is most commonly diagnosed in the 6th and 7th decades of life, but can occur at any age, including childhood. Squamous cell carcinoma is by far the most common malignant disease of the penis, accounting for more than 95% of cases. Malignant melanomas and basal cell carcinomas are less common. Mesenchymal tumours such as Kaposi's sarcoma, angiosarcoma, and epithelioid haemangioendothelioma are very uncommon, with an incidence rate of less than 3%.

In case of penile cancer, imaging is generally not needed for diagnosis because the tumour is usually visible at physical examination. The main purpose of penile imaging is to evaluate the degree of infiltration of the corpora cavernosa. As a matter of fact, tumours involving the foreskin may be treated by circumcision alone, and lesions involving the glans or shaft may be treated by local wedge excision; unfortunately, local recurrence may occur in up to 50% of patients (Narayana et al. 1982). For lesions involving the glans and distal shaft, partial penectomy should leave a residual penile stump suitable for upright micturition and sexual function. Involvement of the proximal shaft requires total penectomy. Extension to the perineal body, pubis, or scrotum in the absence of metastatic disease may require more extensive resection and adjuvant chemotherapy.

Although radical surgery gives excellent control of the primary tumour, it is mutilating and probably unnecessary in case of low-grade and low-stage tumours (Brown et al. 2005). In these cases conservative techniques such as laser therapy, cryotherapy, photodynamic therapy, topical 5-fluorouracil, or local excision (glansectomy and reconstruction) give better cosmetic and functional results (Solsona et al. 2004).

Current guidelines of the European Association of Urology (EAU) on the management of penile cancer strongly recommend a penile-preserving approach for patients with TIS–T1 G1–G2 tumours that can commit to a regular surveillance programme, and the guidelines suggest that a penile-preserving approach may also be an option in very selected patients with T1 G3 and T<2 disease whose tumours occupy less than 50% of the glans (Solsona et al. 2004).

15.3
Erectile Dysfunction

Erectile dysfunction is defined as the consistent inability to achieve or maintain penile erection satisfactory for sexual intercourse. It is estimated that some form of erectile dysfunction will develop in 52% of men between the ages 40 and 70 years (Melman and Gingell 1999).

Non-surgical treatment alternatives for erectile dysfunction include psychological, endocrinological, neurological, and pharmacological therapy, including oral, topical, and intraurethral delivery agents, and external device modalities (Riley and Athanasiadis 1997). For patients in whom none of these therapies have proved to be successful, a variety of surgical procedures have been developed during the years (Rao and Donatucci 2001). Surgical interventions have consisted primarily of penile prosthesis insertion and arterial bypass surgery. Venous leakage surgery for corporeal veno-occlusive dysfunction came later in the mid-1980s to early 1990s (Sharlip 1990).

15.3.1
Penile Prosthesis Implantation

Penile prosthesis implantation is an effective surgical option for treatment of severe vascular erectile dysfunction. However, it remains the third-choice therapeutic option after failure of other less invasive procedures (Wespes et al. 2003; Wespes et al. 2006).

15.3.2
Penile Revascularization Surgery

Penile revascularization is a very useful urological tool in vasculogenic post-traumatic impotence, but correct selection of the patients is mandatory. The ideal candidates for this kind of surgery are young men with no significant vascular risk factors and whose impotence can be related to arterial lesions of the pudendal, common penile, or cavernous arteries due to pelvic bones fractures or blunt perineal trauma (Goldstein and Krane 1992).

Patients with concurrent traumatic veno-occlusive dysfunction following blunt pelvic or perineal trauma should not be considered for revascularization procedures. In fact, this situation is not a rare finding (Munarriz et al. 1995) and would affect patient prognosis unfavourably (Merckx et al. 1992). Moreover, patients with significant vascular risk factors are poor candidates for by-pass surgery and are encouraged to consider other options for treating their impotence (Hatzichristou and Goldstein 1991).

Various penile revascularization techniques have been described in the last 20 years (Newman and Reiss 1982; Shaw and Zorgniotti 1984; Sharlip 1990; Sharaby et al. 1995), but in our opinion each of them should be personalized depending on the pathological findings encountered in each single case. In addition, preference should be given to physiological revascularization procedures whenever possible. Series published in the past 10 years have used a variety of procedures. Long-term successful results in these studies, with admittedly varied patient populations, indications, and techniques, have ranged from 25% to 80% (Rao and Donatucci 2001).

In our opinion, the anastomosis according to the Sharlip technique is the best solution because it envisages a retrograde revascularization of the cavernous artery through the common penile trunk. For this reason we usually anastomosed the epigastric artery on the dorsal artery of the penis end-to-end in the proximal direction (Fig. 15.1). This technique has been associated with the most success and the fewest complications (Wespes et al. 2003).

15.3.3
Penile Venous Surgery

In selected cases, patients with venous leakage can be treated with penile venous dissection and ligation. Penile venous resection decreases the number of channels for venous outflow from the penis and, therefore, increases venous resistance improving erections. Many published series show an important improvement at short-term follow-up, but a poor result at long-term follow-up (Treiber and Gilbert 1989;

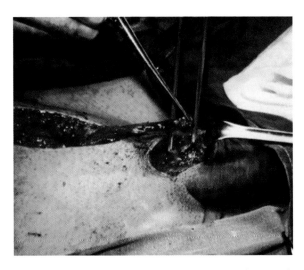

Fig. 15.1. Penile arterial revascularization. Photograph showing the isolated epigastric artery before anastomosis with the dorsal artery at the root of the penis

Wespes et al. 1992; Sasso et al. 1996; Schultheiss et al. 1997; Popken et al. 1999; Da Ros et al. 2000).

Several different factors can account for the important failure rate of penile venous surgery. Inability to accurately diagnose concomitant arterial disease and differences in the extent of venous dissection probably account for many of the early patient failure. With the use of stricter diagnostic inclusion criteria and a more aggressive surgical approach, many of these early failures could have been avoided. The development of collateral venous circulation is the most likely cause of late failure. Finally, another reason for failure is that ligation of penile veins may not address the true underlying pathologic disorder in many patients in whom cavernosal smooth muscle disease reduces compliance of the corpora cavernosa.

15.4
Reconstructive Phallic Surgery

Phalloplasty is considered to be one of the most challenging procedures in reconstructive surgery (Upton et al. 1987). The development of techniques of phalloplasty has paralleled the evolution of flap development in reconstructive surgery itself. Initially, random tubed pedicled flaps were used. Subsequently, pedicled island flaps and myocutaneous flaps have been applied. With the development of the microsurgical techniques, free flaps also were introduced in phalloplasty.

In his review of surgical techniques, Hage reports that for reconstruction of the phallus in non-transsexual men a variety of techniques have been suggested or used (Hage et al. 1993), including bipedicled single abdominal flaps (McIndoe 1948), bipedicled tube-within-tube flaps, infraumbilical pedicled flaps (Hotchkiss et al. 1956), scrotal flaps (Mukherjee 1980), groin flaps (Song 1982), thigh flaps (Orticochea 1972), pedicled myocutaneous gracilis flaps (Devine et al. 1987), pedicled myocutancous rectus abdominis flaps (Chang and Hwang 1984), free microsurgical forearm flaps (Shenaq and Dinh 1989), and free microsurgical upper arm flaps (Jordan et al. 1987).

For phalloplasty in female-to-male transsexuals the following techniques have been described: Bogoras bipedicled abdominal tubed flaps (Bogoras 1936), Maltz-Gillies tube-in-tube bipedicled flaps (Maltz 1946), Stanford inside-out infraumbilical flaps (Hentz et al. 1987), subcutaneous pedicled infraumbilical flaps (Bouman 1987), pedicled groin flaps (Bouman 1987), pedicled thigh flaps (McGregor and Jackson 1972), pedicled myocutaneous flaps (Kaplan 1971) , free microsurgical forearm flaps (Alanis 1969; Kao et al. 1984) and miscellaneous free flaps (Puckett et al. 1982; Gilbert et al. 1987).

The creation of a phallus has been associated with multiple surgical problems, and efforts are ongoing to improve the function and appearance. The older, insensate phallus shrivelled, and efforts to provide stiffness were associated with fistula formation and cutaneous erosions. Generally the initial desire of female-to-male transsexuals is not a functional phallus, but to void while standing in the men's bathroom to elude this closure. Most patients express only a desire for a good appearance in swimsuits, while only some transsexuals would like to be able to use the phallus sexually.

The ideal phalloplasty technique should be a one-stage procedure, be cosmetically acceptable to both patient and partner, construct a neourethra to permit voiding whilst standing, have sufficient rigidity for vaginal penetration, have tactile and erogenous sensitivity, and have minimal scarring in the donor area.

Since the first reported description of phalloplasty (Maltz 1946), a considerable variety of other techniques has been described, but, in our opinion, the gold standard technique for phalloplasty has not been described yet because each of them should be personalised depending on the patient's desires or expectations and surgeon's skill.

The highest priority of most patients is the ability to urinate in public while standing, but this objective is the hardest to reach due the high complications rate. Distal urethral stenosis is the commonest urethral complication and this is due to ischemic necrosis of the most distal part of the labial tube. This would be particularly more common in patients who have a longer phallus and, therefore, need a longer labial tube constructed.

In case of patients who wish a functional phallus to void while standing and to engage in sexual intercourse like a natural man, we think that the forearm free skin flap (SHENAQ and DINH 1989) would be a suitable donor area because it is soft, uniformly thin in subcutaneous tissue, and has a long vascular pedicle (Fig. 15.2).

If on the contrary patients expressed only a desire for a good appearance in swimsuits, pubic phalloplasty (BETTOCCHI et al. 2005) is a simple and relatively quick procedure, leading to minimal scarring or disfigurements in the donor area. It is well accepted by the patient and his partner and occasionally rigid enough for penetrative sexual intercourse (Fig. 15.3).

15.5 Sex Reassignment Surgery Male-to-Female

Ideal surgical procedure to construct female genitalia in a male transsexual should be a one-stage procedure, produce a vagina adequate for intercourse, and have a cosmetic result that is virtually indistinguishable from a normal female subject. The procedure to reconstruct the female genitalia includes bilateral orchiectomy and penectomy and consists of creation of an urethrostomy, neovagina (vaginoplasty), construction of normal-appearing labial structures (labioplasty), and of sensate clitoris (clitoroplasty).

Neovaginal construction in male-to-female transsexuals during sex reassignment surgery may be done by different techniques: inversion of a penile skin flap alone (RUBIN 1993), penile flap combined with a scrotal flap (VAN NOORT and NICOLAI 1993), and bowel neovagina using sigmoid colon (DALTON 1981), and detebularized ileum (BURGER et al. 1989). Up to now not enough long-term data are available to determine which procedure provides the best results.

Complications of sex reassignment surgery are well known. Early postoperative complications are haemorrage or haematoma, infection, rectovaginal, peri-

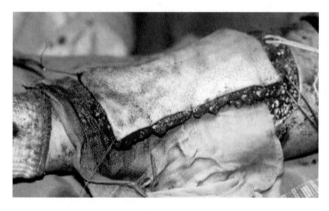

Fig. 15.2. Phalloplasty with forearm free skin flap. Photograph showing the flap completely isolated

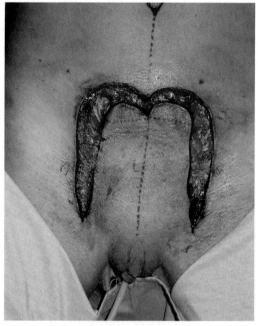

Fig. 15.3. Pubic phalloplasty. The phallus is fashioned from a flap of anterior abdominal wall skin

neal or urethrovaginal fistula, and partial necrosis of the flaps, while late postoperative complications are stenosis of the vagina, prolapse of scrotal flaps, and the presence of a too-long urethral stump (Karim et al. 1996; Eldh et al. 1997; Liguori et al. 2001).

Sex reassignment surgery has been performed on thousands of transsexual patients during the past 30 years and is now coming to the forefront of urology. Although urological treatment of male transsexuals is becoming more common, few follow-up studies have been reported in the literature. Moreover, there is an evident difficulty in objective evaluation of results, and in fact consistent published information is lacking in the international literature.

15.6
Congenital and Acquired Deformity

Congenital penile curvature is caused by a disproportion between the corpora cavernosa and the corpus spongiosum, resulting in dorsal or ventral curvature, or between the two corpora cavernosa, resulting in lateral curvature.

Penile curvature is usually evident only when the penis is in erection. Although the curvature is usually not severe enough to warrant surgical correction, in some cases it may lead to sexual dysfunction or interfere with intercourse due to difficulty in penetration.

Peyronie's disease is the most frequent cause of acquired penile curvature with an estimated prevalence of 0.4% in Caucasian men (Montorsi et al. 2000; Lindsay et al. 1991). No medical therapy is fully effective, and surgery remains the gold standard in patients with severe deformity and/or erectile dysfunction who fail conservative measures. The indications for surgical correction of penile bending include severe curvature, narrowing, or indentation, and severe penile shortening of more than 1 year duration with sexual difficulty or partner discomfort because of deformity (Gholami and Lue 2001).

15.6.1
Shortening Procedures

These reconstructive techniques are performed on the convex surface of the penis at the site opposite to the penile plaque, are the easiest to perform, and require the least expertise. Patient selection is extremely important. Shortening procedures are most appropriate for patients with useful erection, adequate penile length, and without hourglass deformity. Nesbit first described the correction of congenital erectile deformities by shortening the opposite side of the penis by the excision of an ellipse of tunica albuginea. The Nesbit operation is performed by excising one or more ellipsoid wedge resections of the tunica albuginea on the side opposite to the curvature (Fig. 15.4) and closing the albugineal defects with running absorbable sutures. The overall results are satisfactory, with a success rate of 82%. A literature review has confirmed these favourable results (Pryor 1998).

The most common complication of this procedure is loss of penile length. This complication does not preclude most men from having sexual intercourse. Other complications reported include erectile dysfunction, penile hematoma, penile narrowing, and urethral injury (Ralph et al. 1995).

A modification of the Nesbit operation was described by Yachia (1999) in which, instead of removing an ellipse of tunica albuginea, a long longitudinal incision or multiple smaller longitudinal incisions are made in the area of maximum curvature of the corpora cavernosa (Fig. 15.5). These incisions are then closed horizontally to straighten the penis providing equal clinical success with less morbidity. Many surgeons claim a high percentage of good results with this technique, reporting high satisfaction rates (Sassine et al. 1994; Daitch et al. 1999).

Wedge resection or incision of the tunica albuginea requires extensive dissection of the neurovascular bundle or corpus spongiosum. A simplified approach for correcting penile curvature is corporeal plication, in which two or three pairs of nonabsorbable longitudinal plication sutures are placed through the full thickness of the tunica albuginea on the side opposite the curvature. Some investigators describe high recurrence rates and poor results with prolonged follow-up. The literature reports significant variation in the result, ranging from 38% to 100% satisfactory results (Essed and Schroeder 1985; Schultheiss et al. 2000).

15.6.2
Lengthening Procedures

These reconstructive techniques correct penile curvature while restoring the length of the curved shortened penis. Surgery is performed on the convex side of the penis and requires plaque excision or incision with grafting. This procedure is indicated in case of severe curvature and shortened and deformed penis with narrowing or hourglass deformities. Many autologous, cadaveric, and synthetic materials have been described with different results for replacement of the tunica albuginea (KOVAC and BROCK 2007).

In the past excision of the plaque has been the standard approach. Unfortunately there was a great variability in the outcome of plaque excision. The most common problem was erectile dysfunction in case of removal of large areas of tunica albuginea and surrounding cavernosal tissue with the plaque (KENDIRCI and HELLSTROM 2004). In order to reduce the surgery-related traumatism to the erectile tissue, plaque incision and grafting was introduced, rather than excision (Fig. 15.6). Temporalis fascia graft was first described (GELBARD and HAYDEN 1991); nowadays a segment of the long saphenous vein is usually used (BROCK et al. 1993).

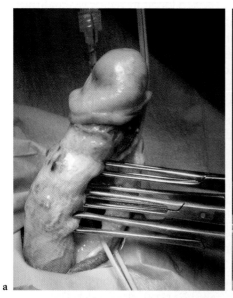
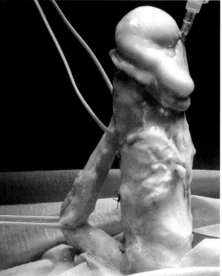

Fig. 15.4a,b. Nesbit operation. **a** Allis clamps are applied contiguously on the longer portion of the tunica albuginea until a complete straightening of the penis is achieved. **b** After closing the albugineal defects with running absorbable sutures, artificial erection confirm the straightening of the penis

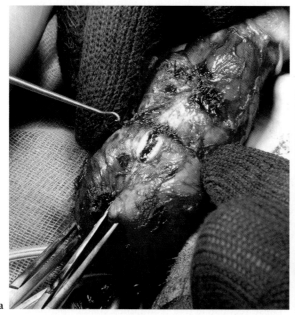
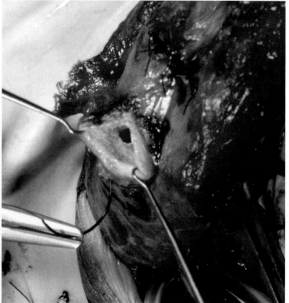

Fig. 15.5a,b. Yachia operation. **a** Multiple longitudinal incisions are made in the area of maximum curvature. **b** Incisions are closed horizontally to straighten the penis

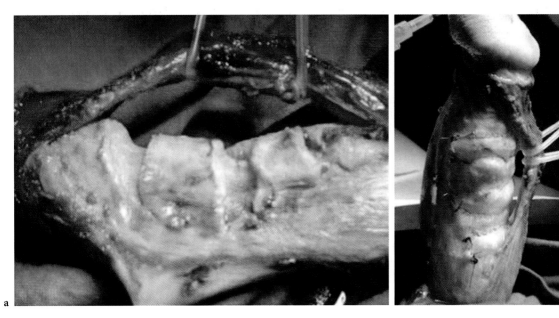

Fig. 15.6a,b. Plaque incision and grafting. **a** Multiple tunical incisions are performed in order to increase the length of incised side. **b** Saphenous grafts are placed over the defect and sewn into place with a continuous 4-0 suture

References

Alanis SZ (1969) An innovation in total penis reconstruction. Plast Reconstr Surg 43:418–422

Bettocchi C, Ralph DJ, Pryor JP (2005) Pedicled pubic phalloplasty in females with gender dysphoria. BJU Int 95:120–124

Bogoras N (1936) Ueber die volle plastische Wiederherstellung eines zum Koitus fähigen Penis (Peniplastica totalis). Zentralbl Chir 63:1271–1276

Bouman FG (1987) The first step in phalloplasty in female transsexuals. Plast Reconstr Surg 79:662–664

Brock G, Kadioglu A, Lue TF (1993) Peyronie's disease: a modified treatment. Urology 42:300–304

Brown CT, Minhas S, Ralph DJ (2005) Conservative surgery for penile cancer: subtotal glans excision without grafting. BJU Int 96:911–912

Burger RA, Riedmiller H, Knapstein PG, et al. (1989) Ileocecal vaginal construction. Am J Obstet Gynecol 161:162–167

Busby JE, Pettaway CA (2005) What's new in the management of penile cancer? Curr Opin Urol 15:350–357

Chang TS, Hwang WY (1984) Forearm flap in one-stage reconstruction of the penis. Plast Reconstr Surg 74:251–258

Da Ros CT, Teloken C, Antonini CC, et al. (2000) Long-term results of penile vein ligation for erectile dysfunction due to cavernovenous disease. Tech Urol 6:172–174

Daitch JA, Angermeier KW, Montague DK (1999) Modified corporoplasty for penile curvature: long-term results and patient satisfaction. J Urol 162:2006–2009

Dalton JR (1981) Use of sigmoid colon in sex reassignment operations. Urology 17:223–227

Devine P, Winslow B, Jordan G, et al. (1987) Reconstructive phallic surgery. In: Libertino J (ed). Williams & Wilkins, Baltimore, pp 552–566

Eldh J, Berg A, Gustafsson M (1997) Long-term follow up after sex reassignment surgery. Scand J Plast Reconstr Surg Hand Surg 31:39–45

Essed E, Schroeder FH (1985) New surgical treatment for Peyronie disease. Urology 25:582–587

Gelbard MK, Hayden B (1991) Expanding contractures of the tunica albuginea due to Peyronie's disease with temporalis fascia free grafts. J Urol 145:772–776

Gholami SS, Lue TF (2001) Peyronie's disease. Urol Clin North Am 28:377–390

Gilbert DA, Horton CE, Terzis JK, et al. (1987) New concepts in phallic reconstruction. Ann Plast Surg 18:128–136

Goldstein I, Krane R (1992) Diagnosis and therapy of erectile dysfunction. In: Walsh P, Gittes R, Perlmutter A, Stamey T (eds) Campbell's Urology. WB Saunders, Philadelphia, pp 3033–3067

Hage JJ, Bloem JJ, Suliman HM (1993) Review of the literature on techniques for phalloplasty with emphasis on the applicability in female-to-male transsexuals. J Urol 150:1093–1098

Hatzichristou D, Goldstein I (1991) Arterial bypass surgery for impotence. Curr Opin Urol 1:144–148

Hentz VR, Pearl RM, Grossman JA, et al. (1987) The radial forearm flap: a versatile source of composite tissue. Ann Plast Surg 19:485–498

Hotchkiss RS, Morales PA, O'Connor JJ, Jr. (1956) Plastic reconstructive surgery after total loss of the penis. Am J Surg 92:403–408

Jordan G, Gilbert D, Winslow B, Devine P (1987) Single-stage phallic reconstruction. World J Urol 5:14–18

Kao XS, Kao JH, Ho CL, et al. (1984) One-stage reconstruction of the penis with free skin flap: report of three cases. J Reconstr Microsurg 1:149–153

Kaplan I (1971) A rapid method for constructing a functional sensitive penis. Br J Plast Surg 24:342–344

Karim RB, Hage JJ, Mulder JW (1996) Neovaginoplasty in male transsexuals: review of surgical techniques and recommendations regarding eligibility. Ann Plast Surg 37:669–675

Kendirci M, Hellstrom WJ (2004) Critical analysis of surgery for Peyronie's disease. Curr Opin Urol 14:381–388

Kovac JR, Brock GB (2007) Surgical Outcomes and Patient Satisfaction after Dermal, Pericardial, and Small Intestinal Submucosal Grafting for Peyronie's Disease. J Sex Med

Liguori G, Trombetta C, Buttazzi L, Belgrano E (2001) Acute peritonitis due to introital stenosis and perforation of a bowel neovagina in a transsexual. Obstet Gynecol 97:828–829

Lindsay MB, Schain DM, Grambsch P, et al. (1991) The incidence of Peyronie's disease in Rochester, Minnesota, 1950 through 1984. J Urol 146:1007–1009

MaItz M (1946) Maltz technic. In: MaItz M (ed) Evolution of Plastic Surgery. Froben Press, New York, pp 278–279

McGregor IA, Jackson IT (1972) The groin flap. Br J Plast Surg 25:3–16

Mclndoe A (1948) Deformities of the male urethra. Br J Plast Surg 1:29–47

Melman A, Gingell JC (1999) The epidemiology and pathophysiology of erectile dysfunction. J Urol 161:5–11

Merckx LA, De Bruyne RM, Goes E, et al. (1992) The value of dynamic color duplex scanning in the diagnosis of venogenic impotence. J Urol 148:318–320

Montorsi F, Salonia A, Maga T, et al. (2000) Evidence based assessment of long-term results of plaque incision and vein grafting for Peyronie's disease. J Urol 163:1704–1708

Mukherjee GD (1980) The rise of surgery: from empiric craft to scientific discipline. Plast Reconstr Surg 65:531

Munarriz RM, Yan QR, A ZN, et al. (1995) Blunt trauma: the pathophysiology of hemodynamic injury leading to erectile dysfunction. J Urol 153:1831–1840

Narayana AS, Olney LE, Loening SA, et al. (1982) Carcinoma of the penis: analysis of 219 cases. Cancer 49:2185–2191

Newman HF, Reiss H (1982) Method for exposure of cavernous artery. Urology 19:61–62

Orticochea M (1972) A new method of total reconstruction of the penis. Br J Plast Surg 25:347–366

Popken G, Katzenwadel A, Wetterauer U (1999) Long-term results of dorsal penile vein ligation for symptomatic treatment of erectile dysfunction. Andrologia 31 Suppl 1:77–82

Pryor J, Akkus E, Alter G, et al. (2004) Peyronie's disease. J Sex Med 1:110–115

Pryor JP (1998) Correction of penile curvature and Peyronie's disease: why I prefer the Nesbit technique. Int J Impot Res 10:129–131

Puckett CL, Reinisch JF, Montie JE (1982) Free flap phalloplasty. J Urol 128:294–297

Ralph DJ, al-Akraa M, Pryor JP (1995) The Nesbit operation for Peyronie's disease: 16-year experience. J Urol 154:1362–1363

Rao DS, Donatucci CF (2001) Vasculogenic impotence. Arterial and venous surgery. Urol Clin North Am 28:309–319

Riley AJ, Athanasiadis L (1997) Impotence and its non-surgical management. Br J Clin Pract 51:99–103, 105

Rubin SO (1993) Sex-reassignment surgery male-to-female. Review, own results and report of a new technique using the glans penis as a pseudoclitoris. Scand J Urol Nephrol Suppl 154:1–28

Sassine AM, Wespes E, Schulman CC (1994) Modified corporoplasty for penile curvature: 10 years' experience. Urology 44:419–421

Sasso F, Gulino G, Di Pinto A, Alcini E (1996) Should venous surgery be still proposed or neglected? Int J Impot Res 8:25–28

Schultheiss D, Meschi MR, Hagemann J, et al. (2000) Congenital and acquired penile deviation treated with the essed plication method. Eur Urol 38:167–171

Schultheiss D, Truss MC, Becker AJ, et al. (1997) Long-term results following dorsal penile vein ligation in 126 patients with veno-occlusive dysfunction. Int J Impot Res 9:205–209

Sharaby JS, Benet AE, Melman A (1995) Penile revascularization. Urol Clin North Am 22:821–832

Sharlip ID (1990) The role of vascular surgery in arteriogenic and combined arteriogenic and venogenic impotence. Semin Urol 8:129–137

Shaw WW, Zorgniotti AW (1984) Surgical techniques in penile revascularization. Urology 23:76–78

Shenaq SM, Dinh TA (1989) Total penile and urethral reconstruction with an expanded sensate lateral arm flap: case report. J Reconstr Microsurg 5:245–248

Solsona E, Algaba F, Horenblas S, et al. (2004) EAU Guidelines on Penile Cancer. Eur Urol 46:1–8

Song R (1982) Total reconstruction of the male genitalia. Clin Plast Surg 9:97–104

Treiber U, Gilbert P (1989) Venous surgery in erectile dysfunction: a critical report on 116 patients. Urology 34:22–27

Upton J, Mutimer KL, Loughlin K, Ritchie J (1987) Penile reconstruction using the lateral arm flap. J R Coll Surg Edinb 32:97–101

van Noort DE, Nicolai JP (1993) Comparison of two methods of vagina construction in transsexuals. Plast Reconstr Surg 91:1308–1315

Wespes E, Amar E, Hatzichristou D, et al. (2006) EAU Guidelines on erectile dysfunction: an update. Eur Urol 49:806–815

Wespes E, Delcour C, Preserowitz L, et al. (1992) Impotence due to corporeal veno-occlusive dysfunction: long-term follow-up of venous surgery. Eur Urol 21:115–119

Wespes E, Wildschutz T, Roumeguere T, Schulman CC (2003) The place of surgery for vascular impotence in the third millennium. J Urol 170:1284–1286

Yachia D (1990) Modified corporoplasty for the treatment of penile curvature. J Urol 143:80–82

US of the Postoperative Penis

Michele Bertolotto, Paola Martingano, Andrea Spadacci, and Maria Assunta Cova

CONTENTS

16.1 Background 133
16.2 Common Postoperative Complications 133
16.3 Straightening Operations 134
16.3.1 Shortening Procedures 134
16.3.2 Lengthening Procedures 134
16.4 Prosthesis Implantation 136
16.5 Vascular Surgery for Impotence 137
16.6 Circumcision 139
16.7 Penile Augmentation Procedures 140
16.8 Shunt Surgery for Ischemic Priapism 140
16.9 Sex Reassignment Surgery 141
16.10 Urethral Surgery 141
16.11 Follow-Up of Patients with Penile Tumors 142
16.12 Diagnostic Role of Other Imaging Modalities 142
References 145

16.1
Background

A variety of surgical procedures has been developed to manage different penile pathologies and malformations. Penile surgery produces anatomical and vascular changes that can be successfully investigated with grey scale and color Doppler ultrasonography. In particular, early and late surgical complications can be identified, and postoperative changes of the normal ultrasound appearance of the penile envelopes, of the penile bodies and of flow characteristics in the penile vessels can be investigated.

M. Bertolotto, MD; P. Martingano, MD; A. Spadacci, MD; M. A. Cova, MD, Professor and Chairman
Department of Radiology, University of Trieste, Ospedale di Cattinara, Strada di Fiume 447, Trieste, 34124, Italy

16.2
Common Postoperative Complications

As occurs in surgical procedures elsewhere, penile hematoma, other postoperative fluid collections and infection are the most common complications of penile surgery. In the course of time, hematomas present with different ultrasound features (Doubilet et al. 1991). Acutely, their content can appear echogenic; then, they become hypoechoic and organize presenting with complex echogenic areas, anechoic regions and septations. Lymphatic and serous collections are uncommon and usually appear anechoic.

Grey-scale ultrasonography allows evaluation of the relationships between postoperative fluid collections and the normal penile anatomical structures (Bertolotto et al. 2005). In particular, the Buck's fascia becomes appreciable as a layer distinct from the tunica albuginea when fluid extravasation accumulates between them. The Colles' fascia is barely visible in pathological conditions as well, but it is possible to assess whether a fluid collection develops in the space between the Buck's and the Colles' fascia when it is identified above the deep dorsal vessels.

High-flow priapism has been reported as a rare complication of penile surgery. Cavernosal artery injury may be produced during insertion of the needle used to obtain the hydraulic erection (Liguori et al. 2005) and, in patients with ischemic priapism, during aspiration of the blood entrapped within the corpora cavernosa (McMahon 2002). Also surgical shunting procedures in patients with ischemic priapism can occasionally complicate with cavernosal artery injury and high-flow priapism. The site and flow characteristics of the arterial cavernosal fistula can be evaluated at color Doppler ultrasound, which demonstrates extravasation of blood from the lacerated artery presenting with a characteristic color blush of variable size. Duplex Doppler interrogation of the lesion shows high-velocity, turbulent flows (Bertolotto et al. 2003).

16.3
Straightening Operations

As described in Chapter 15, surgical correction of penile curvature can be either approached with shortening or with lengthening procedures. In patients with congenital or acquired penile bending, shortening procedures provide excellent results in terms of preservation of erectile function, but the result is loss of penile length because straightening is obtained with excisions or plications of the tunica albuginea at the opposite site of the curvature. Lengthening procedures with grafting are indicated in patients with severe curvature resulting in severe shortening, narrowing or hourglass deformities. In these operations the diseased tunica albuginea is replaced by a variety of autologous tissues, cadaveric tissues and synthetic materials. In patients who underwent straightening surgical procedures, grey-scale and color Doppler ultrasonography allows an excellent evaluation of postoperative anatomical changes and complications (BERTOLOTTO et al. 2005).

16.3.1
Shortening Procedures

As described in Chapter 15, a shortening procedure was first described by Nesbit in 1965 to correct congenital penile curvature and was subsequently used also in patients with Peyronie's disease (NESBIT 1965). Following the Nesbit's operation, grey-scale ultrasound allows identification of the albugineal excisions as interruptions of the echogenic interface of the normal tunica albuginea (BERTOLOTTO et al. 2005). The albugineal sutures are visible as echogenic knots (Fig. 16.1). These features are better visualized in the early postoperative period, because the absorbable sutures are intact and a small amount of fluid is often present that eases their identification. A modification of the Nesbit operation was described by YACHIA (1990). Postoperative ultrasound findings are similar to the Nesbit operation.

In patients with corporeal plication ultrasonography shows small lumps next to the albugineal sutures extending within the corpora cavernosa (BERTOLOTTO et al. 2005). In patients with normal erection before surgery after shortening procedures, postoperative erectile dysfunction is uncommon. When present, color Doppler interrogation allows evaluation of the penile arteries and identification of leakage pathways.

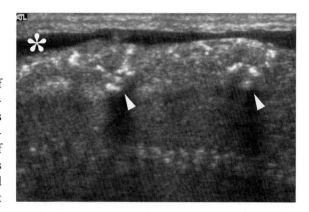

Fig. 16.1. Patient with congenital curvature of the penis who had undergone a Nesbit operation 10 days earlier. Longitudinal image obtained on the side opposite the curvature shows the albugineal sutures as hyperechogenic knots (*arrowheads*). A small amount of fluid (*) above the tunica albuginea eases their identification

16.3.2
Lengthening Procedures

Grey-scale ultrasonography allows identification of albugineal sutures after lengthening operations as well (BERTOLOTTO et al. 2005). As described for shortening operations, their visualization is better in the early postoperative period. In these patients the albugineal patch is usually identified as an interruption of the normally appreciable hyperechoic interface of the tunica albuginea. The appearance of the graft is different depending on its composition (Fig. 16.2). Dermal grafts, for instance, are in general hyperechoic and thicker than the normal tunica albuginea, while the saphenous grafts appear less echogenic (BERTOLOTTO et al. 2005). Also these findings are better appreciable early after the operation. Regardless of composition, albugineal grafts become progressively thinner with time, and their appearance becomes similar to the surrounding native tunica albuginea within 4–6 months.

Causes of surgical failure or complications following lengthening operations can be evaluated with grey-scale and color Doppler ultrasonography. In particular, residual or recurrent plaque can be identified in patients with Peyronie's disease (Fig. 16.3), and epidermoid cysts have been described in dermal grafts (Fig. 16.4) developing from inclusion of surface epithelium (SAVOCA et al. 1999). In patients with postoperative penile narrowing, indentation or bulging, ultrasound allows to confirm contracture or relaxation of the graft with cavernosal tissue herniation.

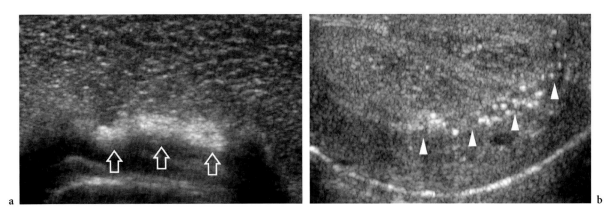

Fig. 16.2a,b. Albugineal patches in patients with Peyronie's disease who had undergone penis lengthening operations. The grafts are identified as interruptions of the normally appreciable hyperechoic interface of the tunica albuginea. **a** Longitudinal image showing a dermal graft that appears as a thick, echogenic interface (*open arrows*). **b** Axial image showing a saphenous vein graft (*arrowheads*) that appears less echogenic than the adjacent tunica albuginea. Sutures are visible as hyperechogenic dots

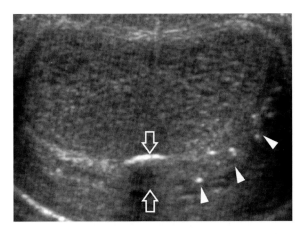

Fig. 16.3. Residual plaque in a patient with Peyronie's disease who had undergone saphenous vein grafting. The patch (*arrowheads*) appears less echogenic than the adjacent tunica albuginea. Sutures are visible as hyperechogenic dots. The residual plaque (*open arrows*) is visible as a localized thickening of the tunica albuginea with a coarse calcification

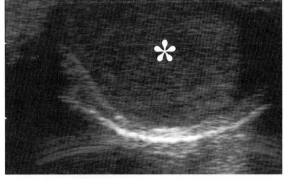

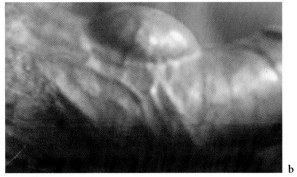

Fig. 16.4a,b. Epidermoid cyst in a patient with Peyronie's disease who had undergone plaque excision with dermal grafting 7 years earlier. **a** Axial ultrasound image showing a well-circumscribed echogenic lesion with acoustic enhancement (*). At histologic analysis, the lesion proved to be an epidermoid cyst arising from the graft, probably originating from accidental inclusion of surface epithelium. **b** Photograph showing an elastic, mobile, painless tumescence that had developed at the site of the graft on the dorsum of the penis. (Reprinted with permission from: Bertolotto M, Serafini G, Savoca G, Liguori G, Calderan L, Gasparini C, Pozzi Mucelli R (2005) Color Doppler US of the Postoperative Penis: Anatomy and Surgical Complications. RadioGraphics 25:731–748)

Color Doppler ultrasonography allows evaluation of postoperative erectile dysfunction. While leakage pathways are commonly observed close to the plaque in patients with severe Peyronie's disease (BERTOLOTTO et al. 2002), after lengthening operations their identification is uncommon. It is conceivable that the scarring process following the operation could produce closure of leakage pathways adjacent to the graft.

16.4 Prosthesis Implantation

Implantation of an inflatable penile prosthesis is usually the surgical treatment of choice after unsuccessful medical therapy. Implantation of other types of prosthesis or other surgical procedures can be considered only in selected cases (Carson et al. 2000).

Ultrasound (Fig. 16.5) provides a good visualization of the corporeal cylinders, scrotal pump and deflation valve of inflatable devices (Bertolotto et al. 2005). Visualization of the abdominal reservoir is usually better when the penis is flaccid since a greater amount of fluid is collected within it. Also tubing is visualized, but not in its whole extent.

Rods of silicone rubber of semi-rigid and malleable penile prosthesis present at ultrasound as echo-poor structures within the corpora cavernosa (Basu et al. 2002). The central metal core of malleable prostheses appears as an echogenic structure with a characteristic comet-tail artifact.

Infection is the most devastating complication of the implant, which usually requires removal of the prosthesis followed by cavernosal fibrosis. Diagnosis is based on clinics (Carson 2001; Montague et al. 2001). Ultrasound can be useful in these patients to evaluate the extent of cavernosal fibrotic changes before prosthesis reimplantation.

Mechanical malfunctions of semi-rigid and malleable prostheses are unusual, and imaging evaluation is seldom necessary. Rupture of a semi-rigid prosthesis can be documented both at ultrasound and with other imaging techniques, but it is usually obvious on physical examination as well (Cohan et al. 1989; Basu et al. 2002). Breaking of the metallic core of malleable prosthesis can be more difficult to evaluate. Mechanical malfunction of inflatable penile prostheses can result from tear or aneurysmal dilatation of the corporeal cylinders, fluid leaks, pump retraction, kinked tubing and erosion. The incidence of these complications has greatly reduced in recent times, thanks to improved prosthesis design. Diagnosis of tear of corporeal cylinders is often obtained at physical examination of the penis with the prosthesis in the inflated state. Diagnosis is confirmed at ultrasound, which shows deformation of the torn cylinder and fluid extravasation (Bertolotto et al. 2005).

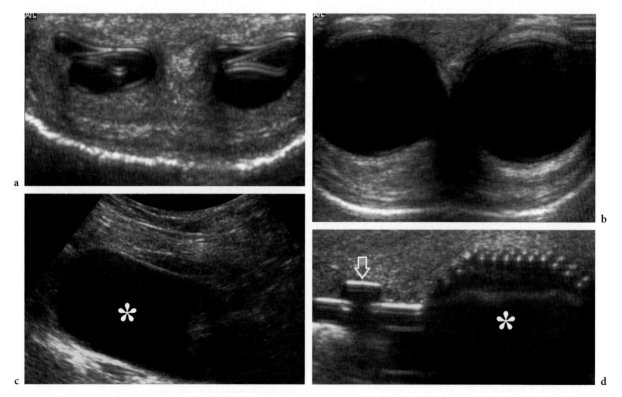

Fig. 16.5a–d. Inflatable penile prosthesis. a,b Axial ultrasound images of the penile shaft obtained before (a) and after (b) inflation of the corporeal cylinders show the cylinders as anechoic structures replacing the cavernosal tissue. c Abdominal reservoir (*). d Scrotal pump (*) and deflation valve (*open arrow*)

16.5
Vascular Surgery for Impotence

Among the organic causes of erectile dysfunction, a variety of pathological conditions can account for impotence of vascular origin (LUE 2000). Arteriogenic causes enclose atherosclerotic or traumatic arterial occlusive disease. Failure of adequate venous occlusion may result from different pathophysiologic processes such as structural alteration of the corpora cavernosa and degenerative changes or traumatic injury to the tunica albuginea. As illustrated in Chapter 15, a series of surgical procedures has been developed in order to restore penile vascular supply in patients with arterial insufficiency or increase penile engorgement reducing venous outflow. The widespread use of oral pharmacotherapy with efficacious drugs has dramatically reduced the indications of these procedures. As a consequence, penile vascular surgery can now be considered in selected cases only (SHARLIP 1990; DEPALMA 1997; HAURI 1998).

In patients undergoing vascular surgery for impotence, preoperative color Doppler ultrasonography is indicated to evaluate cavernosal arterial flows and to assess penile vascular anatomy, with concern for size of the dorsal arteries, for presence of anatomic variations and for collateral arterial vascular pathways (BERTOLOTTO et al. 2005).

Identification of connections between dorsal and cavernosal arteries and between the right and left cavernosal artery is of paramount importance to plan the revascularization procedure. In fact, the size of dorsal penile arteries is often asymmetric, and anastomosis between the inferior epigastric artery to the dorsal artery can be performed only if at least one dorsal artery is present with adequate diameter. Arterial anastomoses between right and left cavernosal arteries can be observed in virtually all patients, while connections between the dorsal and the cavernosal arteries are less common. When these communications exist, epigastric-to-dorsal artery anastomosis can be performed following the physiological direction of flow. The dorsal artery supplies the ipsilateral cavernosal artery through the connections and then the contralateral cavernosal artery through intercavernosal arterial communications. When these communications cannot be demonstrated a retrograde revascularization should be done using the Sharlip technique, in which the blood flows from the epigastric to a dorsal artery with inverted flow towards the common penile trunk, and the origin of the cavernosal arteries (SHARLIP 1990). Several urologists, however, prefer the Sharlip technique in every case (WESPES et al. 2003). If the size of both dorsal arteries is not adequate, deep dorsal vein arterialization could be considered. In the attempt to reduce venous outflow, penile arterial revascularization can be associated with dissection of the superficial dorsal vein and ligation or dissection of the deep dorsal vein.

After the operation, color Doppler ultrasonography allows evaluation of the postoperative vascular anatomy and of blood flow characteristics (BERTOLOTTO et al. 2005). In patients with arterial revascularization, retrograde or anterograde arterial flow is recorded in the dorsal artery, depending on the surgical procedure (Fig. 16.6, Fig. 16.7). The

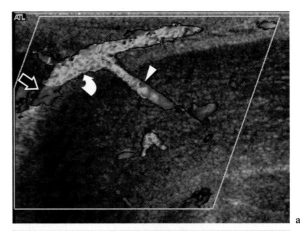

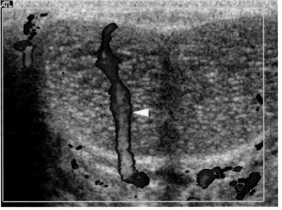

Fig. 16.6a,b. Penile arterial revascularization following the physiological direction of flow. **a** Longitudinal color Doppler image obtained on the dorsal aspect of the base of the penis shows the anastomosis between the epigastric artery (*open arrow*) and the right dorsal artery (*curved arrow*) and an arterial communication connecting the right dorsal artery with the right cavernosal artery (*arrowhead*). **b** Axial image obtained on the ventral aspect of the penile shaft shows another arterial communication (*arrowhead*) connecting the right dorsal artery with the right cavernosal artery

anastomosis between the epigastric and the dorsal artery is identified at the root of the penis. Early in the postoperative period, soft tissue swelling and a small perivascular hematoma are often present. Following cavernosal prostaglandin injection, duplex Doppler interrogation shows increased velocity flow in the epigastric and in the dorsal artery. Abnormal enlargement of the corpus spongiosum can be appreciated due to increased vascular supply via the dorsal artery and, retrogradely, via the urethral arteries. In revascularization following the physiological direction of blood, cavernosal artery flow increases distal to connections with the dorsal artery, while in retrograde arterial revascularization cavernosal artery flow increases from the root of the penis.

In patients with deep dorsal vein arterialization color Doppler ultrasonography allows evaluation of the anastomosis between the inferior epigastric artery and the deep dorsal vein. Following this surgical intervention, the venous wall is thick, with stratified appearance, as a consequence of arterialization changes. The corpus spongiosum and the glans markedly increase in size, with dilated sinusoidal spaces, while only a mild engorgement of the corpora cavernosa is observed. Dilatation of the perispongiosal veins is often detected, as a consequence of the increased pressure in the entire penile venous system (Fig. 16.8).

The major problem of revascularization procedures is early or late closure of the anastomosis (Hauri 1998). Color Doppler ultrasonography is able to identify this complication and to detect blood flow changes that occur in the penile vessels. Rarer complications, such as aneurysmal dilatation of the anastomosis or priapism, can be evaluated as well (Bertolotto et al. 2005).

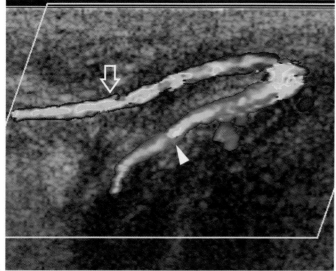

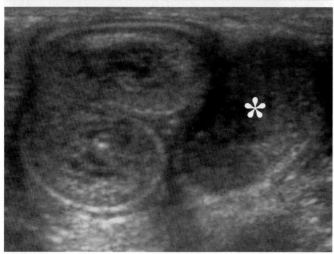

Fig. 16.7a,b. Penile arterial retrograde revascularization (Sharlip technique). a Longitudinal color Doppler image obtained on the dorsal aspect of the base of the penis shows the anastomosis between the epigastric artery (*open arrow*) and the right dorsal artery (*curved arrow*) with retrograde flow. b Axial image of the penile shaft shows abnormal enlargement of the corpus spongiosum (*)

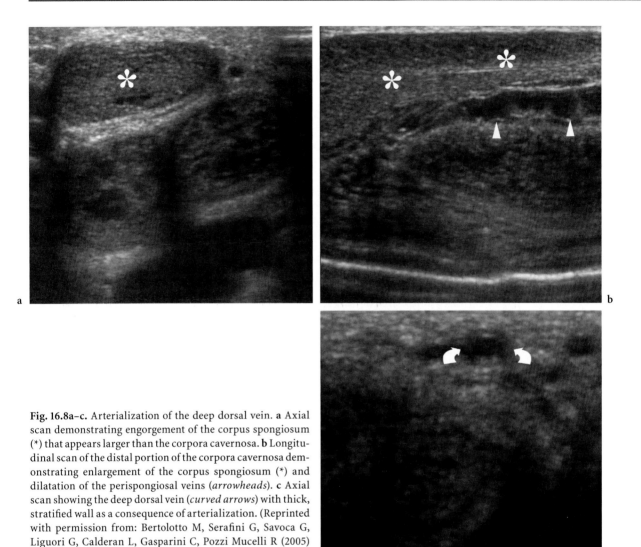

Fig. 16.8a–c. Arterialization of the deep dorsal vein. a Axial scan demonstrating engorgement of the corpus spongiosum (*) that appears larger than the corpora cavernosa. b Longitudinal scan of the distal portion of the corpora cavernosa demonstrating enlargement of the corpus spongiosum (*) and dilatation of the perispongiosal veins (*arrowheads*). c Axial scan showing the deep dorsal vein (*curved arrows*) with thick, stratified wall as a consequence of arterialization. (Reprinted with permission from: Bertolotto M, Serafini G, Savoca G, Liguori G, Calderan L, Gasparini C, Pozzi Mucelli R (2005) Color Doppler US of the Postoperative Penis: Anatomy and Surgical Complications. RadioGraphics 25:731–748)

16.6 Circumcision

Either performed for ritual reasons or associated with other penile surgical maneuvers, circumcision can occasionally lead to complications of varying degrees of severity ranging from minor to fatal (El-Bahnasawy and El-Sherbiny 2002; Ben Chaim et al. 2005; Erdemir 2006). Besides bleeding and infection, skin or meatal injury can occur with formation of inclusion cysts, urethrocutaneous fistulas or meatal stenosis. Partial or complete glans amputation has been rarely reported, as well as ischemia or necrosis of the glans penis. Diagnosis of these complications is based on clinical appearance. Imaging is usually not required. Grey-scale and color Doppler ultrasonography may have a role to characterize inclusion cysts and to evaluate the extent and depth of the ischemic process in patients with ischemia of the glans (Barnes et al. 2006).

Keloids developing after circumcision or degloving from excessive tissue response to skin trauma can be recognized at grey-scale ultrasonography as relatively hyperechoic lesions (Erdemir 2006). Posterior attenuation may be present. Iatrogenic albugineal scars can rarely result from injury of the corporeal tip. They present at ultrasound as a circumscribed thickening of the tunica albuginea, associated or not with corporal deformation (Fig. 16.9).

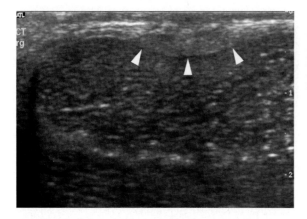

Fig. 16.9. Albugineal scar within the balanopreputial fold (*arrowheads*) following circumcision

16.7
Penile Augmentation Procedures

A variety of procedures have been introduced to obtain augmentation of penile girth and length. The injection of foreign substances into the penis for the purpose of augmentation may result in erectile dysfunction, voiding difficulties and severe deformity (Kalsi et al. 2002). Diagnosis is usually straightforward, and imaging is not required. Ultrasound, however, may be useful to evaluate the extent of acute and chronic inflammatory changes. Surgical division of the suspensory ligament is the most commonly used operation for penile elongation. Postoperative ultrasound is able to document the gap between the pubis and the penile shaft, but usually do not provide clinically useful information (Bertolotto and Pozzi Mucelli 2004).

16.8
Shunt Surgery for Ischemic Priapism

Low-flow, ischemic priapism must be treated as soon as possible because prolonged cavernosal ischemia leads to corporeal fibrosis and permanent erectile dysfunction. If medical management is unsuccessful, surgical management must be considered.

As described in Chapter 15, the principle of surgical correction of ischemic priapism is connecting the engorged corpora cavernosa with the glans, the corpus spongiosum or veins. Glans-cavernosum anastomosis, in particular, can be performed following the Winter technique with a large biopsy needle or a scalpel inserted percutaneously through the glans (Winter 1976), or following the Al-Ghorab technique by excising a piece of the tunica albuginea at the tip of the corpora cavernosa. Proximal shunting may be considered only if more distal shunting procedures have failed to relieve the priapism.

Glans-cavernosum shunts created using the Winter technique can be identified at gray-scale ultrasonography as anechoic tubular structures with irregular margins extending from the glans into the corpora cavernosa. Interruption of the tunica albuginea at the tip of the corporeal bodies is identified in these patients as well as in shunts created with the El-Ghorab technique (Fig. 16.10). No Doppler signals are in general appreciable within the shunts because of very slow flows (Bertolotto et al. 2005). As a consequence, Doppler interrogation cannot help assessing shunt patency. A case of proximal veno-corporeal shunt has been described in which venous blood flow through the shunts was shown at color Doppler ultrasonography (Chiou et al. 1999).

In our experience, high-velocity cavernosal artery flows are recorded early after successful shunt surgery, with variable resistance depending on the degree of deturgescence reached (Lue and Pescatori 2006). Conversely, low-velocity, high-resistance flows, or absence of flows, are observed in cavernosal arteries of patients in whom treatment failed.

Occasionally proximal shunting can complicate with high-flow priapism because of iatrogenic in-

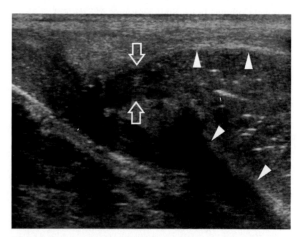

Fig. 16.10. Glans-corpus cavernosum shunt in patients with ischemic priapism. Al-Ghorab technique. The shunt (*open arrows*) appears as an interruption of the tunica albuginea (*arrowheads*) connecting the corpus cavernosum with the glans

jury of the cavernosal arteries during the intervention. We observed this complication also in a patient with a Winter shunt in whom the scalpel produced an arterial injury in the glans with formation of an arterial cavernosal communication (Fig. 16.11). In patients with high-flow priapism after shunting procedures, color Doppler ultrasonography allows evaluation of the vascular lesion and shows high-velocity flows in the cavernosal arteries, consistent with penile hypervascularization.

16.9
Sex Reassignment Surgery

As described in Chapter 15, a variety of surgical procedures for phalloplasty have been developed but, unfortunately, a good substitute for the unique erectile tissue of the penis does not exist. The major complication of phalloplasty is formation of urethral cutaneous fistulas in up to two of three cases, requiring defunctionalization of the urethral anastomosis. Other common postoperative complications are extrusion of the prosthesis and stricture anastomosis between the native urethral stump and the neourethra (Hage et al. 1993).

US appearance of the neophallus is heterogeneous, reflecting the echotexture and echogenicity of the explanted subcutaneous and muscular tissue. The neourethra is visualized after saline instillation as an anechoic tubular structure. Both the arterial and the venous vascular supply of the neophallus can be evaluated with color Doppler ultrasonography. When present, also the prosthesis can be evaluated with the same ultrasonographic appearance described in the native penis. In general, diagnosis of complications after phalloplasty requires imaging in selected cases only. In particular, ultrasonography can be useful to evaluate patients with infection. Urethrosonography can be useful to evaluate fistulas and strictures of the neourethra and to document hair growth in the lumen of the neourethra, which appears at ultrasound as echogenic linear structures (Bertolotto et al. 2005).

Imaging is usually not required in male-to-female gender transition. Ultrasound, however, is able to depict the normal postoperative anatomy of these patients showing the prostate, the urethral stump, the neovagina and remnants of the corpus spongiosum and of the corpora cavernosa. Vascularization of the neoclitoris can be evaluated with Doppler techniques (Fig. 16.12). Complications such as sloughing off of the neovaginal wall, abscess formation and ischemia of the neoclitoris can be identified.

16.10
Urethral Surgery

Urethral strictures can be treated with dilatation, internal urethrotomy or urethroplasty. The male urethra can be accurately studied with ultrasonography either preoperatively or intraoperatively (Morey and McAninch 2000; Pavlica et al. 2003). The posterior tract can be investigated while voiding using linear

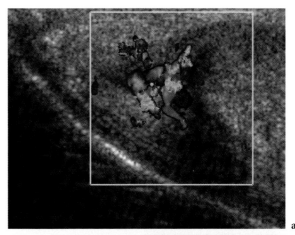

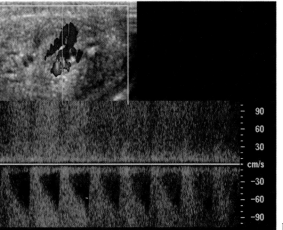

Fig. 16.11a,b. Winter shunting procedure complicated with high-flow priapism. **a** Color Doppler image showing a color blush in the glans displaying aliasing consistent with iatrogenic injury of an arterial vessel. **b** Duplex Doppler interrogation of the vascular lesion confirms diagnosis of arterial-sinusoidal fistula by presence of high velocity, turbulent flows

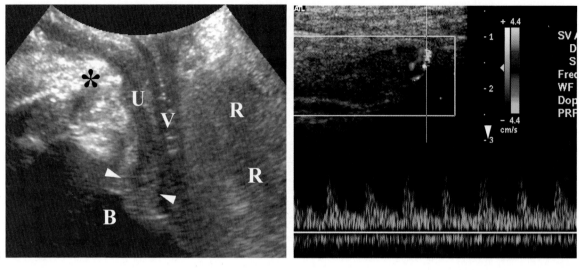

Fig. 16.12a,b. Sex reassignment surgery. Normal postoperative anatomy. **a** Sagittal scan with translabial approach showing neovagina (*V*), prostate (*arrowheads*), urethra (*U*), bladder (*B*), rectum (*R*) and pelvic bones (*). **b** Duplex Doppler interrogation of the neoclitoris

high-frequency endorectal probes; the anterior tract can be explored using high-frequency linear transducers placed to the ventral aspect of the penis, scrotum and perineum while voiding or after distension of the urethal lumen with saline solution or jelly. After urethral surgery, sonourethrography is effective to evaluate restricture, diverticula, fistulas and other complications (Fig. 16.13). Small postoperative anastomotic leaks, however, may not be recognized.

16.11
Follow-Up of Patients with Penile Tumors

Surgical treatment of penile tumors consists of either partial or total penectomy. Ultrasound can be helpful during the follow-up to identify normal postoperative findings, common postoperative complications and recurrence. In particular, grey-scale ultrasonography can be indicated to identify recurrence of tumors arising in the coronal sulcus of the penis since the site of excision is usually covered by skin and postoperative scarring can present as hard at palpation. Moreover, during the postoperative follow-up of glans tumors, ultrasonography is more effective than physical examination alone to evaluate the deep extent of established tumor recurrence and relationship with the urethra and the corpora cavernosa.

16.12
Diagnostic Role of Other Imaging Modalities

If the sonologist is confident with ultrasound penile anatomy and its changes in pathological conditions, other imaging techniques are rarely needed to evaluate patients who had undergone penile surgery. However, conditions exist in which imaging modalities different from ultrasound may provide clinically useful information.

Injury to the metallic core of malleable prostheses can be detected on pelvic radiographs (Cohan et al. 1989; Hovsepian and Amis 1989; Chiou et al. 1999). Despite the excellent radiopacity of the silver core, however, diagnosis is often difficult, and many fractures have been missed or their severity underestimated using standard radiographic technique. Modern inflatable penile prostheses usually contain saline, which cannot be seen radiographically.

Retrograde urethrography and micturition cystourethrography are considered the standard imaging techniques for the morphological and functional study of the urethra after uretral surgery as well. Dynamic infusion cavernosometry and cavernosography have been widely used in the past to evaluate patients with venous leakage before and after venous ligation surgery (Velcek and Evans 1982; Nehra et al. 1996). The role of these techniques faded since venous surgery has been virtually abandoned.

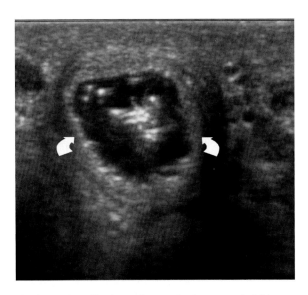 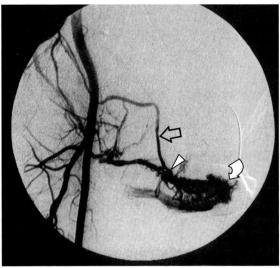

Fig. 16.13. Complications after urethral surgery. Axial image obtained after retrograde distention of the urethra with saline solution shows a hair-bearing ectatic neourethra (*curved arrows*) in a man with bladder exstrophy and urethral duplication corrected during childhood using a scrotal skin flap

Fig. 16.14. Complicated dorsal vein arterialization. Arteriography shows the inferior epigastric artery (*open arrow*) connected to the deep dorsal vein (*arrowhead*) and marked hyperemia of the glans (*curved arrow*) requiring reoperation with ligation of the distal portion of the arterialized vein

Internal pudendal angiography provides precise localization of penile arterial lesions in patients who are candidates for arterial revascularization surgery (Bookstein 1988). The efficacy of such studies requires excellent visualization of the small arteries that constitutes the penile blood supply. In order to achieve this objective, penile arterial inflow must be maximized with pharmacologically induced erection. Also postoperative arterial anatomy and surgical complications can be fully investigated with this technique (Fig. 16.14), but angiography is only rarely required because enough clinically useful information is in general obtained with less invasive procedures.

Using state-of-the art multiple detector-row CT (MDCT) equipment, high-resolution CT angiography examinations are obtained, which allow replacing diagnostic conventional angiography for many clinical applications. In fact, submillimeter section scanning allows production of high-quality MPR images, and reformation images can be created from one helical acquisition with approximately the same spatial resolution as sections from the original acquisition. In our experience MDCT angiography allows preoperative planning and postoperative control of patients undergoing penile vascular surgery providing the same clinically useful information as conventional penile angiography (Fig. 16.15). Similar to angiography, also MDCT angiography requires pharmacologically induced erection to maximize penile arterial inflow in small penile vessels. The advantage of MDCT over color Doppler ultrasonography is evaluation of the entire arterial vascular supply to the penis from the iliac arteries to the cavernosal and dorsal branches. However, small terminal branches and collaterals cannot be usually identified, while they are readily evaluated at color Doppler ultrasonography.

Besides evaluation of penile blood supply to the penis, MDCT can be indicated to evaluate large postoperative fluid collections and complications of urethral surgery such as diverticula, fistulas and postoperative strictures (Chou et al. 2005). Also prosthesis malfunction can be investigated in patients who are not candidates for magnetic resonance imaging. Moreover, in patients with penile and urethral malignancies, CT is often used after the operation to evaluate the pelvis in suspicious postoperative complications extending into the perineum and into the pelvis, such as fistulas and inflammation. Also tumor recurrence and pelvic lymphadenopathies can be evaluated effectively.

MRI has gained acceptance in the last years in evaluation of penile prosthesis (Pretorius et al. 2001; Vossough et al. 2002). However, the characteristics of the prosthesis must be evaluated before the examination because some types of old devices could contain ferromagnetic components that contraindicate this imaging modality (Vossough et al. 2002). The appearance of penile prosthesis at MRI depends on the characteristics of the device. Semi-rigid silicone prostheses will appear as signal void structures within the corpora cavernosa on T1- and T2-weighted images. Inflatable penile prostheses appear as fluid-filled low signal intensity structures. After prosthesis implantation, the corpora cavernosa form a fibrous pseudocapsule around the implant that presents with low signal intensity on both T1- and T2-weighted images.

In patients with penile prosthesis, MRI allows evaluation of penile abscesses and fistulas. Infections in the space between the pseudocapsule and the prosthesis present with low signal intensity on T1-weighted images and high signal intensity on T2-weighted images (Pretorius et al. 2001). Also mechanical penile malfunctioning can be evaluated.

In patients with phallic reconstruction, MRI allows excellent evaluation of normal postoperative anatomy, of urethral pathologies and of prosthesis-related complications. This examination, however, is not commonly used in the clinical practice. MRI allows detailed investigation of postoperative anatomy and surgically related complications also in male-to-female gender transition (Cova et al. 2003). Neovaginal depth and inclination, presence of remnants of the corpus spongiosum and corpora cavernosa, and thickness of the rectovaginal septum can be fully investigated.

In patients who are candidates for penile vascular surgery, magnetic resonance angiography can be used to delineate the internal iliac and proximal pudendal arteries and any associated pelvic abnormality that might cause impotence. Because of limited spatial resolution and artifacts, however, this examination technique cannot adequately assess the pudendal arteries, especially in the pararectal space (John et al. 1999). Moreover, the most distal portions of the penile arterial tree are often obscured by superimposition of signal from penile veins (John et al. 1999). Finally, metallic devices are often present in patients with post-traumatic impotence that produce artifacts and reduce image quality substantially. In fact, preoperative evaluation of patients undergoing penile revascularization procedures cannot be obtained using magnetic resonance angiography alone. Doppler ultrasound, MDCT angiography and conventional digital subtraction angiography remain the imaging modalities of choice.

Visualization of small penile vessels at magnetic resonance angiography can be difficult also during postoperative evaluation of patients. Although evaluation of the anastomosis between the epigastric arteries and the penile vessels is usually possible using superficial coils (Fig. 16.15), metal vascular clips might

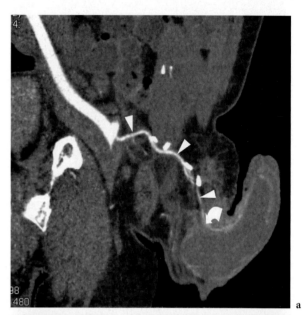

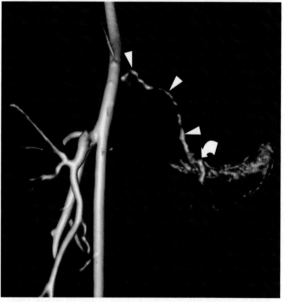

Fig. 16.15a,b. Penile arterial revascularization. **a** MDCT angiography shows the right epigastric artery (*arrowheads*) anastomosed with the right dorsal artery (*curved arrow*). Metallic vascular clips are present along the course of the epigastric artery. **b** Magnetic resonance angiography showing the same vessels (*arrowheads* and *curved arrow*). Compared with CT visualization of the epigastric artery is hampered by artifacts from the metallic vascular clips, presenting as signal void regions, and visualization of the arterial anastomosis is masked in part by superimposition of penile veins

produce artifacts. In the clinical practice enough clinically useful information is usually obtained in these patients with color Doppler ultrasonography.

Due to multiplanar capabilities and excellent soft-tissue contrast resolution magnetic resonance imaging is the imaging modality of choice to evaluate deep tumor recurrence and surgical complications in the pelvis and perineum of patients operated for penile or urethral malignancies (Pretorius et al. 2001). Similar to contrast-enhanced CT, pelvic lymphadenopathies can be identified.

References

Barnes S, Ben Chaim J, Kessler A (2006) Postcircumcision necrosis of the glans penis: Gray-scale and color Doppler sonographic findings. J Clin Ultrasound 35:105–107
Basu S, Biyani CS, Karamuri SS, Shah T (2002) Pseudo-priapism! Forgotten semirigid penile prosthesis. Int J Impot Res 14:418–419
Ben Chaim J, Livne PM, Binyamini J et al (2005) Complications of circumcision in Israel: a 1-year multicenter survey. Isr Med Assoc J 7:368–370
Bertolotto M, de Stefani S, Martinoli C et al (2002) Color Doppler appearance of penile cavernosal-spongiosal communications in patients with severe Peyronie's disease. Eur Radiol 12:2525–2531
Bertolotto M, Pozzi Mucelli R (2004) Nonpenetrating penile traumas: sonographic and Doppler features. AJR Am J Roentgenol 183:1085–1089
Bertolotto M, Quaia E, Mucelli FP et al (2003) Color Doppler imaging of posttraumatic priapism before and after selective embolization. Radiographics 23:495–503
Bertolotto M, Serafini G, Savoca G et al (2005) Color Doppler US of the postoperative penis: anatomy and surgical complications. Radiographics 25:731–748
Bookstein JJ (1988) Penile angiography: the last angiographic frontier. AJR Am J Roentgenol 150:47–54
Carson CC (2001) Penile prosthesis implantation and infection for Sexual Medicine Society of North America. Int J Impot Res 13 [Suppl 5]:S35–38
Carson CC, Mulcahy JJ, Govier FE (2000) Efficacy, safety and patient satisfaction outcomes of the AMS 700CX inflatable penile prosthesis: results of a long-term multicenter study. AMS 700CX Study Group. J Urol 164:376–380
Chiou RK, Henslee DL, Anderson JC, Wobig RK (1999) Colour doppler ultrasonography assessment and a saphenous vein-graft penile venocorporeal shunt for priapism. BJU Int 83:138–139
Chou CP, Huang JS, Wu MT et al (2005) CT voiding urethrography and virtual urethroscopy: preliminary study with 16-MDCT. AJR Am J Roentgenol 184:1882–1888
Cohan RH, Dunnick NR, Carson CC (1989) Radiology of penile prostheses. AJR Am J Roentgenol 152:925–931
Cova M, Mosconi E, Liguori G et al (2003) Value of magnetic resonance imaging in the evaluation of sex-reassignment surgery in male-to-female transsexuals. Abdom Imaging 28:728–732
DePalma RG (1997) Vascular surgery for impotence: a review. Int J Impot Res 9:61–67
Doubilet PM, Benson CB, Silverman SG, Gluck CD (1991) The penis. Semin Ultrasound CT MR 12:157–175
El-Bahnasawy MS, El-Sherbiny MT (2002) Paediatric penile trauma. BJU Int 90:92–96
Erdemir F (2006) A rare complication after circumcision: Keloid of the penis. Int Urol Nephrol 38:609–611
Hage JJ, Bout CA, Bloem JJ, Megens JA (1993) Phalloplasty in female-to-male transsexuals: what do our patients ask for? Ann Plast Surg 30:323–326
Hauri D (1998) A critical review of penile revascularization procedures. Urol Int 60:133–146
Hovsepian DM, Amis ES Jr (1989) Penile prosthetic implants: a radiographic atlas. Radiographics 9:707–716
John H, Kacl GM, Lehmann K et al (1999) Clinical value of pelvic and penile magnetic resonance angiography in preoperative evaluation of penile revascularization. Int J Impot Res 11:83–86
Kalsi JS, Arya M, Peters J et al (2002) Grease-gun injury to the penis. J R Soc Med 95:254
Liguori G, Garaffa G, Trombetta C et al (2005) High-flow priapism (HFP) secondary to Nesbit operation: management by percutaneous embolization and colour Doppler-guided compression. Int J Impot Res 17:304–306
Lue TF (2000) Erectile dysfunction. N Engl J Med 342:1802–1813
Lue TF, Pescatori ES (2006) Distal cavernosum-glans shunts for ischemic priapism. J Sex Med 3:749–752
McMahon CG (2002) High flow priapism due to an arterial-lacunar fistula complicating initial veno-occlusive priapism. Int J Impot Res 14:195–196
Montague DK, Angermeier KW, Lakin MM (2001) Penile prosthesis infections. Int J Impot Res 13:326–328
Morey AF, McAninch JW (2000) Sonographic staging of anterior urethral strictures. J Urol 163:1070–1075
Nehra A, Goldstein I, Pabby A et al (1996) Mechanisms of venous leakage: a prospective clinicopathological correlation of corporeal function and structure. J Urol 156:1320–1329
Nesbit RM (1965) Congenital curvature of the phallus: Report of three cases with description of corrective operation. J Urol 93:230–232
Pavlica P, Barozzi L, Menchi I (2003) Imaging of male urethra. Eur Radiol 13:1583–1596
Pretorius ES, Siegelman ES, Ramchandani P, Banner MP (2001) MR imaging of the penis. Radiographics 21 Spec No:S283–298; discussion S298–289
Savoca G, Ciampalini S, De Stefani S et al (1999) Epidermoid cyst after dermal graft repair of Peyronie's disease. BJU Int 84:1098–1099
Sharlip ID (1990) The role of vascular surgery in arteriogenic and combined arteriogenic and venogenic impotence. Semin Urol 8:129–137
Velcek D, Evans JA (1982) Cavernosography. Radiology 144:781–785
Vossough A, Pretorius ES, Siegelman ES et al (2002) Magnetic resonance imaging of the penis. Abdom Imaging 27:640–659
Wespes E, Wildschutz T, Roumeguere T, Schulman CC (2003) The place of surgery for vascular impotence in the third millennium. J Urol 170:1284–1286

Winter CC (1976) Cure of idiopathic priapism: new procedure for creating fistula between glans penis and corpora cavernosa. Urology 8:389–391

Yachia D (1990) Modified corporoplasty for the treatment of penile curvature. J Urol 143:80–82

Penile Inflammation

Giovanni Serafini, Michele Bertolotto, Francesca Lacelli, Luca Scofienza, and Nadia Perrone

CONTENTS

17.1 Background 147
17.2 Cellulitis 147
17.3 Balanitis and Balanoposthitis 147
17.3.1 Infective Balanitis 147
17.3.2 Non-Infectious Balanitis 148
17.4 Cavernositis 148
17.5 Penile Abscesses 148
17.6 Penile Mondor's Phlebitis 148
17.7 Ultrasonographic Features 148
17.8 Diagnostic Role of Other Imaging Modalities 149

References 151

17.1
Background

Penile inflammations caused by infections of the glans and foreskin are common pathological entities that occur in about 11% of male genitourinary clinics attendees. This group of pathologies, however, has a poor radiological relevance except in cases of severe inflammation with involvement of the corpora cavernosa or abscess formation (Pearle and Wendel 1993).

G. Serafini, MD; F. Lacelli, MD; L. Scofienza, MD; N. Perrone, MD
U.O. Radiologia, Ospedale S. Corona, Via XXV Aprile, Pietra Ligure, 17027, Italy
M. Bertolotto, MD
Department of Radiology, University of Trieste, Ospedale di Cattinara, Strada di Fiume 447, Trieste, 34124, Italy

17.2
Cellulitis

Cellulitis is an inflammation of the connective tissue underlying the penile skin that can be caused by normal skin flora or by exogenous bacteria, and often occurs where the skin has previously been broken: cracks in the skin, cuts, burns, insect bites and surgical wounds. The mainstay of therapy is treatment with appropriate antibiotics.

17.3
Balanitis and Balanoposthitis

Balanitis is defined as an inflammation of the glans penis; when inflammation involves the prepuce it is called balanoposthitis. Balanitis and balanoposthitis are collections of disparate conditions with similar clinical presentation and different aetiologies, which can be classified into infective, irritant and traumatic, premalignant, malignant and idiopathic (Janier et al. 2006). Diagnosis is based on clinics, laboratory and microbiological findings. Usually imaging is not required.

17.3.1
Infective Balanitis

Candida albicans is the most frequent cause of balanitis and usually follows intercourse with an infected sexual partner. However, infection may occur without sexual contact, usually in those patients suffering from diabetes or under antibiotic therapy (Huuskonen and Aaltomaa 2006).

The pathogenicity of the yeast depends on the host factors, in particular on the immunological condition. The clinical features include severe itching and pain, presence of red patches and blisters in the glans and around the foreskin, a non-purulent skin surface, slightly scaling edge and eroded satellites pustules. The groin may also be affected.

Trichomonal infection occurs more commonly in the prepuce and presents as a superficial or erosive balonoposthitis. Phimosis may occur. In this case, it is possible to detect severe cancer-like lesions or penile abscesses.

Chlamidial balanitis is a non-specific form of irritation that comes from a contiguous urethritis. Balanitis and balanoposthitis caused by anaerobes may be severe, with superficial erosions, oedema of the prepuce, foul smelling discharge and inguinal lymphoadenopathy (Palacios et al. 2006).

17.3.2
Non-Infectious Balanitis

Poor hygiene, retained soap, detergents, retained smegma or inadequate drying may cause an irritant dermatitis. Frictional traumas and accidental wounds can cause fissures, erosions or localised area of erythema and oedema. Post-coital frenal erosions, in particular, are common.

Whenever an unresolving balanitis is in progress, premalignant conditions should be taken into consideration, such as Queyrat erythroplasia, extramammary Paget's disease, Lichen planus and balanitis xerotica obliterans (Palacios et al. 2006).

17.4
Cavernositis

Infection of the corpora cavernosa can be a serious life-threatening complication of intracavernosal drug injection. Other causes include spreading of perineal inflammatory processes and complicated penile cellulitis or balanitis. Cavernous tissue ischaemia represents a predisposing factor, in particular, in diabetic patients.

Treatment includes antibiotics, bilateral corporotomy, debridement and placement of intracorporeal irrigation and suction drains. Acute purulent cavernositis often fails to respond to conservative therapy and requires penile amputation. In case of recovery, severe fibrotic cavernosal changes usually develop producing irreversible erectile dysfunction.

17.5
Penile Abscesses

Penile abscesses are uncommon. They usually result as a complication of an advanced or untreated superficial balanitis or cellulitis, from infection of the corpora cavernosa, or following a systemic infection with lymphatic or haematogenous dissemination (Sater and Vandendris 1989). Immuno-compromised patients are at high risk of developing a penile abscess. Diabetic patients may develop penile infections after surgical manoeuvres or prosthesis implantation.

Clinical features of penile abscesses include both systemic (fever, leucocytosis) and local symptoms such as redness, oedema and painful swelling of the foreskin and purulent discharge with or without inguinal lymphadenopathy. Persistent inflammation can cause urethral narrowing, with urine retention or post-flogistic stenosis (Koksal et al. 1999; Sommerauer et al. 2006; Nielson et al. 2007).

17.6
Penile Mondor's Phlebitis

Thrombophlebitis of the deep dorsal vein, also known as penile Mondor's phlebitis, is an inflammatory reaction of the involved vessel associated with thrombus formation. Other causes of thrombosis of the deep superficial vein have been illustrated elsewhere.

Clinically, the patients present with a rod-like painful induration in the dorsal aspect of the shaft. Clinical signs and symptoms suggestive for thrombophebitis, such as fever and local pain, can be present. The disease is usually treated with fibrinolytics and anticoagulation, associated with discontinuance of sexual activity. Spontaneous resolution usually occurs within 6–8 weeks.

17.7
Ultrasonographic Features

The role of ultrasonography in balanitis and balanoposthitis is exclusively to rule out complications, such as involvement of the erectile bodies or abscess formation.

Cellulitis presents at colour Doppler ultrasonography with superficial tissue thickening, inhomogeneous echotexture and hypervascularization at colour Doppler interrogation (Fig. 17.1). No alteration of the erectile bodies is appreciable. During the follow-up a progressive restoration of the normal appearance of the penile tissues is appreciable.

Cavernositis presents at colour Doppler ultrasonography with markedly increased vascularity of the cavernosal bodies (Fig. 17.2). Echotexture of the corpora cavernosa may be altered. Oedema produces increased echogenicity, while microabscesses present as hypoechoic areas. Usually the inflammatory process involves the superficial tissues as well, which present thickened, inhomogeneous and hyperhaemic.

Penile abscesses present at ultrasonography as hypoechoic collections with corpuscolated content and internal debris. As occurs for abscesses elsewhere, a thick wall can be present with vascular signals at Doppler interrogation. Thrombosis of the dorsal vessels can be associated.

Ultrasonography is able to define the abscess location, evaluate the relationships with the adjacent structures and guide drainage. In fact, most penile abscesses are confined within the superficial layers, outside the tunica albuginea, while other spread deeply in the tissues surrounding the corpora cavernosa or involve the corpora cavernosa themselves (Fig. 17.3).

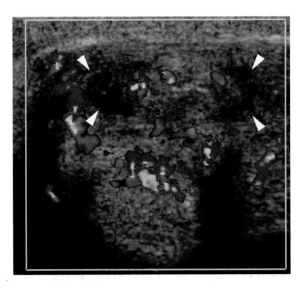

Fig. 17.2. Cavernositis. Axial colour Doppler image showing hypervascularity of the corpora cavernosa and of the corpus spongiosum. A small fluid collection (*arrowheads*) consistent with abscess formation surrounds the corpus spongiosum

In patients with thrombophlebitis of the dorsal vein (Fig. 17.4), grey-scale and colour Doppler ultrasonography show thickened vessel wall and complete or segmental thrombosis (Dicuio et al. 2005; Abaci et al. 2006; Shamloul and Kamel 2006), which can be occasionally associated with thrombosis of the circumflex veins. In complete thrombosis, no Doppler signal is recorded.

17.8
Diagnostic Role of Other Imaging Modalities

CT and magnetic resonance imaging has a limited role in the management of inflammatory processes confined to the penis. These imaging modalities, however, can have a role in widespread inflammatory processes involving the pelvis and the perineum. Magnetic resonance imaging, in particular, has the advantage of a wider field of view and better contrast resolution compared with ultrasound (Kickuth et al. 2001). Consequently, extension of the inflammatory process to the perineum, abdominal wall, fascial planes and buttocks can be fully evaluated.

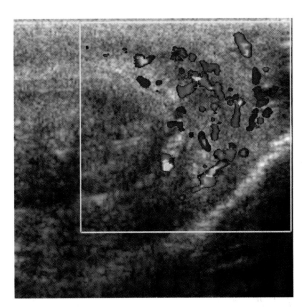

Fig. 17.1. Penile cellulitis. Axial colour Doppler image showing thickening and hypervascularity of the soft tissues surrounding the corpora cavernosa

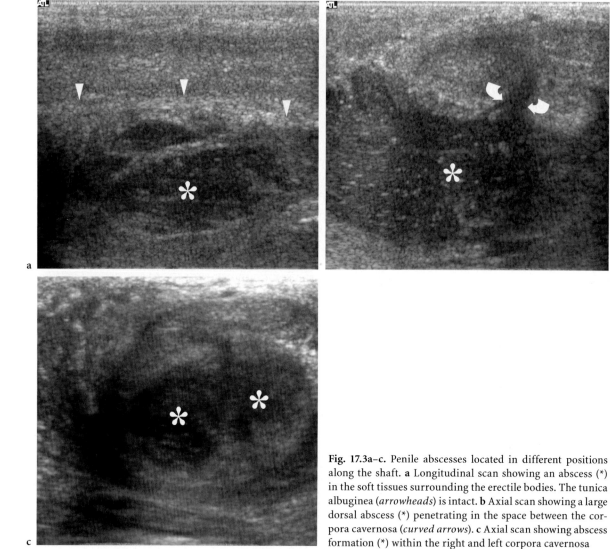

Fig. 17.3a–c. Penile abscesses located in different positions along the shaft. a Longitudinal scan showing an abscess (*) in the soft tissues surrounding the erectile bodies. The tunica albuginea (*arrowheads*) is intact. b Axial scan showing a large dorsal abscess (*) penetrating in the space between the corpora cavernosa (*curved arrows*). c Axial scan showing abscess formation (*) within the right and left corpora cavernosa

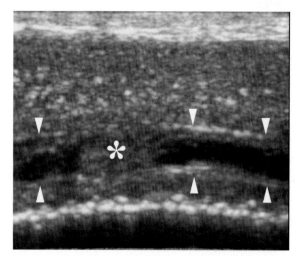

Fig. 17.4. Thrombophlebitis of the deep penile dorsal vein. Patient presenting with painful induration of the dorsal aspect of the penis. Longitudinal scan showing wall thickening of the dorsal vein (*arrowheads*) and echogenic material within the lumen (*) consistent with partial thrombosis

References

Abaci A, Makay B, Unsal E et al (2006) An unusual complication of dorsal penile nerve block for circumcision. Paediatr Anaesth 16:1094–1095

Dicuio M, Pomara G, Ales V et al (2005) Doppler ultrasonography in a young patient with penile Mondor's disease. Arch Ital Urol Androl 77:58–59

Huuskonen J, Aaltomaa S (2006) Candida sepsis originating from bulbar abscess of the penis. Scand J Urol Nephrol 40:347–349

Janier M, Dupin N, Milpied B et al (2006) [Balanitis]. Ann Dermatol Venereol 133:2S56–52S57

Kickuth R, Adams S, Kirchner J et al (2001) Magnetic resonance imaging in the diagnosis of Fournier's gangrene. Eur Radiol 11:787–790

Koksal T, Kadioglu A, Tefekli A et al (1999) Spontaneous bacterial abscess of bilateral cavernosal bodies. BJU Int 84:1107–1108

Nielson CM, Flores R, Harris RB et al (2007) Human papillomavirus prevalence and type distribution in male anogenital sites and semen. Cancer Epidemiol Biomarkers Prev 16:1107–1114

Palacios A, Masso P, Versos R et al (2006) [Penile abscess. Case report]. Arch Esp Urol 59:809–811

Pearle MS, Wendel EF (1993) Necrotizing cavernositis secondary to periodontal abscess. J Urol 149:1137–1138

Sater AA, Vandendris M (1989) Abscess of corpus cavernosum. J Urol 141:949

Shamloul R, Kamel I (2006) Early treatment of cavernositis resulted in erectile function preservation. J Sex Med 3:320–322

Sommerauer M, Walden O, Doehn C, Jocham D (2006) [Penile skin necrosis after application of a ring and defect coverage by a skin mesh graft]. Aktuelle Urol 37:376–378

Penile Scar and Fibrosis

Michele Bertolotto, Paola Martingano, and Maja Ukmar

CONTENTS

18.1 Background 153
18.2 Diffuse Cavernosal Fibrosis 154
18.3 Circumscribed Fibrosis 155
18.4 Distal Segmental Fibrosis 155
18.5 Proximal Segmental Fibrosis 155
18.6 Grey-Scale Ultrasonography 155
18.7 Color Doppler Ultrasound 158
18.8 Differential Diagnosis 159
18.9 Diagnostic Role of Other Imaging Modalities 160
References 160

18.1 Background

The corpora cavernosa consist of smooth muscle cells, loose areolar tissue, blood vessels, nerves and collagen fibers. All these components play a role in the complex physiologic event of erection, together with endocrinal, vascular, neural and psychogenic factors (Jevtich et al. 1990).

The balance between different components of the cavernous tissue varies with age. In normal potent young men collagen fibers constitute about 48% of cavernosal tissue (Lin et al. 2000), while smooth muscle cells constitute about 46% of them (Wespes 2002). Corporeal fibrosis results from reduction of smooth muscle fibers and increase of collagen deposition (Dahiya et al. 1999). Increased stiffness of the corpora cavernosa restricts their expansion during tumescence causing erectile dysfunction (Lin et al. 2000). In fact, between 41 and 60 years the percentage of smooth muscle cells reduces at 40%, and over 60 years of age is about 35% (Wespes 2002); this decrease in smooth muscle content may be responsible for the decline in potency of older men. Histological specimens of the senescent penis demonstrate an abundance of collagen fibers and larger lacunars spaces if compared to the adult penis (Wespes 2000).

Penile fibrosis is a histological diagnosis. Urologists, however, usually use this term in a non-specific way to describe increased penile consistency at physical examination. While localized corporeal fibrosis is usually firm at palpation, diffuse fibrosis is not always recognized.

Clinicians should be aware that most of patients with penile stiffness at palpation actually have Peyronie's disease. Differential diagnosis is clinically relevant because important fibrosis constitutes an end organ failure, may explain ineffectiveness of oral medications (Basar et al. 2001) and prevents unsuccessful surgery for veno-occlusive or arteriogenic diseases (Yaman et al. 2003). Also, when the implantation of a prosthesis is considered, preoperative identification of severe cavernosal fibrotic changes is needed for the choice of the more appropriate surgical technique (Ghanem et al. 2000; Montague and Angermeier 2006).

In fact, major clinical questions remain unsolved since specific definition of cavernosal fibrosis is lacking, and no established diagnostic test is available. Biopsy is the most accurate method to establish cavernosal fibrosis (Wespes et al. 1994), but it is very invasive and not well accepted as a routine preoperative procedure (Basar et al. 1998). Moreover, even when a bioptic specimen is available, there is no widely accepted histological standard to assess and grade the disease (Sattar et al. 1994).

M. Bertolotto, MD; P. Martingano, MD; M. Ukmar, MD
Department of Radiology, University of Trieste, Ospedale di Cattinara, Strada di Fiume 447, Trieste, 34124, Italy

18.2
Diffuse Cavernosal Fibrosis

Experimental studies have demonstrated that low oxygen tension induces transforming growth factor β1 (TGF-β1) mRNA expression in cavernosal tissue (Moreland et al. 1998). Increased TGF-β1 production induces connective tissue synthesis and is correlated to renal, hepatic and pulmonary fibrosis (Border and Noble 1994). On the contrary, type E prostaglandins, which are synthesized by an oxygen-dependent reaction, suppress collagen synthesis (Moreland 1998). These experimental data suggest that diffuse cavernosal fibrosis is correlated to hypoxemia. Smoking and several pathologic conditions associated with a low cavernosal oxygen tension, such as diabetes mellitus, hypertension, hypercholesterolemia and atherosclerosis, may complicate with cavernosal fibrosis, as well as traumatic or iatrogenic lesions resulting in severe reduction of the penile arterial supply (Moreland 1998).

Erections play an important role in cavernosal tissue oxygenation, which is essential to preserve normal erectile function. While in the flaccid penis partial pressure of oxygen in the cavernosal blood (pO_2) is 25–40 mmHg, during erection oxygenated arterial blood inflow increases pO_2 up to 90–100 mmHg. Cavernosal tissue oxygenation while flaccid is consistent with TGF-β1 induction, but prostaglandin synthesis during sexual activity or during nocturnal penile tumescence counteracts its action maintaining connective tissue/smooth muscle balance (Moreland 1998).

A variety of clinical situations can result in diffuse cavernosal fibrotic changes. Low-flow priapism is a well-known cause of cavernosal tissue fibrosis with resulting venous occlusive deficiency. It is commonly accepted that prompt treatment is mandatory because recovery of erectile function becomes increasingly unlikely over time (El-Bahnasawy et al. 2002). Cavernosal tissue damage leading to fibrotic changes can occasionally occur also in patients with stuttering priapism and with arterial priapism (Hakim et al. 1996; Bertolotto et al. 2003).

A significant association was found between penile fibrosis and diabetes mellitus. This may be explained by the fact that diabetes mellitus produces microangiopathy of the small blood vessels, leading to defective oxygenation to the cavernous tissue and subsequently helping in fibrosis development (Moreland 1998). Systemic connective tissue disorders, such as systemic sclerosis, are associated to erectile dysfunction in as much as 80% of patients due to combined arterial insufficiency and collagenization of corporeal smooth muscle (Lotfi et al. 1995).

Experimental studies in rabbits suggest that environmental pollutants, such as dioxin, might have a role in cavernous fibrosis through inhibition of testosterone synthesis (Moon et al. 2004), and experimental studies in rats (Shen et al. 2003) demonstrate a high degree of cavernosal fibrosis following castration, and a lower degree of cavernosal fibrosis after inhibition of dihydrotestosterone. These results, however, cannot be easily extrapolated to men because androgens regulate erection in rodents while in man they have a less precise role (Moreland 1998).

Radical prostatectomy is associated with increased cavernosal fibrous content even after nerve-sparing surgery. In fact, User et al. (2003) have demonstrated in a rat model that even unilateral cavernous neurotomy causes apoptosis of smooth muscle cells in both corpora, in particular just beneath the tunica albuginea, and Iacono et al. (2005) have proven that iatrogenic denervation alone or with hemodynamic alterations, resulting from surgical prostate ablation, causes cavernous fibrosis, and consequent erectile deficiency, often refractory to symptomatic therapy. Hypoxia-induced tissue damage could be temporarily prevented by the use of intracorporeal prostaglandin injection (Montorsi et al. 1997) or phosphodiesterase-5 inhibitors (Ferrini et al. 2006).

In patients with prostate cancer undergoing external beam radiotherapy, penile irradiation results in cavernosal damage. In particular, patients receiving at least 70 Gy to the 70% or more of the bulb of the penis have a high risk of developing a radiotherapy-induced erectile dysfunction (Fisch et al. 2001).

Intracavernous injection of vasoactive drugs can rarely complicate with diffuse cavernosal fibrosis following low-flow priapism and/or cavernositis (Schwarzer and Hofmann 1991; Chew et al. 1997).

In particular, the superficial dorsal vein of the penis is occasionally used by parenteral drug abusers as injection site. When heroin and cocaine spread within the corpora cavernosa, this can produce cavernositis and priapism, evolving into corporal fibrosis (Mireku-Boateng and Nwokeji 2004).

Recently, a new syndrome has been identified as "hypoactive corpus cavernosum." In this pathological condition degenerative changes of the corpora cavernosa are observed on histopathologic examination such as fragmented collagen and elastic fibers, degenerated muscle fibers and areas of fibrosis (SHAFIK et al. 2006). Patients who do not respond to any form of treatment including sildenafil citrate or papaverine intracavernosal injection have erectile dysfunction. Penile implants are the only treatment.

18.3
Circumscribed Fibrosis

Most of patients with circumscribed cavernosal fibrosis or scar have had penile surgery or traumas. Postraumatic fibrosis usually results from healing of intracavernosal hematoma (BERTOLOTTO and POZZI MUCELLI 2004; MUNARRIZ et al. 2005) or rupture of the tunica albuginea from sudden bending of the erect penis. A recent report (BRANT et al. 2007) describes a subset of patients with penile induration who were found to have only a circumscribed septal fibrotic change on penile ultrasonography. About 36% of these patients had a significant history of penile trauma.

Intracavernosal injection of vasoactive drugs is another frequent cause of circumscribed penile fibrosis. In fact, focal fibrotic changes in the subcutaneous tissue, in the tunica albuginea or into the cavernosal sinusoids have been reported as high as 57% and 15% after papaverine and prostaglandin injection, respectively (CHEW et al. 1997). Most fibrotic nodules occur in patients who inject themselves frequently and in those who do not compress the injection site for a sufficient time with the subsequent development of intracavernous hematomas. It is conceivable that cavernosal tissue damage results from multiple microtraumas to the corporeal tissue, or begins as a localized vasculitis of subtunical tissues eventually resulting in fibrotic nodules (CHEW et al. 1997).

18.4
Distal Segmental Fibrosis

A 10% incidence of distal penile fibrosis has been reported following long-term use of intracavernous prostaglandin injection (MUMTAZ et al. 1998). This complication is not related to the injection site as the lesions occur distally. Suggested explanation is speculative. It is conceivable that during pharmacologically induced erection reduction of elastic fibers in the tunica albuginea, especially in aging and diabetic men, could make the corpora unable to tolerate the high intracavernosal pressures, and relative ischemia, in the distal part of the penis. This situation could result in microvascular damage, especially in men with arteriogenic erectile dysfunction.

18.5
Proximal Segmental Fibrosis

Recently, increasing concern is rising that penile fibrotic changes either diffuse or, more often, localized at the corporal crura can develop in equestrians, long-distance bikers and racing cyclists. Different causes contribute to this pathological condition. First, direct cavernosal tissue injury can result from microtraumas when the crura are compressed against the pubic bone by the saddle. Second, cavernosal arteries are compressed along their perineal course determining a recordable decrease of penile blood flow and, thus, of cavernous PO_2 (NAYAL et al. 1999). Third, a poorly fitting saddle that irritates the pudendal nerve can occasionally result in pudendal neuritis, which usually presents with paresthesia or scrotal and penile numbness, but can occasionally complicates with priapism. These andrologic problems are more often found when narrow seats are used with nose-extension (SCHWARZER et al. 2002).

18.6
Grey-Scale Ultrasonography

Although findings are often not specific in patients with cavernosal fibrosis, ultrasound represents the imaging modality of choice to evaluate patients that present with increased stiffness of the corpora cavernosa. In fact, grey-scale ultrasonography allows differential diagnosis between various causes of penile induration and, in particular, between pathologies of the tunica albuginea and of the corpora cavernosa.

The diagnostic capabilities of ultrasound to detect diffuse fibrotic changes of the corpora cavernosa depend on the underlying cause and extent of tissue damage. Patients with hypoactive corpus cavernosum or alteration of the connective tissue/smooth muscle balance secondary to diabetes, smoking, prostatectomy or advanced age usually present with normal appearance of the corpora cavernosa or subtle alterations. In particular, a slight increase in echogenicity can be observed, and larger lacunar spaces with thickened wall have been described in the senescent penis with age-related fibrosis of smooth muscle fibers (Wespes 2000). Recognition of these subtle changes, however, is highly subjective, and particular attention should be paid to avoid misinterpretation of normal features as initial fibrosis. In fact, sinusoidal spaces at the base of the penis are normally larger than in the remaining portions of the shaft.

Diffuse fibrosis that develops after priapism, after infection and in patients with systemic sclerosis is usually recognized at ultrasound as ill-defined hyperechogenic areas replacing the sinusoid of the corpora cavernosa, which are often prevailing around the cavernosal arteries. Little changes are usually appreciable after prostaglandin injection, and patients usually do not reach erection also following high intracavernosal doses of vasoactive drugs. Less frequently, the corpora cavernosa present coarse echotexture because of large, irregular sinusoidal spaces with thick, echogenic wall. In this case distension of the sinusoids is prevalent around the cavernosal arteries and in the proximal portion of the shaft, while the remaining portions of the corpora cavernosa usually remain undistended, reflecting poor erectile response and veno-occlusive dysfunction (Fig. 18.1).

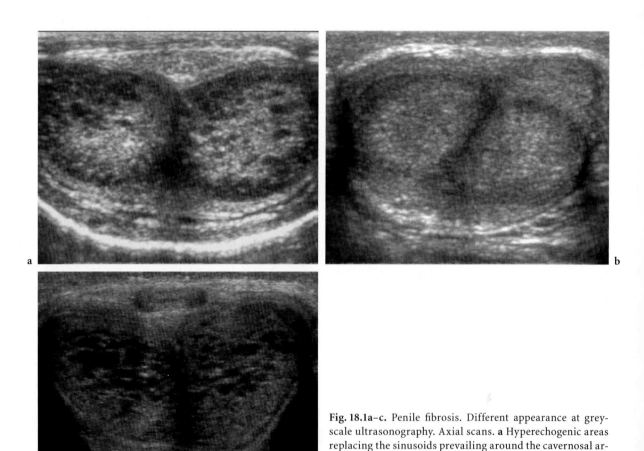

Fig. 18.1a–c. Penile fibrosis. Different appearance at grey-scale ultrasonography. Axial scans. **a** Hyperechogenic areas replacing the sinusoids prevailing around the cavernosal arteries. **b** Widespread involvement of the corpora that appear diffusely hyperechoic. **c** Large, irregular sinusoidal spaces with thick, echogenic wall. Distension of the sinusoids is prevalent around the cavernosal arteries

Other authors report the presence of diffuse hyperechoic and hypoechoic foci within the corpora cavernosa of patients with systemic sclerosis and penile fibrosis (Aversa et al. 2006). However, air bubbles that can be incidentally injected in the corpora cavernosa along with the vasoactive substance may mimic these features.

Focal fibrotic changes within the corpora cavernosa present at ultrasound as hyperechogenic areas or nodules with variable ultrasound beam attenuation (Fig. 18.2). Small or coarse calcifications can be occasionally present. Penile bending or indentation can be present.

Occasionally, cavernosal tissue injury from a blunt perineal trauma can result in a fibrotic scar encompassing the entire circumference of a corpus cavernosum. Ultrasound shows a hyperechogenic stripe with acoustic shadow dividing the corpus in two portions. The cavernosal artery can be obliterated or warped at the level of the scar (Fig. 18.3). Since the penile septum is usually nearly complete at the base of the penis, the proximal portion of the injured corpus remains hemodinamically isolated from the other portions (Horger et al. 2005).

Circumscribed septal fibrosis presents at ultrasound as an alteration of the normal ultrasonographic appearance of the penile septum (Fig. 18.4), which is replaced by inhomogeneous echogenic tissue (Brant et al. 2007).

Distal segmental fibrosis presents at grey-scale ultrasonography as hyperechogenic tissue prevailing around the cavernosal arteries at the tip of the penis (Fig. 18.5). The diameter of the distal portion of the penis is usually reduced, compared to the base of the shaft. Clinically turgidity of the penile tip is reduced compared to the base.

Proximal segmental fibrosis usually presents at grey-scale ultrasonography as an alteration of the appearance of the penile crura with coarse echotexture because of large, irregular sinusoidal spaces displaying thick, echogenic wall (Fig. 18.6). More circumscribed echogenic fibrotic changes may be present.

There is no accordance in the literature on the sensitivity of ultrasound in detecting corporeal fibrosis. Some authors do not find ultrasound a sensible technique to diagnose or confirm penile fibrosis, reporting a positivity in less than 60% of patients with clinically evident penile fibrosis, consequent to prostaglandin intracavernous injection (Chew et al. 1997). Other authors, however, suggest that ultrasound could be helpful in demonstrating subclinical fibrosis (Moemen et al. 2004).

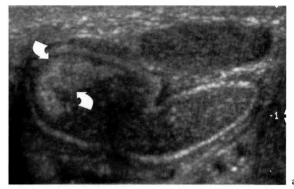

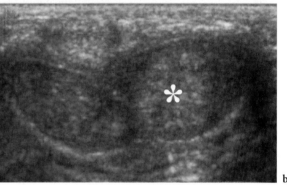

Fig. 18.2a,b. Circumscribed fibrosis. Axial scans. a Focal fibrotic area in the right corpus cavernosum (*curved arrows*) following repeated intracavernosal injection of vasoactive drugs. b Postraumatic fibrotic scar (*) in the left corpus cavernosum

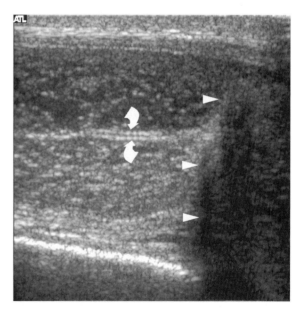

Fig. 18.3. Postraumatic fibrotic scar encompassing the entire circumference of a corpus cavernosum. Longitudinal scan showing a stripe with acoustic shadow (*arrowheads*) dividing the corpus in two portions. The cavernosal artery (*curved arrows*) is encased by the scar

18.7
Color Doppler Ultrasound

Diffuse fibrotic changes of the corpora cavernosa are invariably associated with erectile dysfunction. Even after cavernosal administration of high prostaglandin doses, incomplete erection is reached. Doppler interrogation of the cavernosal arteries usually shows pathological waveform changes in these patients consistent with veno-occlusive dysfunction. Peak systolic velocity is variable, depending of the cause leading to penile fibrosis, severity of damage of the peripheral vascular tree and underlying systemic vascular status. In general, the higher the degree of fibrosis is, the lower the changes of arterial inflow after prostaglandin injection. Also, end diastolic velocity is variable depending on the degree of penile turgidity and on the degree of corporal fibrosis. In our experience, severe fibrosis is usually associated with high resistance flow. Since the corpora cavernosa are stiff at palpation in these patients, and only a limited turgescence is reached after prostaglandin injection, it is conceivable that

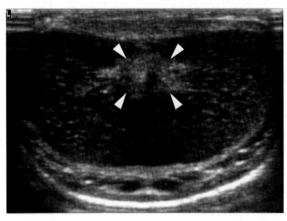

Fig. 18.4. Circumscribed septal fibrosis. Axial scan showing inhomogeneous echogenic tissue (*arrowheads*) within the penile septum

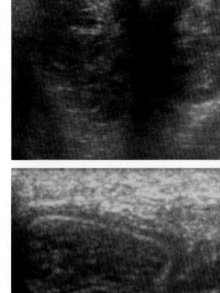

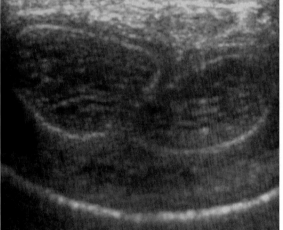

Fig. 18.5. Distal segmental fibrosis. Longitudinal scan showing echogenic areas with irregular margins at the tip of the corpora cavernosa (*arrowheads*), consistent with fibrotic changes. The diameter of the distal portion of the penis is reduced compared to the base of the shaft

Fig. 18.6a,b. Fibrosis of the penile crura following repeated saddle microtraumas. a Axial scan to the penile crura shows coarse echotexture of the corpora cavernosa with echogenic areas and large, irregular sinusoidal spaces. b Transverse scan to the middle penile shaft of the same patient shows normal echotexture of the corpora cavernosa

high resistance flows reflect decreased compliance of the corpora cavernosa, rather then blood pressure within the cavernosal bodies.

In patients with diffuse cavernosal fibrosis associated with severe impairment of the cavernosal artery inflow, small peripheral vessels can be demonstrated at color Doppler ultrasonography feeding the outer portions of the corpora cavernosa through small collaterals from extraalbugineal vessels (Fig. 18.7).

In patients with circumscribed fibrotic changes leakage pathways are often identified as color Doppler ultrasound adjacent to the region in which the cavernosal tissue is replaced by a fibrotic scar (Fig. 18.8). Scar-related arterial insufficiency can be associated when cavernosal arteries are encased by the scar. In these patients Doppler interrogation of the cavernosal arteries shows high velocity flows proximal and markedly lower velocity flows distal to the scar.

18.8 Differential Diagnosis

During ultrasound evaluation of patients with clinically suspicious cavernosal fibrosis, other causes of penile induration must be considered. In fact, most of patients with penile induration actually have Peyronie's disease. Other less common con-

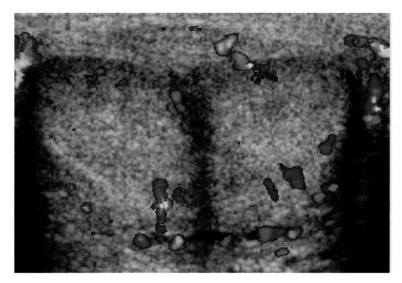

Fig. 18.7. Diffuse penile fibrosis following prolonged ischemic priapism. Color Doppler axial image obtained after prostaglandin injection shows small peripheral vessels feeding the outer portion of the corpora cavernosa. Cavernosal arteries are obliterated

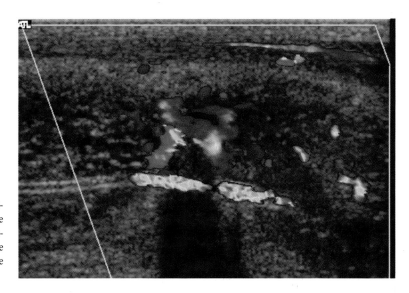

Fig. 18.8. Posttraumatic penile deformation following untreated penile fracture. Color Doppler US shows venous leak at the level of the scar due to incomplete distension of the erectile tissue

ditions that enter in the differential diagnoses include: posttraumatic albugineal scar, penile dorsal vein thrombosis, benign or malignant primary or secondary tumors and fibrosis of the corpus spongiosum caused by urethral manipulation (Kelamy syndrome). The ultrasound features of these different pathologies are described in detail in other chapters.

18.9
Diagnostic Role of Other Imaging Modalities

Dynamic infusion cavernosometry and cavernosography have been widely used to evaluate erectile function in patients with cavernosal fibrosis. This procedure is an effective mean to obtain objective information on the presence of abnormal venous drainage, either diffuse or localized at the site of circumscribed cavernosal scars. When complete smooth muscle relaxation is obtained using a sufficiently high intracavernous dose of vasoactive drugs, venous occlusive dysfunction resulting from alteration in the trabecular fibroelastic structure can be differentiated from dysfunction resulting from functional inability to relax trabecular smooth muscle tone completely (Hatzichristou et al. 1995). In patients with diffuse fibrosis, cavernosography demonstrates heterogeneous opacification of the corpora cavernosa and multiple irregular filling defects (Velcek and Evans 1982; El-Bahnasawy et al. 2002). Circumscribed fibrosis presents as a filling defect within normally enhancing bodies (Abrahamy and Leiter 1980). Dynamic infusion cavernosometry and cavernosography, however, are not longer performed in most centers because of the invasiveness and relatively high risks of complications.

Magnetic resonance imaging is as effective as ultrasonography in evaluation of fibrous changes in the corpora cavernosa, with the advantage of panoramic view and better contrast resolution. In patients with severe and diffuse fibrotic changes, heterogeneous areas of low signal intensity are appreciable in T2-weighted images especially around the cavernosal arteries, while the peripheral portion of the corpora cavernosa can present with high signal intensity (Fig. 18.9).

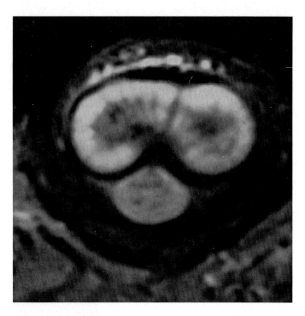

Fig. 18.9. Penile fibrosis. Axial T2-weighted MR image showing low signal intensity around the cavernosal arteries and high signal intensity under the tunica albuginea (courtesy of Pietro Pavlica, Bologna, Italy)

After intravenous gadolinium administration, inhomogeneous signal intensity is appreciable with non-enhancing areas often prevailing around the cavernosal arteries. Microscopic fibrotic changes can present with normally appearing corpora cavernosa at both T1-weighted and T2-weighted images, but markedly reduced enhancement after gadolinium administration (Fig. 18.10).

References

Abrahamy R, Leiter E (1980) Post-traumatic segmental corpus cavernosum fibrosis: the diagnostic value of cavernosography and the surgical correction by cavernosum-cavernosum shunt. J Urol 123:289–290

Aversa A, Proietti M, Bruzziches R et al (2006) The penile vasculature in systemic sclerosis: A duplex ultrasound study. J Sex Med 3:554–558

Basar M, Sargon MF, Basar H et al (1998) Electron microscopic findings of penile tissues in veno-occlusive dysfunction: is penile biopsy necessary? Int Urol Nephrol 30:331–338

Basar M, Tekdogan UY, Yilmaz E et al (2001) The efficacy of sildenafil in different etiologies of erectile dysfunction. Int Urol Nephrol 32:403–407

Bertolotto M, Pozzi Mucelli R (2004) Non-penetrating penile traumas: sonographic and Doppler features. AJR Am J Roentgenol 183:1085–1089

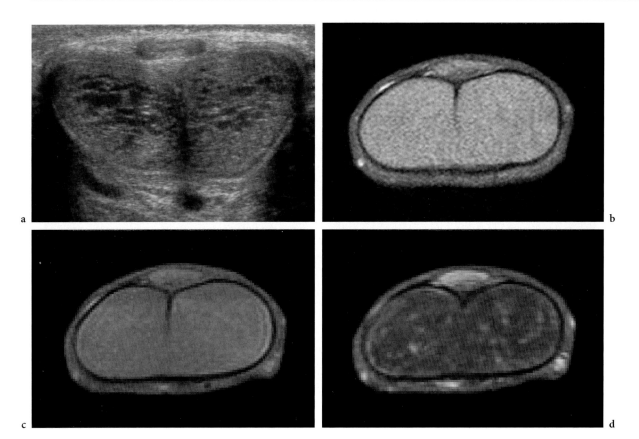

Fig. 18.10a–d. Patient who developed posttraumatic erectile dysfunction 5 years before. a Grey-scale ultrasound image of the shaft showing insufficient distension of the cavernosal sinusoids. b–c Magnetic resonance imaging of the same patient showing normally appearing T1-weighted (b) and T2-weighted (c) images. d After gadolinium administration the enhancement of the corpora cavernosa is markedly reduced, suggesting microvessel injury and diffuse microscopic fibrotic changes

Bertolotto M, Quaia E, Pozzi Mucelli F et al (2003) Color Doppler imaging of posttraumatic priapism before and after selective embolization. Radiographics 23:495–503

Border WA, Noble NA (1994) Transforming growth factor beta in tissue fibrosis. N Engl J Med 331:1286–1292

Brant WO, Bella AJ, Garcia MM et al (2007) Isolated septal fibrosis or hematoma-atypical Peyronie's disease? J Urol 177:179–182; discussion 183

Chew KK, Stuckey BG, Earle CM et al (1997) Penile fibrosis in intracavernosal prostaglandin E1 injection therapy for erectile dysfunction. Int J Impot Res 9:225–229; discussion 229–230

Dahiya R, Chui R, Perinchery G et al (1999) Differential gene expression of growth factors in young and old rat penile tissues is associated with erectile dysfunction. Int J Impot Res 11:201–206

El-Bahnasawy MS, Dawood A, Farouk A (2002) Low-flow priapism: risk factors for erectile dysfunction. BJU Int 89:285–290

Ferrini MG, Davila HH, Kovanecz I et al (2006) Vardenafil prevents fibrosis and loss of corporal smooth muscle that occurs after bilateral cavernosal nerve resection in the rat. Urology 68:429–435

Fisch BM, Pickett B, Weinberg V, Roach M (2001) Dose of radiation received by the bulb of the penis correlates with risk of impotence after three-dimensional conformal radiotherapy for prostate cancer. Urology 57:955–959

Ghanem H, Ghazy S, El-Meliegy A (2000) Corporeal counter incisions: a simplified approach to penile prosthesis implantation in fibrotic cases. Int J Impot Res 12:153–156

Hakim LS, Kulaksizoglu H, Mulligan R et al (1996) Evolving concepts in the diagnosis and treatment of arterial high flow priapism. J Urol 155:541–548

Hatzichristou DG, Saenz de Tejada I, Kupferman S et al (1995) In vivo assessment of trabecular smooth muscle tone, its application in pharmaco-cavernosometry and analysis of intracavernous pressure determinants. J Urol 153:1126–1135

Horger DC, Wingo MS, Keane TE (2005) Partial segmental thrombosis of corpus cavernosum: case report and review of world literature. Urology 66:194

Iacono F, Giannella R, Somma P et al (2005) Histological alterations in cavernous tissue after radical prostatectomy. J Urol 173:1673–1676

Jevtich MJ, Khawand NY, Vidic B (1990) Clinical significance of ultrastructural findings in the corpora cavernosa of normal and impotent men. J Urol 143:289–293

Lin JS, Lin YM, Chow NH et al (2000) Novel image analysis of corpus cavernous tissue in impotent men. Urology 55:252–256

Lotfi MA, Varga J, Hirsch IH (1995) Erectile dysfunction in systemic sclerosis. Urology 45:879–881

Mireku-Boateng AO, Nwokeji C (2004) Sequelae of parenteral drug abuse involving the external genitalia. Urol Int 73:302–304

Moemen MN, Hamed HA, Kamel II et al (2004) Clinical and sonographic assessment of the side effects of intracavernous injection of vasoactive substances. Int J Impot Res 16:143–145

Montague DK, Angermeier KW (2006) Corporeal excavation: new technique for penile prosthesis implantation in men with severe corporeal fibrosis. Urology 67:1072–1075

Montorsi F, Guazzoni G, Strambi LF et al (1997) Recovery of spontaneous erectile function after nerve-sparing radical retropubic prostatectomy with and without early intracavernous injections of alprostadil: results of a prospective, randomized trial. J Urol 158:1408–1410

Moon DG, Lee KC, Kim YW et al (2004) Effect of TCDD on corpus cavernosum histology and smooth muscle physiology. Int J Impot Res 16:224–230

Moreland RB (1998) Is there a role of hypoxemia in penile fibrosis: a viewpoint presented to the Society for the Study of Impotence. Int J Impot Res 10:113–120

Moreland RB, Watkins MT, Nehra A et al (1998) Oxygen tension modulates transforming growth factor β1 expression and PGE productionin human corpus cavernosum smooth muscle cells. Mol Urol 2:41–47

Mumtaz FH, Khan MA, Mikhailidis DP, Morgan RJ (1998) Intracavernosal PGE1-related penile fibrosis: possible mechanisms. Int J Impot Res 10:195

Munarriz R, Huang V, Uberoi J et al (2005) Only the nose knows: penile hemodynamic study of the perineum-saddle interface in men with erectile dysfunction utilizing bicycle saddles and seats with and without nose extensions. J Sex Med 2:612–619

Nayal W, Schwarzer U, Klotz T et al (1999) Transcutaneous penile oxygen pressure during bicycling. BJU Int 83:623–625

Pavlica P, Barozzi L (1998) Ultrasound of penile tumors and trauma. Ultrasound Quarterly 14:95–109

Sattar AA, Wespes E, Schulman CC (1994) Computerized measurement of penile elastic fibres in potent and impotent men. Eur Urol 25:142–144

Schwarzer JU, Hofmann R (1991) Purulent corporeal cavernositis secondary to papaverine-induced priapism. J Urol 146:845–846

Schwarzer U, Sommer F, Klotz T et al (2002) Cycling and penile oxygen pressure: the type of saddle matters. Eur Urol 41:139–143

Shafik A, Ahmed I, El Sibai O, Shafik AA (2006) The hypoactive corpora cavernosa with degenerative erectile dysfunction: a new syndrome. BMC Urol 6:13

Shen ZJ, Zhou XL, Lu YL, Chen ZD (2003) Effect of androgen deprivation on penile ultrastructure. Asian J Androl 5:33–36

User HM, Hairston JH, Zelner DJ et al (2003) Penile weight and cell subtype specific changes in a post-radical prostatectomy model of erectile dysfunction. J Urol 169:1175–1179

Velcek D, Evans JA (1982) Cavernosography. Radiology 144:781–785

Wespes E (2000) Erectile dysfunction in the ageing man. Curr Opin Urol 10:625–628

Wespes E (2002) Smooth muscle pathology and erectile dysfunction. Int J Impot Res 14 [Suppl 1]:S17–21

Wespes E, Moreira de Goes P, Sattar AA, Schulman C (1994) Objective criteria in the long-term evaluation of penile venous surgery. J Urol 152:888–890

Yaman O, Yilmaz E, Bozlu M, Anafarta K (2003) Alterations of intracorporeal structures in patients with erectile dysfunction. Urol Int 71:87–90

US Imaging of the Male Urethra

Libero Barozzi, Pietro Pavlica, Massimo Valentino, and Massimo De Matteis

CONTENTS

19.1 Background 163

19.2 Normal Anatomy 163
19.2.1 Posterior Urethra 164
19.2.2 Anterior Urethra 164

19.3 Ultrasound Anatomy and Technique 164

19.3 Urethral Pathology 166
19.3.1 Malformations 166
19.3.2 Stenosis 167
19.3.3 Diverticula 169
19.3.4 Stones 170
19.3.5 Fistulae 171
19.3.6 Trauma 171
19.3.7 Cysts 171
19.3.8 Tumors 171

19.4 Diagnostic Role of Other Imaging Modalities 172

References 173

19.1 Background

The urethra is a tubular structure through which urine is expelled after accumulating in the physiological reservoir called the bladder. In men, this canal is also used by the seminal ducts and carries the sperm from the veru montanum all the way to the external urethral orifice.

Traditional radiological exams such as retrograde urethrography and micturition cystourethrography are considered the standard imaging techniques for the morphological and functional study of the urethra. They do however present certain limitations and only provide images of the urethral lumen similar to those obtained by urethroscopy (Merchant et al. 1997). With a view to reducing doses and exposure to the gonads, ultrasonography imaging is increasingly used even though its diagnostic role has not been fully tested.

Male urethral imaging and pathology are not widely covered in the radiological literature since this part of the urinary tract is easily studied by urologists with clinical or endoscopic examinations. Ultrasonography is used in association with voiding cystourethrography and retrograde urethrography.

Voiding cystourethrography is used to study the posterior urethra allowing the detection of bladder neck pathologies, post-surgical stenosis and neoplasms. The functional aspects of micturition can be monitored in patients with neuromuscular dysfunction of the bladder using digital radiographic imaging.

Retrograde urethrography is commonly used to explore the anterior urethral anatomy and pathologies, but recently sonourethrography has been increasingly proposed. The latter is able to study the urethral mucosa and the periurethral tissues possibly involved in urethral pathologies such as strictures, diverticula, trauma and tumors, which cannot be detected radiographically or at urethroscopy.

19.2 Normal Anatomy

The male urethra has a mean length of 16–18 cm and is divided into a posterior and an anterior portion. The posterior urethra, which stretches from

---

L. Barozzi, MD; P. Pavlica, MD; M. Valentino, MD; M. De Matteis, MD
Department of Radiology, University Hospital S. Orsola-Malpighi, Via Massarenti 9, Bologna, 40138, Italy

the bladder neck to the lower edge of the urogenital diaphragm, includes the prostatic and the membranous portions. The anterior urethra is 14–15 cm long and is divided into the bulbar and into the penile or pendulous portions.

On account of its complex embryological origin, the urethral epithelial lining differs depending on the tract under consideration. In particular, transitional epithelium is found from the bladder neck to the veru montanum, the cylindrical epithelium as far as the fossa navicularis and squamous epithelium up to the external meatus.

19.2.1
Posterior Urethra

The prostatic urethra is about 3–4 cm long in the young male, but reaches 8–10 cm in cases of benign prostatic hyperplasia. It begins at the vesical neck, passes through the prostate gland assuming an arcuate course up to the prostate apex. Two parts can be identified: the supramontanal tract from which the periurethral gland ducts emerge and the submontanal tract where the excretory ducts of the peripheral gland are located. The submontanal urethra is surrounded by the striated sphincter.

The membranous urethra, about 1–2 cm long, passes through the uro-genital diaphragm, which contains the Cowper glands. In this tract the urethra is surrounded by the striate sphincter and the perineal muscles.

19.2.2
Anterior Urethra

The bulbar urethra is surrounded by the bulb of the corpus spongiosum; it is larger than the other portions (1.5–2 cm), does not have stiff fascia and extends from the perineal area to the suspensor ligament of the penis.

The penile or pendulous urethra is of relatively uniform diameter, about 1 cm, stretching from the penile ligament to the external urethral meatus. Before its emergence at the meatus, there is an ampullar dilatation called the fossa navicularis.

Many small glands (of Littré) are to be found at the lumen of the anterior urethra, which are more numerous in the bulbar portion and near the fossa navicularis.

19.3
Ultrasound Anatomy and Technique

Because of its complex morphology and course, the male urethra can be accurately studied using different approaches and probes (DESSER et al. 1999).

The posterior urethra can be investigated using high frequency endorectal probes at rest, which can depict the normal anatomy of the collapsed posterior urethra identifying the mucosa and the posterior urethral musculature (Fig. 19.1). The voiding phase is well studied with linear endorectal probes (Fig. 19.2), which are commonly employed in the study of the prostate and the anal canal (MERKLE and WAGNER 1988; MOREY and MCANINCH 1997). The technique is not different from voiding cystourethrography, even though it does offer a smaller field of view. The bladder is distended physiologically and does not require the application of a catheter or the use of contrast medium. Some problems may be observed in patients suffering from incontinence or renal failure with reduced urine output, but the main drawback is the difficulty patients have voiding in the lateral position with the probe in the rectum (MCANINCH et al. 1988). The problem can be sometimes resolved by placing the patient in an upright position or by using a special stool with a hole at the centre through which the probe can be inserted into the rectum (simil-urodynamic stool). The images are recorded continuously on videotapes or electronically on CD and can be reviewed later with the urologist or neurologist.

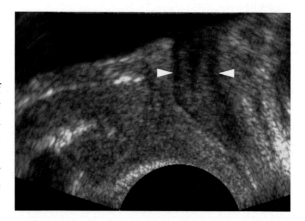

Fig. 19.1. Normal posterior urethra during rest in a young male. Endorectal end-fire probe in sagittal scan. The collapsed urethra is hypoechoic (*arrowheads*) with respect to the surrounding prostatic tissue, and a linear hyperechoic structure corresponds to the mucosa; the hypoechoic outer line is due to the muscular layers

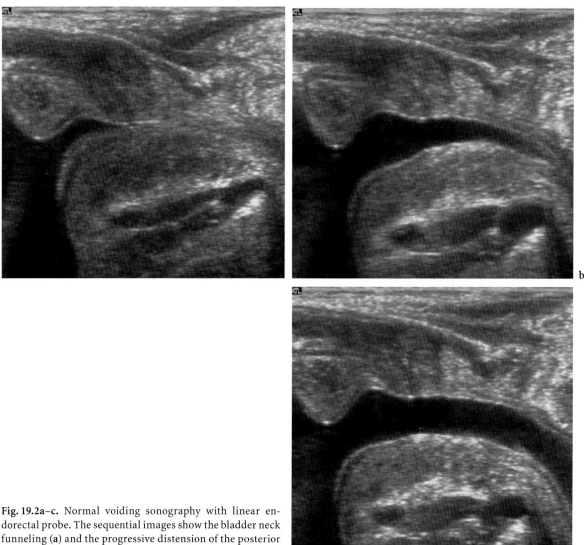

Fig. 19.2a–c. Normal voiding sonography with linear endorectal probe. The sequential images show the bladder neck funneling (a) and the progressive distension of the posterior urethra from the bladder neck to the perineal plane (b,c)

Voiding sonography may be combined with urodynamic studies (US-videourodynamics), requiring the collaboration of a urodynamist and the right equipment to ensure simultaneous reproduction of urodynamic tracing and ultrasound imaging. It is a complex procedure that takes about 1 h to perform and is indicated in patients with urinary complaints secondary to central or peripheral neurological disorders.

The anterior urethra can be explored using high frequency linear probes that are able to examine the penile and perineal tract and the structures of the surrounding corpus spongiosum (GLUCK et al. 1988; NASH et al. 1995). This exam consists of scanning performed after a saline solution is introduced through the external urethral meatus (Fig. 19.3). After cleaning the gland and urethral meatus with antiseptic material, a small Foley catheter is placed in the distal urethra, and the balloon is slowly distended in the fossa navicularis until the patient complains of the onset of pain.

Overly rapid or excessive distension can cause laceration of the mucosa, prompting intense and long-lasting pain. In order to avoid air bubbles in the urethra, which can cause artifacts, it is advisable to allow the saline solution to slowly seep out of the catheter as it is being introduced into the urethra, holding the penis upwards. When the fluid comes out of the meatus, the Foley balloon is distended by saline solution. Distension of the urethra occurs

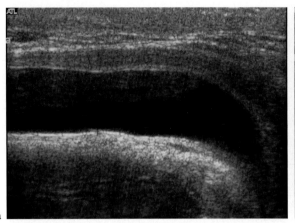 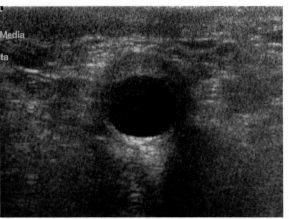

Fig. 19.3a,b. Sonourethrography. Normal appearance of the urethra in sagittal (a) and transversal (b) scans. The urethra distended by the saline solution appears as an anechoic tubular structure well depicted with linear array transducer using direct skin contact on the ventral surface of the penis and with trans-scrotal and perineal scanning for bulbar urethra

slowly, allowing the solution to drip down through a bottle located at a height of 40–50 cm so as to avoid periurethral spill from hyperpression (which however soon resolves by itself). The saline solution can sometimes be delivered via a syringe placed directly in the urethral meatus. Its low viscosity makes urethral distension difficult to maintain, and securing the Foley catheter in position with the balloon in the distal urethra can be difficult because the balloon often slips from the urethral meatus. Catheter-tip syringes are not ideal because they do not fit perfectly with the urethral meatus.

An intraluminal lubricant and anesthetic jelly were recently used instead of saline solution as a contrast medium for distending the urethra in sonourethrography. It is injected directly into the meatus until the urethra appears fully distended on sonographic observation. To avoid jelly reflux from the external meatus and maintain urethral distension, a flexible penile clamp is employed to occlude the urethra. The use of jelly, however, has the disadvantage that distension is less marked, especially during scanning, provoking compression of the urethral canal. Many artifacts can be observed due to the non-homogeneous composition of the jelly, which contains small air bubbles that cause reverberations (BEARCROFT and BERMAN 1994). Sonourethrography with jelly is nevertheless particularly useful in tight distal urethral stenosis and meatus stenosis when it is not possible to introduce the Foley catheter.

The bulbar urethra can be studied by placing the probe on the ventral surface or transperineally after having lifted the scrotum. The most useful scans are longitudinal since they reproduce the urethral canal. Because of the narrower field of view, transversal scans are used to explore focal lesions that have already been identified. Real time US observation allows targeted investigation by using the best scanning planes.

19.3
Urethral Pathology

The male urethra can be the site of frequent and serious primitive diseases that may affect the quality of life of patients. Diagnostic imaging has an important role to play since it can detect lesions that are inaccessible to urethroscopy and can help identify the extraurethral spread of the process. Ultrasonography, in particular, provides adjunct information that cannot be obtained either by traditional radiological examination, urethroscopy or urodynamics (PAVLICA et al. 2003b; YEKELER et al. 2004; SEPULVEDA et al. 2005; SALAM 2006).

19.3.1
Malformations

These are generally to be found in children and can cause serious damage to the bladder and upper urinary tract due to chronic obstruction, which is well documented with abdominal ultrasonography. Malformations of the posterior urethra mainly affect the urethral valves, which can be studied by voiding cystourethrography, even though some cases have been explored with trans-perineal sonography with high frequency probes (COHEN et al. 1994).

Malformations of the anterior urethra (DAS 1992; CHIOU et al. 1996) are due to complete or incomplete stenoses or segmentary atresia, duplications and congenital dilatations (megalourethra). Other malformations include hypospadia and epispadia, which are associated with enlargement of the prostatic utricle and müllerian duct remnants. All these malformations can be better examined by retrograde urethrography or sonourethrography, while cross-sectional imaging provides information on associated paraurethral malformations such as uretheral ectopic emptying and disorders of the seminal tracts.

19.3.2
Stenosis

Obstruction of the lower urinary apparatus can be caused by primitive lesions of the urethra or lesions secondary to compression by an enlarged prostate or perineal masses. The most frequent cause of non-prostatic obstructive dysuria is acquired stenosis, which can be divided into post-inflammatory, post-traumatic and post-surgical.

Posterior urethral stenoses can be studied with voiding cystourethrography and voiding cystourethrosonography and may be divided into vesical neck obstructive syndrome and post-prostatectomy stenosis.

Vesical neck obstructive syndrome or vesical neck disease becomes evident only during urination (GUPTA et al. 1993). It may be attributed to hypertrophy of the vesical neck muscle, hyperplasia of the paraurethral glands or a detrusor-bladder neck dyssynergia, as can be seen in patients with congenital or acquired neurogenic bladder. It can be observed in both children and adults and can be accurately diagnosed by videourodynamic examination combined with electromyography of the extrinsic urethral sphincter.

Ultrasonography using an endorectal linear probe can be used as an alternative to voiding cystourethrography in that it provides diagnostic images without exposing the patient or examiner to radiation and obviates some of the problems these patients have during voiding (SHABSIGH et al. 1987). Ultrasonography typically reveals a rounded protrusion at the bladder neck, which does not disappear even in advanced phases of urination, and the absence of the funnel-shaped feature that can normally be seen in the cervical area, with prominence of the posterior bladder neck, prolonged voiding time, bladder wall thickening and marked post-voiding residue. The posterior urethra is only slightly distended since the flow is very reduced (Fig. 19.4).

Much more common in clinical practice are post-surgical stenoses following suprapubic or endoscopic prostatectomy. The stenosis can occur at the vesical neck, may affect the whole of the prostate cavity or may be localized only at its distal zone (Fig. 19.5).

The site and importance of the stenosis can be easily monitored using transrectal sonography.

Bladder neck stenosis is characterized by the absence of neck distension, and US shows hyperechogenic spots reflecting post-surgical scarring. The prostatic cavity is normally small since the flow is reduced. When the scarring process affects the prostatic cavity extensively, the posterior urethra appears thin, irregular and difficult to visualize. Sonographic images are however more diagnostic when the stenosis is located in the distal part of the post-prostatectomy cavity, near the urethral striated sphincter. The prostatic cavity is wide and distended, and full of urine at sonography. The urethra below is narrow or not detectable since there is little distension due to markedly reduced flow.

Acquired stenoses of the anterior urethra on the other hand are more often caused by inflammatory or traumatic processes. In clinical practice they are the more frequent and can be divided into post-inflammatory, post-traumatic and iatrogenic.

Post-inflammatory stenoses are the result of urethritis, normally of blenorrhagic origin. The stenotic process takes several years to develop before any serious obstruction ensues, which means that diagnosis is often made many years after actual infection. These stenoses are normally multiple and affect those parts of the anterior urethra with the greatest number of glandular structures (the final destination of germs), triggering a chronic inflammatory process that in turn provokes fibrotic scarring extending to the urethral submucosa and corpus spongiosum. Voiding cystourethrography and retrograde urethrography are always necessary since the number, site and extent of the stenoses have to be defined before deciding on therapy (GIUDICI et al. 1991; CALLEA et al. 1997).

Voiding cystourethrography allows identification of the dynamically most important stenosis as well as

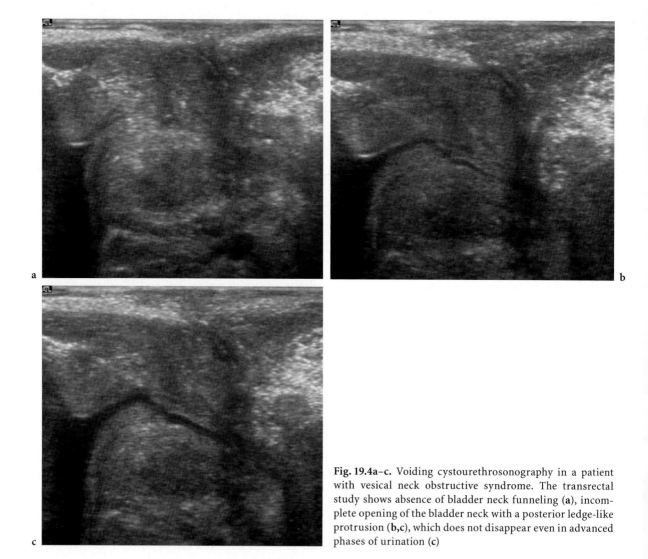

Fig. 19.4a–c. Voiding cystourethrosonography in a patient with vesical neck obstructive syndrome. The transrectal study shows absence of bladder neck funneling (**a**), incomplete opening of the bladder neck with a posterior ledge-like protrusion (**b,c**), which does not disappear even in advanced phases of urination (**c**)

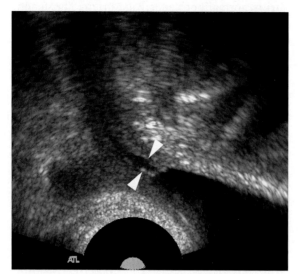

Fig. 19.5. Post-surgical stenosis after prostatectomy. Voiding sonography shows a stenosis (*arrowheads*) at the distal end of the prostatic urethra

evaluation of the functional involvement of the upper urinary tract above that point. Stenoses located below the main one are not easy to identify due to reduced flow and to detect them retrograde urethrography is usually required. Since 1989 sonourethrography (Fig. 19.6) has been increasingly used by urethra surgeons since from a diagnostic point of view it is just as reliable as retrograde urethrography and facilitates the evaluation of two key diagnostic elements for the surgeon: the extent of the stenosis and the involvement of the periurethral spongy tissue (PERKASH and FRIEDLAND 1987; FRIEDLAND 1990; MOREY et al. 1998). Many surgeons perform the exam in the operating theatre immediately before incision for urethrotomy or reconstruction (HOEBEKE et al. 1997).

At sonourethrography stenoses appear as urethral lumen reduction. The submucosa is initially thickened and hypoechoic, and finally becomes hyperecogenic and thin (Fig. 19.7). The morphologic changes may extend and involve the adjacent spongy tissue with extensive fibrosis.

Since radiological and ecographic techniques cannot detect the state or extent of the inflammatory process (a key element for the surgeon), magnetic resonance imaging with contrast agent can be useful. When the inflammatory process is active, the peristenotic scarred areas, hypointense at T1- and T2-weighted imaging, show uptake of the contrast agent with hyperintense signals at T1.

Post-traumatic stenoses occur after direct trauma or rupture of the urethral canal due to pelvic fracturing, with laceration of the perineal muscles. They differ from inflammatory stenoses to the extent that they affect different areas of the urethral tract and are normally one-off short-lived episodes.

Stenoses caused by the use of instruments (catheterization, endoscopic resection) are usually located in three areas: the external meatus, suspensor ligament of the penis and just below the urethral sphincter (BLAIVAS and NORLEN 1984).

Stenoses due to pelvic fracturing, on the other hand, affect almost exclusively the membranous urethra. They can be easily investigated with retrograde urethrography and voiding cystourethrography, but are difficult to explore with sonourethrography.

19.3.3
Diverticula

This term refers to diverticula and pseudodiverticular dilatations. Congenital diverticula are very

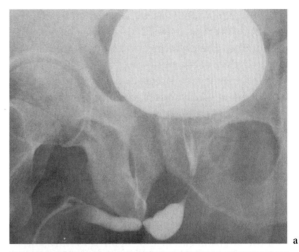
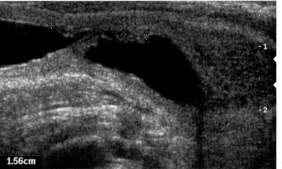

Fig. 19.6a,b. Post-inflammatory urethral stenosis. a Voiding cystourethrography in association with retrograde urethrography shows posterior urethral dilatation with severe stenosis at the level of the bulbar urethra. b Sonourethrography is more accurate for measuring stricture size and length for a better preoperative assessment of the bulbar stricture because the scanning probe is aligned directly in the mid sagittal plane

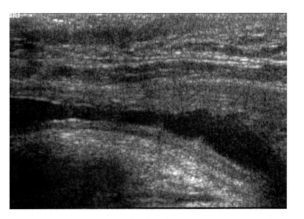

Fig. 19.7. Distal urethral stenosis studied with sonourethrography. Long stenosis of the bulbo-perineal urethra. The mucosa is hyperechoic with strong spots due to fibrotic strictures. The corpus spongiosum is thinned and hyperechoic due to chronic inflammation

rare and are usually associated with other malformations of the urethra. They are normally to be found in the distal urethra and are diagnosed by retrograde urethrography or sonouretrography, which show a dilatation of the urethral lumen. The advantage of ultrasonography is the possibility to analyze the surrounding soft tissues that are commonly involved.

Syringocele or cystic dilatation of Cowper's gland ducts is a lesion of uncertain origin, though probably congenital since it is commonly found in young patients with negative clinical history.

According to the classification of MAIZELS et al. (1983), four radiological types can be recognized, and this division can also be applied to ultrasonography:
1. simple syringocele, presenting as modest dilatation of the bulbourethral duct;
2. imperforate or cystic syringocele, when the duct does not communicate with the urethra and prompts a submucosal cystic dilatation that at urethrography appears as a filling defect or a cystic lesion of the urethral wall;
3. perforate syringocele, when the dilated excretory ducts communicate with the bulbar urethra allowing reflux and opacification of the bulbourethral glands;
4. ruptured syringocele, when the thin, frail membrane remaining in the bulbous urethra after the syringocele has ruptured can be seen.

Syringocele can be easily diagnosed by sonourethrography using transperineal scanning, which shows a thin septation in the bulbar urethra dividing the distended lumen into two parts. The part nearest the probe corresponds to the dilated Cowper's duct, the more distal part to the urethral lumen distended by saline solution (Fig. 19.8). Transversal scanning normally shows a double channel tubular image. In bilateral syringocele a triple lumen channel can be observed.

Acquired diverticula are usually the result of inflammation of the periurethral glands, with the formation of abscesses that burst within the urethral lumen. A cavity communicates with the urethra, lined by a transitional epithelium and presenting a pseudodiverticulum image.

Ultrasound examination identifies the urethrocele, located most often in the anterior urethra or the penile-scrotal ligament. The cavity appears as a single saccular image with clear edges and opens into the urethral lumen. Similar diverticular cavities can also be observed in the prostatic urethra due to spontaneous or post-surgical intraglandular abscesses communicating with the urethral lumen. These can be easily detected during transrectal sonography.

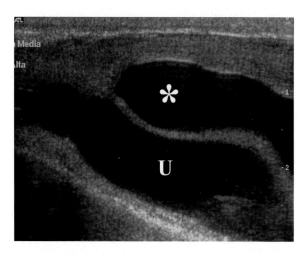

Fig. 19.8. Syringocele studied with sonourethrography. Sagittal scan showing double-channel image corresponding to duct dilatation (*) and urethral distention (*U*)

19.3.4
Stones

Urethral stones are rare and originate from the upper urinary tracts or the bladder. Primary stones are caused only when there are stenoses or cavities with urine stasis and salts precipitation.

Sonography is a useful technique since urethral stones can be easily identified by high ultrasound beam absorption and typical hyperechoic features (Fig. 19.9).

Stones located in the posterior urethra should be distinguished from intraprostatic calcifications, which are normally to be found periurethrally or in the pseudocapsule. A voiding sonography is normally required for the exact definition of posterior urethral stones since the non-distended intraprostatic urethra is usually unclear. When the stone is located in the penile urethra, basal sonography reveals a hyperechoic image with shadowing enclosed in the spongy tissue that should not be confused with phleboliths or other calcifications. Sonourethrography is always necessary to locate the site of the stone and to establish the reasons why it has not been expelled.

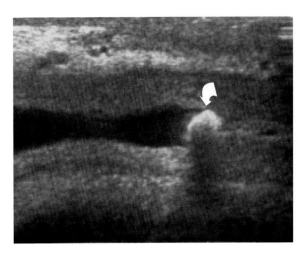

Fig. 19.9. Urethral stone studied with sonourethrography. Longitudinal scan of the urethra after fluid distension with saline solution reveals the stone (*curved arrow*) producing occlusion of the urethral lumen

19.3.5
Fistulae

Fistulae are divided into congenital or acquired and, depending on their site, into urethro-rectal and urethro-cutaneous. Urethro-rectal fistulae are usually caused by inflammation or surgery. Iatrogenic fistulae following catheterization or surgery have also been reported. In urethro-cutaneous fistulae, the fistula can open in the perineal area or on the ventral surface of the penis. Most cases are the result of urethral inflammation with secondary paraurethral abscesses that open externally. More rarely fistulae may be caused by direct or penetrating trauma and surgery of the urethra.

Sonography is generally not useful since it is unable to provide complete images of the fistulous tract, though it can visualize prostatic or urethral lesions.

Retrograde urethrography is the best way to study fistulae located under the striate sphincter of the urethra since it can visualize the fistula, the concomitant cavities and passage of the contrast agent into adjacent organs.

Fistulae developing in the posterior urethra are better detected using voiding cystourethrography. CT is used for monitoring and identifying the extent of the periurethral and periprostatic fluid collections.

19.3.6
Trauma

Because of its length, the male urethra is vulnerable to traumatic lesions that may cause acute urinary retention and sudden onset of urethrorrhagia and even late stenosis. Urethral trauma can be divided into external trauma, either contusive or penetrative, and internal or endourethral trauma. Internal traumas usually follow iatrogenic maneuvers. External traumas are frequent events and can occur in the penile urethra as a result of road or work accidents, sporting activities or sex. The urethra can be compressed by subcutaneous or intraspongiosal hematomas and may present complete or incomplete mucosal interruption.

Retrograde urethrography is the most diffuse exam to detect compression of the urethra in cases of bruising or mucosa damage, with iodate contrast agent diffused into the periurethral area or the spongy tissue with subsequent spongiography and visualization of the drainage veins.

Sonography is very useful to detect lesions of the periurethral tissues and particularly the small fluid collections that compress or communicate with the urethral lumen. The procedure is commonly performed in all patients with perineo-scrotal trauma when testicular rupture is suspected. CT and MR imaging can be used to evaluate the extension of fluid collections and bone fractures, while MR imaging shows a very high sensitivity in the detection of tunica albuginea ruptures (CHANG and YEH 1992; BARBAGLI et al. 1995).

19.3.7
Cysts

Paraurethral cysts of non-traumatic origin are very rare with only a few cases described in the literature (HAKENBERG et al. 2000; BUJONS et al. 2006). They are usually secondary to submucosal gland distension and appear at ultrasound as lesions with typical anechoic appearance (Fig. 19.10) that adject in the distended urethral lumen. Sonourethrography is indicated to locate the lesion and to assess the relationships with the urethra.

19.3.8
Tumors

Primitive benign or malignant lesions of the male urethra account for only 1% of urological tumors

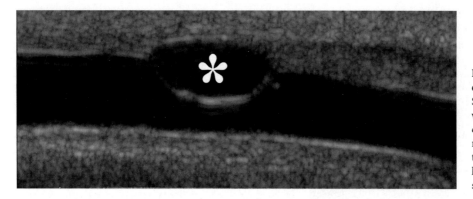

Fig. 19.10. Mucosal cyst of the penile urethra. Sonourethrography with sagittal scan. The cyst (*) is anechoic with regular margin and protrudes into the urethral lumen distended with saline solution

(FELLOWS et al. 1987). Therapy and prognosis depend very much on the site of onset. Depending on their origin they show different histological structures, which may be transitional or malpighian cells. Secondary tumors are much more frequent and are generally caused by seeding of urothelial vesical neoplasms repeatedly treated with endoscopy. These secondary metastases are more common at the bladder neck and in the posterior urethra (Fig. 19.11) and are sometimes located at the level of a post-inflammatory longstanding stenosis. Primary tumors located in the prostatic urethra are usually transitional cell carcinoma and can be differentiated from prostatic carcinoma that have infiltrated the posterior urethra.

Tumors of the penile urethra are more often epidermoidal and are not particularly aggressive or malignant. Neoplasms of the external meatus are usually papillomas or acuminate condylomata. In papillary lesions, radiological examination and sonourethrography show a single or multiple endoluminal filling defects or a growing mass, usually associated with stenosis. Infiltrating tumors on the other hand trigger extensive and tight stenoses, which often prevent opacification of the urethral lumen lying above the lesion. In these cases sonourethrography (PAVLICA et al. 2003a) is particularly useful since it can detect the spread into the surrounding periurethral tissue (Fig. 19.12). Neoformations of the posterior urethra can be better studied with transrectal sonography. When they spread to the urethra, acuminate condylomata present as multiple endoluminal masses that do not allow retrograde distension of the penile urethra.

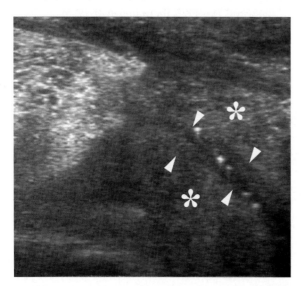

Fig. 19.11. Metastatic involvement of the urethra. Patient presenting with blood discharge 1 year after cistectomy and radical prostatectomy for bladder cancer. Transrectal sagittal scan showing encasement of the urethral stump (*arrowheads*) by recurrent tumor tissue (*)

19.4
Diagnostic Role of Other Imaging Modalities

CT has a limited role in the evaluation of the urethra. Certain urethral abnormalities such as calculi or diverticula may be incidentally discovered at CT performed for other indications. CT is useful in patients with pelvic trauma (CHOU et al. 2005) and associated urethral injuries and for staging of urethral carcinoma. CT virtual cystoscopy and voiding urethrography can be indicated in patients with complex urethral strictures and malformations.

Magnetic resonance imaging is not widely used to evaluate the urethra. The technique is complex and

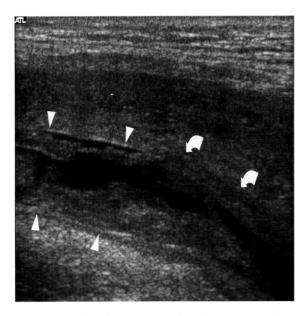

Fig. 19.12. Infiltrating transitional cell carcinoma of the bulbous urethra. Sonourethrography in sagittal scan. The sonogram shows the lesion protruding in the urethral lumen (*arrowheads*) with secondary stenosis. The surrounding spongiosa is involved (*curved arrows*)

offers little extra information that cannot be obtained by radiographic urethrography and sonourethrography. However, due to multiplanar capability and excellent tissue contrast, it provides excellent anatomical detail of both the urethra and periurethral tissues (Ryu and Kim 2001). Distension of the urethra is obtained with saline solution after a small Foley catheter is placed in the fossa navicularis. Imaging is performed using a surface coil that employs a small field of view with multiplanar T1- and T2-weighted sequences. The exam is indicated for evaluation of complex malformations, for staging of tumors, assessment of traumas and for the diagnosis of spongiofibrosis, which is associated with inflammatory urethral stenosis (Kawashima et al. 2004). Contrast medium is injected to evaluate tumors and the degree of activity in inflammatory lesions (Pavlica et al. 2003a; Pavlica et al. 2003b).

References

Barbagli G, Azzaro F, Menchi I et al (1995) Bacteriologic, histologic and ultrasonographic findings in strictures recurring after urethrotomy. A preliminary study. Scand J Urol Nephrol 29:193–195

Bearcroft PW, Berman LH (1994) Sonography in the evaluation of the male anterior urethra. Clin Radiol 49:621–626

Blaivas JG, Norlen LJ (1984) Primary bladder neck obstruction. World J Urol 2:191–195

Bujons A, Ponce de Leon X, Baez C et al (2006) [Paraurethral cyst of the Littre's gland: an exceptional case]. Arch Esp Urol 59:624–626

Callea A, Macchia R, Balacco G et al (1997) [Echodynamics of the cervical ureter junction]. Arch Ital Urol Androl 69:185–187

Chang SC, Yeh CH (1992) The applications of dynamic transrectal ultrasound in the lower urinary tract of men and women. Ultrasound Quarterly 10:185–223

Chiou RK, Anderson JC, Tran T et al (1996) Evaluation of urethral strictures and associated abnormalities using high-resolution and color Doppler ultrasound. Urology 47:102–107

Chou CP, Huang JS, Wu MT et al (2005) CT voiding urethrography and virtual urethroscopy: preliminary study with 16-MDCT. AJR Am J Roentgenol 184:1882–1888

Cohen HL, Susman M, Haller JO et al (1994) Posterior urethral valve: transperineal US for imaging and diagnosis in male infants. Radiology 192:261–264

Das S (1992) Ultrasonographic evaluation of urethral stricture disease. Urology 40:237–242

Desser TS, Nino-Murcia M, Olcott EW, Terris MK (1999) Advantages of performing sonourethrography with lidocaine hydrochloride jelly in a prepackaged delivery system. AJR Am J Roentgenol 173:39–40

Fellows GJ, Cannell LB, Ravichandran G (1987) Transrectal ultrasonography compared with voiding cystourethrography after spinal cord injury. Br J Urol 59:218–221

Friedland GW (1990) The urethra-imaging and intervention in the 1990s. Clin Radiol 42:157–160

Giudici L, Costato C, Ricci-Barbini V (1991) [Transrectal echographic micturitional evaluation of bladder neck pathology]. Arch Ital Urol Nefrol Androl 63 [Suppl 2]:69–71

Gluck CD, Bundy AL, Fine C et al (1988) Sonographic urethrogram: comparison to roentgenographic techniques in 22 patients. J Urol 140:1404–1408

Gupta S, Majumdar B, Tiwari A et al (1993) Sonourethrography in the evaluation of anterior urethral strictures: correlation with radiographic urethrography. J Clin Ultrasound 21:231–239

Hakenberg OW, Froehner M, Wirth MP (2000) Symptomatic paraurethral corpus spongiosum cyst in a male patient. Urology 55:590

Hoebeke PB, Van Laecke E, Raes A et al (1997) Membranobulbo-urethral junction stenosis. Posterior urethra obstruction due to extreme caliber disproportion in the male urethra. Eur Urol 32:480–484

Kawashima A, Sandler CM, Wasserman NF et al (2004) Imaging of urethral disease: a pictorial review. Radiographics 24 [Suppl 1]:S195–216

Maizels M, Stephens FD, King LR, Firlit CF (1983) Cowper's syringocele: a classification of dilatations of Cowper's gland duct based upon clinical characteristics of eight boys. J Urol 129:111–114

McAninch JW, Laing FC, Jeffrey RB Jr (1988) Sonourethrography in the evaluation of urethral strictures: a preliminary report. J Urol 139:294–297

Merchant SA, Amonkar PP, Patil JA (1997) Imperforate syringoceles of the bulbourethral duct: appearance on urethrography, sonography, and CT. AJR Am J Roentgenol 169:823–824

Merkle W, Wagner W (1988) Sonography of the distal male urethra–a new diagnostic procedure for urethral strictures: results of a retrospective study. J Urol 140:1409–1411

Morey AF, McAninch JW (1997) Role of preoperative sono-urethrography in bulbar urethral reconstruction. J Urol 158:1376–1379

Morey AF, McAninch JW, Duckett CP, Rogers RS (1998) American Urological Association symptom index in the assessment of urethroplasty outcomes. J Urol 159:1192–1194

Nash PA, McAninch JW, Bruce JE, Hanks DK (1995) Sono-urethrography in the evaluation of anterior urethral strictures. J Urol 154:72–76

Pavlica P, Barozzi L, Menchi I (2003a) Imaging of male urethra. Eur Radiol 13:1583–1596

Pavlica P, Menchi I, Barozzi L (2003b) New imaging of the anterior male urethra. Abdom Imaging 28:180–186

Perkash I, Friedland GW (1987) Ultrasonographic detection of false passages arising from the posterior urethra in spinal cord injury patients. J Urol 137:701–702

Ryu J, Kim B (2001) MR imaging of the male and female urethra. Radiographics 21:1169–1185

Salam MA (2006) Posterior urethral valve: Outcome of antenatal intervention. Int J Urol 13:1317–1322

Sepulveda W, Elorza C, Gutierrez J et al (2005) Congenital megalourethra: outcome after prenatal diagnosis in a series of four cases. J Ultrasound Med 24:1303–1308

Shabsigh R, Fishman IJ, Krebs M (1987) The use of transrectal longitudinal real-time ultrasonography in urodynamics. J Urol 138:1416–1419

Yekeler E, Suleyman E, Tunaci A et al (2004) Contrast-enhanced 3D MR voiding urethrography: preliminary results. Magn Reson Imaging 22:1193–1199

Miscellaneous Benign Diseases

20

Michele Bertolotto, Pietro Pavlica, and Manuel Belgrano

CONTENTS

20.1 Penile Cysts 175
20.1.1 Median Raphe Cysts 175
20.1.2 Epidermoid Cysts 175
20.1.3 Sebaceous Cysts 177
20.1.4 Dermoid Cysts 177
20.1.5 Paraurethral Cysts and Syringocele 177

20.2 Sclerosing Lymphangitis of the Penis 177

20.3 Fibrous Hamartoma of the Corpus Cavernosum 178

20.4 Idiopathic Deep Dorsal Vein Thrombosis 178

20.5 Partial Segmental Thrombosis of the Corpus Cavernosum 179

20.6 Penile Calciphylaxis 180

20.7 Parasitic Infection of the Penis 180

20.8 Urethral Manipulation Syndrome 182

References 182

20.1 Penile Cysts

A variety of cystic lumps can be recognized in the penis, either congenital or acquired. Diagnosis of most of them is straightforward based on clinical appearance, but imaging can be required, especially in large lesions, to confirm diagnosis and to assess relationships with adjacent penile structures.

M. Bertolotto, MD; M. Belgrano, MD
Department of Radiology, University of Trieste, Ospedale di Cattinara, strada di Fiume 447, Trieste, 34124, Italy
P. Pavlica, MD
Department of Radiology, University Hospital S. Orsola-Malpighi, Via Massarenti 9, Bologna, 40138, Italy

20.1.1 Median Raphe Cysts

These uncommon benign lesions are due to entrapment of epithelial cells during fusion of the labial scrotal folds. They can occur anywhere along the penile or scrotal raphe from the anus to the urinary meatus and are usually asymptomatic, but can get secondarily infected (Cardoso et al. 2005). When located on the border of the urethral meatus, which is the predominant site, they are also known as parameatal cysts (Otsuka et al. 1998). Most are present from birth and remain undetectable until adolescence or adulthood, occurring as a solitary freely movable nodule on the ventral surface of the penis.

Histopathologically, the luminar surface wall of all cysts consists of pseudostratified columnar epithelium with large polygonal cells developing apocrine metaplasia in the free border. The content of all cysts was clear mucinous fluid. At ultrasound they usually appear as simple cysts, with typically anechoic content (Pavlica 1998).

20.1.2 Epidermoid Cysts

These lesions result from the proliferation of epidermal cells within a circumscribed space of the dermis. They are composed of keratin producing epithelium and can be distinguished from dermoid cysts, which contain skin and skin appendages, and from sebaceous cysts.

Clinically, epidermoid cysts appear as firm, oval or lobulated nodules of variable size located either on the dorsum of the penis or, less frequently, on the ventral aspect of the penile shaft (Rattan et al. 1997). They are more often encountered in childhood, but can occur also in middle age and in the elderly.

These lesions are usually slowly growing and asymptomatic, but occasionally can grow rapidly and get inflamed. Large epidermoid cysts may interfere with intercourse and cause problems with walking or wearing underwear. They can also interfere with urination.

Therapy consists of surgical removal of the mass. Imaging is often required in patients with large, rapidly growing epidermoid cysts to confirm the cystic nature of the lesion and assess the relationship with adjacent organs.

At ultrasound (Fig. 20.1) epidermoid cysts appear as ovoid or lobulated masses with well-defined margins, with relatively echogenic content with hypoechoic foci. Calcifications are occasionally identified. No vascularity is recognized at color Doppler interrogation.

Ruptured cysts may have more lobulated contours and show perilesional Doppler signals. Calcified cysts appear as solid hypoechoic masses with multiple calcified foci associated with dense digital acoustic shadowing.

At magnetic resonance imaging (Fig. 20.1), epidermoid cysts present with well-circumscribed masses lacking internal contrast enhancement. On T1-weighted images signal intensity is similar or higher compared to muscle, while signal intensity is high on T2-weighted images. Irregular low-signal intensity areas are recognized on both T1- and T2-weighted images.

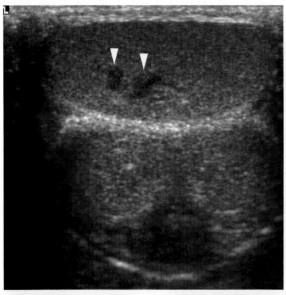

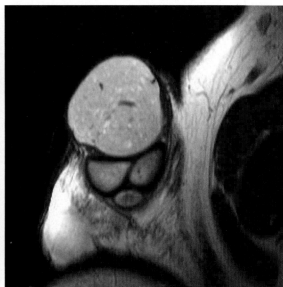

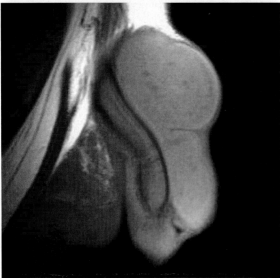

Fig. 20.1a–c. Epidermoid cyst of the penis. **a** Axial ultrasound scan showing a well-circumscribed mass with echogenic content containing hypoechoic foci (*arrowheads*). **b,c** Magnetic resonance imaging. **b** Axial T2-weighted image showing a high signal intensity lesion with irregular low signal intensity foci. **c** Sagittal T1-weighted image showing an intermediate signal intensity mass containing low signal intensity foci

20.1.3
Sebaceous Cysts

These lesions are formed by an abnormal sac of retained excretion from the sebaceous follicles and appear as tender, painless flesh-colored or whitish-yellow lumps underneath the skin.

Sebaceous cysts are found most commonly on the scrotum, but can be found on the penile shaft as well. Usually they do not require treatment. Surgical excision can be indicated when they continue to grow or become unsightly, painful and infected. Infected cysts may require oral antibiotics or other treatment before excision.

At ultrasound sebaceous cysts present as homogeneously hypoechoic or relatively echogenic nodules within the dermis, with well-defined margins (Fig. 20.2). No vascular signals are recorded at color Doppler interrogation. Infected sebaceous cysts may present with increased vascularity of the surrounding soft tissue.

20.1.4
Dermoid Cysts

These lesions are extremely rare in the penis with only few cases reported in the literature (AIDAROV and ZOLOTAREV 1962; TOMASINI et al. 1997). In contrast to epidermoid cysts, dermoid cysts are lined by an epidermis that possesses various fully mature epidermal appendages. Hair follicles containing hairs that project into the lumen are often present. The dermis usually contains sebaceous glands, eccrine glands and, in many patients, apocrine glands.

The appearance of penile dermoid cysts at ultrasound and magnetic resonance imaging has not been described, but it is conceivable that it should be similar to that of dermoid cysts in the scrotum (DOGRA et al. 2001).

20.1.5
Paraurethral Cysts and Syringocele

These lesions have been described in Chapter 19. In brief, paraurethral cysts are usually secondary to submucosal gland distension and appear at ultrasound with a typical anechoic appearance. Syringocele presents at sonourethrography as a tubular image at the bulbous urethra, parallel to the urethral canal, with a "double tube" appearance.

20.2
Sclerosing Lymphangitis of the Penis

Sclerosing lymphangitis of the penis is a rare condition involving the distal lymphatics that is characterized by a cord-like lesion just proximal to the

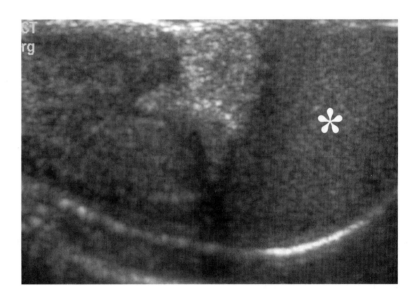

Fig. 20.2. Axial scan. Sebaceous cyst of the penis presenting as a homogeneously echogenic lesion (*)

coronal sulcus. It is most commonly associated with vigorous sexual activity, but it is also seen with infections including gonorrhea, syphilis, chlamydia and herpes (LEE et al. 2003).

Histological study reveals hypertrophy and sclerosis of lymphatic vessel walls and, in some cases, thrombus formation within the dilated vessels (LEE et al. 2003). Most cases are self-limited, lasting only a few weeks, and conservative management is indicated. Treatment has traditionally consisted of avoidance of vigorous sexual activity until the lesion disappears. In a few rare cases in which there are persistent symptomatic lesions, surgery is indicated.

Diagnosis is based on typical clinical presentation. Ultrasonography confirms the diagnosis showing a dilated serpiginous structure with anechoic content resembling rosary beads (Fig. 20.3). No color signals are appreciable at Doppler interrogation.

20.3
Fibrous Hamartoma of the Corpus Cavernosum

As occurs for fibrous amartomatous lesions elsewhere in the body, this extremely rare, probably dysembriogenetic lesion is characterized by the presence of tissue maintaining the same histological features of the normal cavernosal bodies, but with altered architecture by the presence of increased fibrotic component and reduced vascular and smooth muscle components.

Clinically, the lesion presents as a palpable mass in patients with congenital penile curvature and erectile dysfunction. Ultrasound features are indistinguishable from those of a classic fibrotic lesion (BERTACCINI et al. 2004). A mostly hyperechoic lesion is identified, displaying no vascularity at color Doppler interrogation. At magnetic resonance imaging the lesion presents with low signal intensity on T2-weighted images (Fig. 20.4).

20.4
Idiopathic Deep Dorsal Vein Thrombosis

Thrombosis of the deep dorsal vein can be associated with thrombophilia (SCHMIDT et al. 2000), can result from reduced penile blood outflow in patients with pelvic malignancies and infiltration of the cavernosal veins or may results from trauma, inflammation or following vigorous intercourse. This pathological condition, however, may also

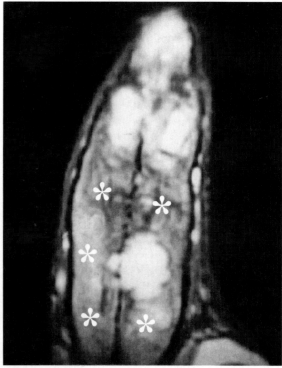

Fig. 20.4. Fibrous hamartoma of the corpora cavernosa. Coronal T2-weighted image showing relatively low signal intensity tissue (*) replacing wide portions of the normal hyperintense cavernosal tissue

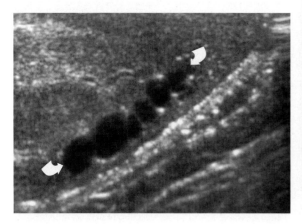

Fig. 20.3. Sclerosing lymphangitis of the penis. Axial scan showing a serpiginous anechoic structure (*curved arrows*) proximal to the coronal sulcus resembling rosary beads

present spontaneously in patients without known risk factors.

Clinically, the patients present with a rod-like painless induration in the dorsal aspect of the shaft. Clinical signs and symptoms suggestive for thrombophebitis, such as fever and local pain, are not associated with the idiopathic form.

Grey-scale and color Doppler ultrasonography show complete and segmental thrombosis of the deep dorsal penile vein, isolated or associated with thrombosis of the circumflex veins, by the presence of echogenic material within the vessels (Fig. 20.5), which does not change in shape following compression with the transducer.

The disease is usually treated with fibrinolytics and anticoagulation, associated with discontinuance of sexual activity. Spontaneous resolution usually occurs within 6–8 weeks.

20.5
Partial Segmental Thrombosis of the Corpus Cavernosum

This uncommon clinical situation, often inaccurately called partial segmental priapism, is characterized by thrombosis of an isolated portion of a corpus cavernosum, either idiopathic or associated with a traumatic event. In particular, crural segmental thrombosis may result from chronic perineal saddle trauma in patients with a history of extensive bicycle riding.

Thrombus formation has been associated with the presence of a membrane isolating the involved crus, which prevents the usual free communication of blood among the crura and the remainder of the corpora cavernosa. Although a congenital origin for this cavernosal web has been initially suggested, increasing evidence shows that it is in most cases a posttraumatic scar.

Clinically, the patients present with persistent painful swelling of the involved cavernosal crus (HORGER et al. 2005). Physical examination reveals a firm mass. Complete resolution of symptoms and resumption of normal erectile function are reported in most cases; conservative management is therefore advocated (GOEMAN et al. 2003; HORGER et al. 2005).

Imaging allows differential diagnosis between partial segmental thrombosis and other penile masses. At ultrasound a heterogeneously echogenic mass is identified, replacing the affected portion of the corpus cavernosum (Fig. 20.6). No vascular signals are recognized at color Doppler ultrasonography (THIEL et al. 1998; GOEMAN et al. 2003).

At CT the penile thrombus presents as a tubular-shaped mass of fluid density with no internal enhancement and mild peripheral enhancement (BURKHALTER and MORANO 1985; PTAK et al. 1994).

The appearance of a thrombus at magnetic resonance imaging characteristically varies with time on both T1-weighted and T2-weighted images depending on the oxygenation and degradation of its contained hemoglobin (UNGER et al. 1986). No enhancement is recognized after gadolinium administration (KIMBALL et al. 1988; PTAK et al. 1994; THIEL et al. 1998; GOEMAN et al. 2003; HORGER et al. 2005).

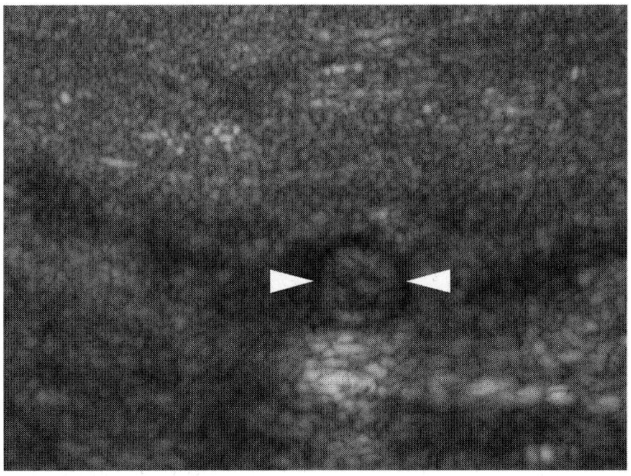

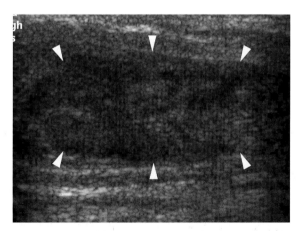

Fig. 20.5. Idiopathic deep dorsal vein thrombosis. Axial scan showing echogenic material within the deep dorsal vein (*arrowheads*)

Fig. 20.6. Partial segmental thombosis of the corpus cavernosum. Longitudinal scan showing the thrombus (*arrowheads*) replacing the crus of the left corpus cavernosum

20.6 Penile Calciphylaxis

Calciphylaxis is a rare life-threatening disorder characterized by progressive vascular calcification and ischemic tissue loss in patients with end-stage renal disease (Wood et al. 1997; Hafner et al. 1998; Karpman et al. 2003; Guvel et al. 2004). The pathogenesis is poorly understood; it is likely the result of a multiplicity of co-morbid factors or events. Disorders that are most often implicated include chronic renal failure, hypercalcemia, hyperphosphatemia, an elevated calcium-phosphate product and secondary hyperparathyroidism. Very rare cases of calciphylaxis not associated with chronic renal failure have been reported with breast cancer, hyperparathyroidism and alcoholic cirrhosis.

Histological characteristics of calciphylaxis include small-vessel calcifications of the skin, subcutaneous tissue and visceral organs. These vascular changes promote tissue ischemia that often results in tissue necrosis.

While systemic calciphylaxis affects 1% of patients with end-stage renal disease, penile involvement has rarely been reported (Wood et al. 1997; Karpman et al. 2003; Guvel et al. 2004). The disease results from medial calcification and fibrosis of penile blood vessels. The co-morbidity and mortality associated with this disease are extremely high (Guvel et al. 2004). The disease results in penile infection and gangrene. Most cases are associated with systemic calciphylaxis. Ischemia may be circumscribed to the glans or may involve the entire shaft. Treatment may be either surgical or conservative, depending on the extent of the ischemia and on the patient's general condition (Guvel et al. 2004).

Clinically, the patients usually present with penile induration and severe pain that are unresponsive to narcotics. This situation may be misinterpreted, leading to incorrect diagnosis of low-flow priapism and inappropriate management.

Grey-scale and color Doppler ultrasonography characteristically show widespread calcification (Fig. 20.7) of the tunica albuginea, of the cavernosal arteries and obliteration of the distal segments of the penile vessels. In patients with severe presentation, the entire penile vascular tree may be calcified. Small calcifications can be occasionally identified within the cavernosal tissue as well.

Pudendal angiography and contrast-enhanced CT confirm occlusion of the vascular supply to the penis (Guvel et al. 2004), but are usually not indicated in these severely ill patients with end-stage renal disease. Plain film radiographs and non-contrast CT (Fig. 20.7) demonstrate severe calcification in the penile arteries and in the tunica albuginea (Karpman et al. 2003).

20.7 Parasitic Infection of the Penis

Most of the parasitic infestations of the penis are of dermatologic interest and recognized based on clinical appearance alone. Imaging is usually not required. Among the most common situations, scabies and pediculosis pubis should be considered. In scabies, in particular, multiple typical scabetic

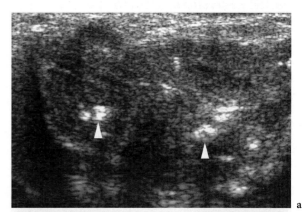

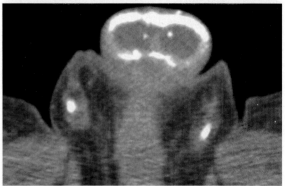

Fig. 20.7a,b. Penile calciphylaxis. a Axial ultrasound scan showing diffuse calcification of the tunica albuginea and of the cavernosal arteries (*arrowheads*). b Calcifications are better appreciable at non-contrast TC

burrows and papules are often present on the glans penis, scrotum and penis shaft.

Some parasitic diseases, however, can present with penile lumps and cause problems in diagnosis. Imaging could be indicated for better definition before surgical removal, especially when these lesions are recognized far from the endemic geographic areas. In fact, with the continuing increase in international travel, these diseases can manifest almost anywhere in the world.

Onchocerchiasis is caused by a parasitic roundworm transmitted by the bite of the black fly endemic to tropical Africa, Yemen, Mexico, Guatemala, Venezuela, Brazil and Colombia. Humans, gorillas and chimpanzees are the only hosts of this disease. Adult worms are typically found as nodules in subcutaneous tissues. Microfilariae are present in the skin, where they may be asymptomatic or cause a variety of dermatological manifestations. Ocular involvement is the most severe complication, which can lead to blindness.

A case of penile onchocerchiasis has been reported, presenting as a painless nodule in the mid portion of each crus of the corpus cavernosum, which increased in size and became painful within 14 months. Imaging was not performed in this case (MEYER and NOSANCHUK 1996).

Sparganosis is a rare parasitic disease that is caused by the plerocercoid, sparganum, or various tapeworms of the genus Spirometra. The cycle of the parasite requires two intermediate hosts. The first is a copepod, a planktonic crustacean that ingests embryos that develop from the tapeworm's eggs when they reach the water with the feces of dogs or cats (the worm's normal host). The infected copepod is then ingested by one of many vertebrates, including humans.

Human infection can occur by drinking water contaminated with copepods infected with the procercoid larval stage of the parasite, through ingestion of undercooked meat infected with the plerocercoids and by placing poultices of frog or snake flesh on open wounds, other lesions, or the eyes. This practice is common in many Asian cultures.

Sparganosis is reported sporadically around the world; a higher prevalence of the disease occurs in several Asian countries. The highest endemicity of sparganosis is in Korea and Japan, mostly because of dietary customs.

The clinical manifestations of sparganosis depend on which organs or tissues are involved. Subcutaneous tissues, superficial muscles and fascia are most likely to be infected, but the parasite has been recovered on any part of the body, including the scrotum (KIM et al. 2007) and penis (KIM 2001). The larval worms usually grow slowly into irregular nodules. A local tissue reaction results in an itchy, inflamed and painful lump.

There are no specific treatments, but the spargana may be removed surgically. Prevention involves avoiding eating potentially infected foods and drinking contaminated water.

A typical ultrasound appearance of spargana has been described (KIM 2001; KIM et al. 2007). A poorly defined inflammatory mass is identified, containing multiple elongated tubular hypoechoic structures and serpiginous echogenic lesions, consistent with empty tracts caused by the migration of the sparganum larvae, and with presence of the larvae themselves. Intermittent whirling movements can be observed during the ultrasound examination (Fig. 20.8).

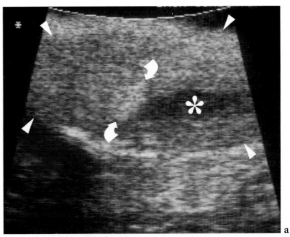

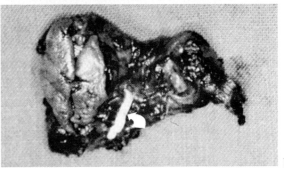

Fig. 20.8a,b. Penile sparganosis. **a** Longitudinal scan showing an ill-defined lesion (*arrowheads*) containing an elongated hyperechoic area (*curved arrows*) and a hypoechoic tubular structure (*). **b** Photograph of the removed mass showing a white live worm (*curved arrow*). [Reprinted with permission from: Kim SH (2001) Imaging for evaluation of erectile dysfunction. J Korean Soc Med Ultrasound 20:1-13]

20.8 Urethral Manipulation Syndrome

Ventral penile deviation following any kind of urethral manipulation is known by the name of urethral manipulation syndrome or Kelami syndrome (KELAMI 1984). This condition is due to fibrosis and scarring of the corpus spongiosum. Ventral penile deviation is noticed only in sexually active patients. Partial, gradual disappearance of glans engorgement and irregularities palpable along the penile urethra are constant findings. Surgical treatment is indicated when the deformity interferes with sexual intercourse or is accompanied by severe urethral strictures.

Diagnosis of Kelami syndrome is based on clinics and the history of iatrogenic urethral manipulation and confirmed by identification at ultrasonography of circumscribed fibrotic changes within the corpus spongiosum (Fig. 20.9).

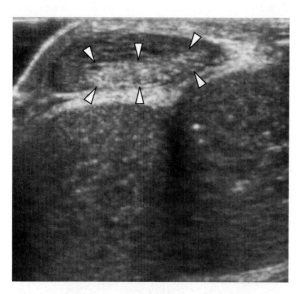

Fig. 20.9. Kelami syndrome. Patient with a history of repeated endourethral maneuvers presenting with ventral penile curvature. Axial ultrasound scan showing an area of circumscribed fibrosis (*arrowheads*) at the middle portion of the corpus spongiosum

References

Aidarov AA, Zolotarev MA (1962) [Dermoid cyst of the penis.]. Urol Mosc 27:71

Bertaccini A, Marchiori D, Giovannini C et al (2004) Fibrous hamartoma of corpus cavernosum: a rare cause of congenital penile curvature associated with erectile dysfunction. J Urol 172:642–643

Burkhalter JL, Morano JU (1985) Partial priapism: the role of CT in its diagnosis. Radiology 156:159

Cardoso R, Freitas JD, Reis JP, Tellechea O (2005) Median raphe cyst of the penis. Dermatol Online J 11:37

Dogra VS, Gottlieb RH, Rubens DJ, Liao L (2001) Benign intratesticular cystic lesions: US features. Radiographics 21 Spec no:S273–281

Goeman L, Joniau S, Oyen R et al (2003) Idiopathic partial thrombosis of the corpus cavernosum: conservative management is effective and possible. Eur Urol 44:119–123

Guvel S, Yaycioglu O, Kilinc F et al (2004) Penile necrosis in end-stage renal disease. J Androl 25:25–29

Hafner J, Keusch G, Wahl C, Burg G (1998) Calciphylaxis: a syndrome of skin necrosis and acral gangrene in chronic renal failure. Vasa 27:137–143

Horger DC, Wingo MS, Keane TE (2005) Partial segmental thrombosis of corpus cavernosum: case report and review of world literature. Urology 66:194

Karpman E, Das S, Kurzrock EA (2003) Penile calciphylaxis: analysis of risk factors and mortality. J Urol 169:2206–2209

Kelami A (1984) Urethral manipulation syndrome. Description of a new syndrome. Urol Int 39:352–354

Kim S (2001) Imaging for evaluation of erectile dysfunction. J Korean Soc Med Ultrasound 20:1–13

Kim YJ, Lee MW, Jeon HJ et al (2007) Sparganosis in the scrotum: sonographic findings. J Ultrasound Med 26:129–131

Kimball DA, Yuh WT, Farner RM (1988) MR diagnosis of penile thrombosis. J Comput Assist Tomogr 12:604–607

Lee S, Moon Y, Kim D et al (2003) Three cases of sclerosing lymphangitis of the penis. Korean J Androl 21:48–51

Meyer R, Nosanchuk J (1996) Parasitic infection of the penis. J Urol 155:2030–2031

Otsuka T, Ueda Y, Terauchi M, Kinoshita Y (1998) Median raphe (parameatal) cysts of the penis. J Urol 159:1918–1920

Pavlica PB, L. (1998) Ultrasound of penile tumors and trauma. Ultrasound Q 14:95–109

Ptak T, Larsen CR, Beckmann CF, Boyle DE Jr (1994) Idiopathic segmental thrombosis of the corpus cavernosum as a cause of partial priapism. Abdom Imaging 19:564–566

Rattan J, Rattan S, Gupta DK (1997) Epidermoid cyst of the penis with extension into the pelvis. J Urol 158:593

Schmidt BA, Schwarz T, Schellong SM (2000) Spontaneous thrombosis of the deep dorsal penile vein in a patient with thrombophilia. J Urol 164:1649

Thiel R, Kahn T, Vogeli TA (1998) Idiopathic partial thrombosis of the corpus cavernosum. Urol Int 60:178–180

Tomasini C, Aloi F, Puiatti P, Caliendo V (1997) Dermoid cyst of the penis. Dermatology 194:188–190

Unger EC, Glazer HS, Lee JK, Ling D (1986) MRI of extracranial hematomas: preliminary observations. AJR Am J Roentgenol 146:403–407

Wood JC, Monga M, Hellstrom WJ (1997) Penile calciphylaxis. Urology 50:622–624

Contrast-Enhanced US of the Penis

Michele Bertolotto, Stefano Bucci, and Roberta Zappetti

CONTENTS

21.1 Background 183
21.2 Microbubble Contrast Agents 184
21.3 Examination Technique 184
21.4 Normal Penile Anatomy 184
21.5 Penile Malformations 187
21.6 Impotence 187
21.7 Peyronie's Disease 187
21.8 Traumas 187
21.9 Penile Malignancies 188
21.10 Acute Penile Ischemia 189
21.11 Cavernosal Tissue Scar and Fibrosis 190
21.12 Urethral Pathology 191
References 191

21.1 Background

Contrast-enhanced ultrasonography of superficial organs has long been considered unlikely because the main resonance frequency of these agents, which depends mainly on the size of microbubbles, is in the range of abdominal ultrasound applications. It has been suggested that microbubble contrast agents would not produce useful non-linear signals at the frequencies needed to provide the spatial resolution required for evaluation of superficial structures (Cosgrove 2004).

Ultrasound contrast agents, however, contain microbubbles of different sizes whose resonance frequency range covers the whole range of frequencies used for ultrasound imaging (Greis 2004). In particular, in microbubble distribution there is a substantial tail of small bubbles, which resonate at high frequencies, making possible contrast-specific imaging at high frequencies as well.

However, contrast-specific modes have been implemented in small-part probes only recently. High-performance contrast-specific modes are needed to obtain images of diagnostic quality since the amount of microbubbles that resonates at high frequencies is relatively low, and signal from small resonating particles is much lower than for larger bubbles. While relatively low insonation frequencies of approximately 4–5 MHz have been initially used in small-part probes as well to collect signal from a larger percent of resonating bubbles, transducers operating with frequencies of 7 MHz or higher are now available for clinical use (Cosgrove 2004).

Preliminary investigations on superficial structures show that contrast-enhanced ultrasonography may prove useful for assessing superficial lymph nodes (Rubaltelli et al. 2004), thyroid and parathyroid disease (Cosgrove 2004), muscle and joint pathologies (Krix et al. 2005; Weber et al. 2006), and breast masses (Cassano et al. 2006).

Little has been written on contrast-enhanced ultrasonography of penile disease. Only few preliminary investigations have been done in which first generation microbubble contrast agents and conventional Doppler techniques have been used. To the best of our knowledge, use of the latest generation microbubble contrast agents with contrast-specific ultrasound modes has been reported in a very limited number of cases.

M. Bertolotto, MD; R. Zappetti, MD
Department of Radiology, University of Trieste, Ospedale di Cattinara, Strada di Fiume 447, Trieste, 34124, Italy
S. Bucci, MD
Department of Urology, University of Trieste, Ospedale di Cattinara, Strada di Fiume 447, Trieste, 34124, Italy

21.2
Microbubble Contrast Agents

Contrast agents for ultrasound are microbubbles, 1–7 μm in diameter, which are mainly used as intravascular contrast media, though other ways of administration exist. For instance, these agents can be instilled into the urinary bladder to look for ureteric reflux and into the uterus to check for tubal patency. Though detectable with Doppler systems, special multipulse insonating sequences have been developed that selectively display their presence, whether in large vessels or in the microvasculature (Cosgrove 2006).

The choice of size for clinical microbubbles is determined by the diameter of the pulmonary capillaries, since they must be able to cross the lung bed to produce systemic enhancement after intravenous injection. In practice, this means that they must be smaller than 7 μm in diameter.

Gas microbubbles are by far the most effective scatterers to use in an ultrasound contrast agent, due to their large differences in acoustic impedance compared with the surrounding blood. However, free bubbles smaller than 7 μm can only persist intact for a few seconds in the blood. This is much less than the required time to reach the target organ from the site of injection. In order for the agent to achieve sufficiently long persistence, gas bubbles have to be stabilized with an outer shell.

All ultrasound contrast agents are encapsulated microbubbles. Both stabilizing shell properties and the gas contained in the microbubbles are critical to their effectiveness as contrast agents and to rendering them sufficiently stable (Cosgrove 2006).

Contrast-enhanced ultrasonography is safe (Piscaglia and Bolondi 2006), fast, and easy to perform. What contrast agents really do is to modify the characteristic signature of the echo from blood. When properly insonated, microbubbles work by resonating, rapidly contracting and expanding in response to the pressure changes of the sound wave. Multiple harmonic signals are produced, which can be recorded using specialized "non-destructive" modes. Since signal intensity does not depend on the speed of blood, but only on the amount of microbubbles that are insonated, also very slow flows, and stationary blood can be evaluated.

Levovist (Shering, Berlin) was the first agent approved for general clinical use. It is made of galactose microcrystals whose surfaces provide nidation sites on which air bubbles form when they are suspended in water; they are then stabilized by a trace of palmitic acid, which acts as a surfactant. Perfluorocarbon or octafluoropropane gas-containing agents such as SonoVue (Bracco, Milan, Italy) and Definity (Bristol-Meyers Swibb, Billerica, NJ) are the most currently used in the clinical practice. These agents use phospholipids as a stabilizing membrane.

21.3
Examination Technique

Different examination techniques should be used to image penile vasculature with microbubble contrast agents. While patients with penile malformations, primary penile tumors, and Peyronie's disease are evaluated after cavernosal injection of vasoactive drugs to obtain erection, patients with trauma, ischemic priapism, and penile metastases are examined in basal condition.

Microbubbles can be injected intravenously or directly into the corpora cavernosa. In our clinical practice, we use SonoVue (BR1, Bracco, Milan, Italy), a sulfur hexafluoride-filled microbubble contrast agent licensed for liver imaging in most European countries. When SonoVue is injected intravenously, a bolus of 4.8 ml is needed to image the penis with currently available small-part probes. When SonoVue is injected into the corpora cavernosa, a much lower dose of microbubbles is needed. Typically, 200 μl of contrast agent is diluted to a total volume of 20 ml, and about 0.5 ml of this microbubble suspension is injected in one corpus cavernosum by using a 27-gauge needle. Digital cine clips should be registered during contrast-enhanced ultrasonography to allow accurate retrospective evaluation of the entire study.

21.4
Normal Penile Anatomy

When microbubble contrast agents are injected intravenously, enhancement of the corpora cavernosa depends on penile inflow and intracavernosal pressure.

In patients with normal erection, maximum enhancement is obtained during the onset of erection, when penile blood inflow is maximum, and blood pressure within the corpora cavernosa is still low. In this phase the entire cavernosal artery tree can be evaluated. Cavernosal arteries and their branches enhance within 15–30 s, followed by rapid refill of the cavernosal sinusoids starting from the central portion towards the periphery (Fig. 21.1).

During rigid erection, penile blood inflow is limited, and blood pressure within the corpora cavernosa is high. When microbubbles are injected in this phase, cavernosal arteries and the most proximal portions of their branches enhance, while only limited enhancement of the corpora cavernosa is observed (Fig. 21.2). Homogeneous enhancement of the glans and of the corpus spongiosum is obtained both during penile turgescence and when the penis is fully erect. In patients with erectile dysfunction, enhancement of the corpora cavernosa is less dependent on the phase of erection.

When microbubble contrast agents are injected directly within one corpus cavernosum, enhancement of both corpora is obtained (Fig. 21.3). Microbubbles spread from the site of injection filling the entire corpus, and then the contralateral corpus. Homogeneous enhancement is obtained faster in the tumescent penis, while penile manipulation may be necessary to obtain homogeneous distribution of microbubbles in patients with full erection. The glans and the corpus spongiosum do not enhance.

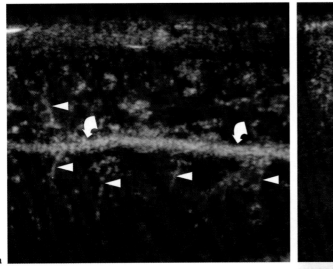

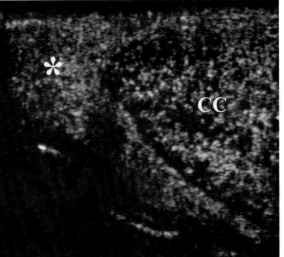

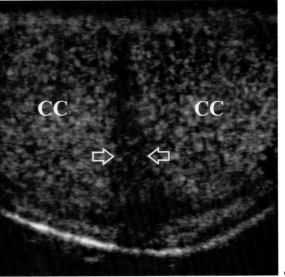

Fig. 21.1a–c. Normal penile anatomy at contrast-enhanced ultrasonography during the onset of erection after intravenous injection of SonoVue microbubbles. a Sagittal scan obtained 30 s after microbubble injection shows enhancement of the cavernosal arteries (*curved arrows*) and helicine arterioles (*arrowheads*). b Sagittal scan on the tip of the penis obtained 160 s after microbubble injection shows enhancement of the corpora cavernosa (*CC*) and of the glans (*). c Axial scan on the midshaft obtained 220 s after microbubble injection shows homogeneous enhancement of both corpora cavernosa (*CC*). The penile septum (*open arrows*) is identified by the presence of acoustic shadow

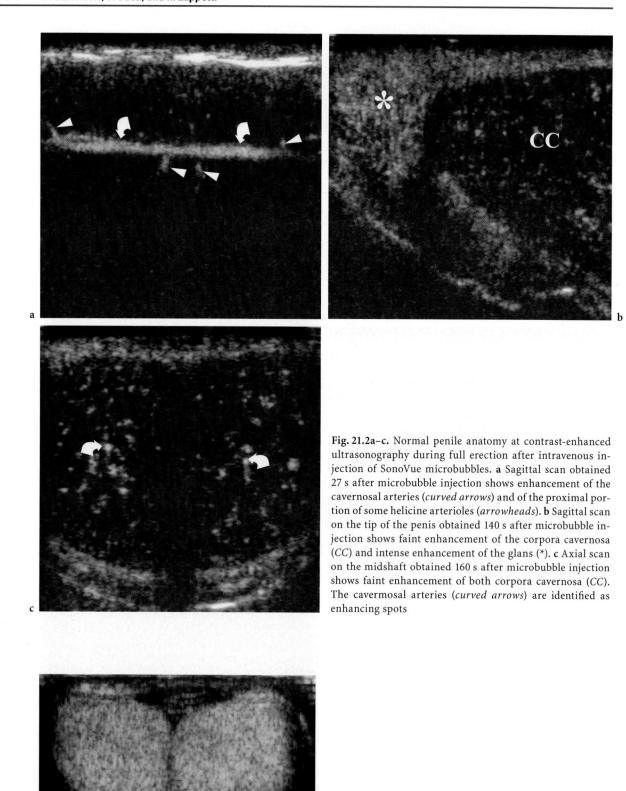

Fig. 21.2a–c. Normal penile anatomy at contrast-enhanced ultrasonography during full erection after intravenous injection of SonoVue microbubbles. **a** Sagittal scan obtained 27 s after microbubble injection shows enhancement of the cavernosal arteries (*curved arrows*) and of the proximal portion of some helicine arterioles (*arrowheads*). **b** Sagittal scan on the tip of the penis obtained 140 s after microbubble injection shows faint enhancement of the corpora cavernosa (*CC*) and intense enhancement of the glans (*). **c** Axial scan on the midshaft obtained 160 s after microbubble injection shows faint enhancement of both corpora cavernosa (*CC*). The cavermosal arteries (*curved arrows*) are identified as enhancing spots

Fig. 21.3. Normal penile anatomy at contrast-enhanced ultrasonography after intracavernosal injection of SonoVue microbubbles showing homogeneous enhancement of the corpora cavarnosa. The corpus spongiosum (*) does not enhance

21.5
Penile Malformations

Complete penile corporeal septation is a rare malformation in which the corpora cavernosa are completely isolated. Although asymmetrical penile turgescence after prostaglandin E1 injection strongly suggests complete penile corporeal septation, other pathologies such as localized fibrosis or hypoplasia of the corpora cavernosa should be considered. Final diagnosis is usually accomplished with cavernosography, which demonstrates that injection of iodinated contrast agent in one corpus cavernosum fails to fill the contralateral cavernosal body. Contrast-enhanced ultrasonography is as effective as cavernosography to obtain the final diagnosis of complete penile corporeal septation showing unilateral enhancement after cavernosal injection of microbubbles (Fig. 21.4).

21.6
Impotence

Contrast-enhanced US was used to evaluate helicine arterioles in subjects with normal erection and with erectile dysfunction (Lencioni et al. 1998). Conventional Doppler techniques have been used. After Levovist injection distal ramifications of helicine arterioles were betted evaluated. Visibility of helicine arteries is reduced in patients with arteriogenic erectile dysfunction and arteriolar damage, such as heavy smokers, diabetic patients, and patients with severe hypertension. As occurs for non-enhanced color Doppler and power Doppler evaluation, however, visibility of helicine arteries strongly depends on penile arterial inflow and on corporeal pressure (Bertolotto and Neumaier 1999). In fact, this evaluation has a limited clinical value.

21.7
Peyronie's Disease

Microbubble contrast agents have been temptatively used to obtain information on the inflammatory state of the albugineal plaques in patient with Peyronie's disease (Carbone et al. 1999). A preliminary study performed with conventional Doppler techniques after intravenous administration of Levovist microbubbles suggests that contrast-enhanced ultrasonography could improve detection of color signals around and within the plaque. Evidence of microvascularization around the plaque should be a sign of active inflammation and evolving disease, while absence of flow signal should be a sign of disease stabilization. Other investigators, however, failed to confirm these findings (Sarteschi et al. 2003). In fact, conventional Doppler techniques are not able to evaluate signals from microvessels (Bruce et al. 2004). Signal from leakage pathways and emissary veins passing through the plaque, blooming, and twinkling artifacts produced by small plaque calcifications may be mistaken for plaque vascularization. It is conceivable that these limitations could be overcome using contrast-specific modes that allow evaluation of very low flow in microvessels as well (Cosgrove 2006). In fact, using these modes, enhancement can be occasionally demonstrated in painful plaques (Fig. 21.5). Differentiation of these signals from those of adjacent vessels, however, remains problematic.

21.8
Traumas

In patients with penile fracture, ultrasonography is able to detect the site of the tear as an interruption of the echogenic line of the tunica albuginea. Small defects, however, could be overlooked. In case of doubt,

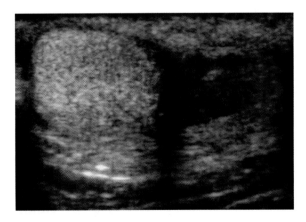

Fig. 21.4. Complete penile corporeal septation. Microbubble injection in the right corpus cavernosum produces unilateral corporeal enhancement

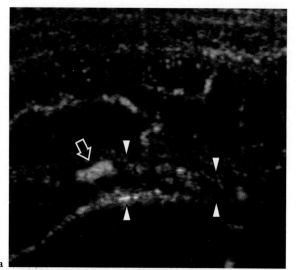

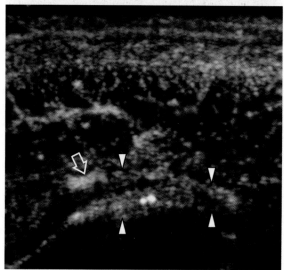

Fig. 21.5a,b. Patient with Peyronie's disease and painful erection. Sagittal scans at the level of a large dorsal plaque (*arrowheads*) obtained during the maximum erection phase reached by the patient after intravenous microbubble administration. **a** At 32 s after microbubble injection arterial vessels enhance. Note a portion of the dorsal artery (*open arrow*) that must be differentiated by plaque enhancement. **b** At 40 s after microbubble injection enhancement of the plaque and surrounding tissue is appreciable.

alone when microbubbles are detected outside the urethral lumen. No investigation is currently available, however, confirming this hypothesis.

21.9 Penile Malignancies

Contrast-enhanced ultrasonography allows differentiation between enhancing solid tumors of the penis and non-enhancing masses, such as complex cystic lesions. Evaluation of patients with penile masses improves when the penis is turgescent, because the relationship between the lesion and the surrounding structures is better delineated. Full erection is not recommended, because enhancement of the corpora cavernosa reduces. Most malignant penile tumors are squamous-cell carcinomas. After intravenous microbubble administration, tumor tissue usually displays early inhomogeneous enhancement, usually less intense than the corporal bodies, and rapid wash out. When a good enhancement of the corpora cavernosa is obtained, tumor spreading within the corpora cavernosa can be evaluated as areas with poor contrast enhancement starting from 1–2 min after microbubble injection. Similar information can be obtained after cavernosal microbubble administration (Fig. 21.6).

Metastatic involvement of the penis can present with distinct tumor nodules or diffuse infiltration of the penile shaft. In patients with diffuse secondary involvement of the shaft, the lesions can be barely visible at ultrasound except for mild alteration of the penile echotexture, diffuse or focal infiltration of the tunica albuginea, or irregular bulking of the penis. Occasionally, isoechoic distinct nodules cannot be identified at grey-scale ultrasonography. After intravenous microbubble administration, patients with secondary involvement of the penis present with profound alteration of penile vasculature. A variable early arterial enhancement is followed by a washout phase in which the corpora cavernosa present with inhomogeneous enhancement. Distinct isoechoic nodules may become appreciable after microbubble administration (Fig. 21.7) because they present with different enhancement characteristics, compared with cavernous tissue (BERTOLOTTO et al. 2005).

contrast-enhanced ultrasonography after cavernosal microbubble injection can be useful to confirm diagnosis and to identify the site of the albugineal tear when contrast extravasation from the corpora cavernosa is observed. It is conceivable that associated urethral injury could be detected by retrograde contrast-enhanced sonourethrography with increased sensitivity compared to grey-scale ultrasonography

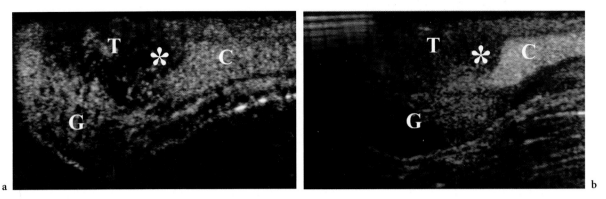

Fig. 21.6a,b. Penile cancer involving the tip of the corpora cavernosa. **a** Sagittal scan obtained on the right corpus cavernosum after intravenous microbubble injection showing enhancement of the glans (*G*) and of the corpus cavernosum (*C*). Tumor (*T*) enhancement is lower compared with enhancement of the erectile bodies. The tip of the right corpus cavernosum (*) presents with irregular borders and poor enhancement by presence of tumor infiltration. **b** Sagittal scan of the same corpus cavernosum obtained after intracavernosal injection of microbubbles confirms infiltration of the corporeal tip (*)

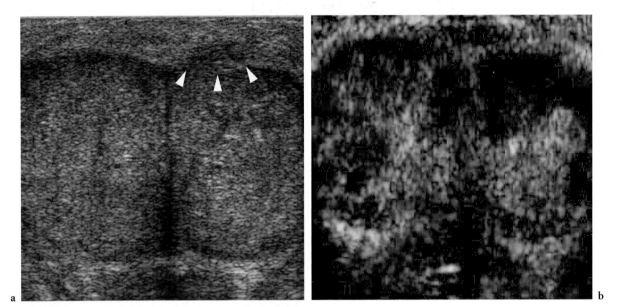

Fig. 21.7a,b. Advanced prostate cancer spreading in the penile shaft. Axial scans. **a** Conventional grey-scale ultrasonography showing infiltration of the corpora cavernosa. The tumor tissue is isoechoic to the cavernous tissue, but can be identified by focal infiltration (*arrowheads*) of the tunica albuginea. **b** Contrast-enhanced ultrasonography. Axial scan obtained after intravenous microbubble injection demonstrates distinct secondary nodules as areas displaying poor contrast enhancement within the cavernosal bodies

21.10
Acute Penile Ischemia

No enhancement of the cavernosal arteries or filling of the central portion of the corpora cavernosa is detected in patients with ischemic priapism. Occasionally, the outer portion of the corpora cavernosa may enhance via collateral pathways. Conversely, enhancement of the glans, of the corpus spongiosum, and of the soft tissues surrounding the corpora cavernosa is usually appreciable (Fig. 21.8).

Cavernosal blood aspiration followed by intracavernous microbubble injection allows identification of non-enhancing cavernosal blood clots. In patients who had undergone shunting procedure, shunt patency can be evaluated when microbubbles injected in the corporal bodies are observed flowing outside the corpora cavernosa (Fig. 21.9).

Acute penile ischemia secondary to calciphylaxis in end-stage renal disease (BARTHELMES et al. 2002), vasculitis, metabolic disease, iatrogenic procedures or trauma is very rare. In fact, collateral circulation usually prevents cavernosal tissue ischemia, also after bilateral occlusion. We observed a patient with Fabry's disease who developed acute penile ischemia. After intravenous microbubble injection, no enhancement of the corpora cavernosa was observed, while only mild enhancement of the soft tissues surrounding the corpora occurred, reflecting compromise of the general circulation.

21.11 Cavernosal Tissue Scar and Fibrosis

Contrary to gadolinium-based and to iodinated contrast agents, microbubbles do not diffuse out of the blood circulation. As a consequence, after intravenous microbubble administration fibrotic tissue shows no enhancement in all vascular phases. At contrast-enhanced ultrasonography, localized cavernosal tissue fibrosis presents as a circumscribed perfusion defect. Diffuse fibrotic changes present with inhomogeneous enhancement of the corpora cavernosa. Contrary to the normal cavernosal tissue, delayed peripheral enhancement of variable degree is often appreciable, probably by the presence of viable subalbugineal cavernosal tissue fed by peripheral vascular pathways, while poor or no contrast enhancement is appreciable in the central portion of the corpora cavernosa (Fig. 21.10).

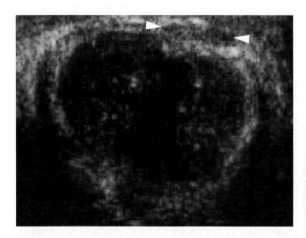

Fig. 21.8. Acute penile ischemia in a patient with low flow priapism and bilateral cavernosal artery occlusion. After intravenous microbubble injection, no enhancement of the corpora cavernosa and of the cavernosal arteries is appreciable, while enhancement of the corpus spongiosum (*arrowheads*) and of the soft tissues surrounding the corpora cavernosa is appreciable

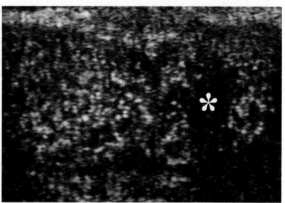

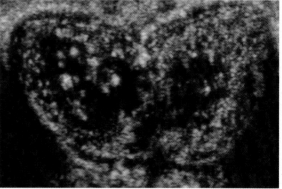

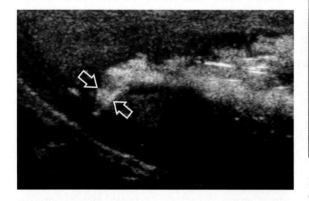

Fig. 21.9. Al-Ghorab shunting in a patient with ischemic priapism. Patency of the shunt is assessed at contrast-enhanced ultrasonography after intracavernosal contrast injection by presence of microbubbles flowing via the shunt (*open arrows*) towards the glans

Fig. 21.10a,b. Cavernosal tissue scar and fibrosis. Axial scans obtained after intravenous microbubble injection. **a** Cavernosal tissue scar within the left corpus cavernosum presenting as a circumscribed area (*) in which contrast enhancement is lacking. **b** Diffuse penile fibrosis following ischemic priapism. Peripheral enhancement of the corpora cavernosa is appreciable, while the central portion does not enhance

21.12 Urethral Pathology

Usually microbubble administration is not required for evaluation of the anterior urethra because sonourethrography after introduction of normal saline solution provides enough clinically useful information (Pavlica et al. 2003). Use of sonographic contrast medium intra-urethrally, however, can be indicated in selected cases to improve the definition of long narrow strictures (Babnik Peskar and Visnar Perovic 2004) and reduce artifacts such as those produced by shadowing caused by severe fibrosis.

Cystosonography with microbubble contrast agents has proved to be a reliable method for the identification and grading of vesicoureteral reflux without the use of ionizing radiation (Berrocal et al. 2001). The main limitation of contrast-enhanced cystosonography compared with conventional voiding cystourethrography was considered to be its difficulty in accurately imaging the urethra (Mentzel et al. 1999). In the latest studies, however, it has been demonstrated that voiding ultrasonography can adequately assess the female, as well as the male, urethra (Berrocal et al. 2005).

Ultrasound evaluation of the posterior urethra is obtained during the voiding phase of contrast-enhanced cytosonography by using a 3.5- or 5-MHz sector array or a 7.5-MHz linear transducer. The examination is often performed in conventional grey-scale ultrasound (Berrocal et al. 2005) using the tissue harmonic mode, when available, but contrast-specific modes, either destructive or non-destructive, can be used as well (Mate et al. 2003; Ascenti et al. 2004) with the advantage of increased sensitivity in detection of signal from microbubbles. The entire procedure is videotaped to allow review of the complete examination in real time. Using this approach, posterior urethral valves are diagnosed at voiding ultrasonography when a dilated posterior urethra is observed with poor distention of the valve area and a reduced caliber of the anterior urethra. A urethral stenosis is diagnosed when a difference in caliber of at least one-third is observed between the pre- and post-stenotic areas (Berrocal et al. 2005). Retrograde contrast-enhanced sonourethrography can be useful for evaluation of complex strictures of the anterior urethra, especially in the bulbar portion (Fig. 21.11).

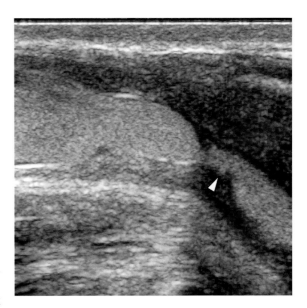

Fig. 21.11. Sagittal scan obtained after SonoVue microbubble administration showing a stenosis of the bulbar urethra (*arrowhead*)

References

Ascenti G, Zimbaro G, Mazziotti S et al (2004) Harmonic US imaging of vesicoureteric reflux in children: usefulness of a second generation US contrast agent. Pediatr Radiol 34:481–487

Babnik Peskar D, Visnar Perovic A (2004) Comparison of radiographic and sonographic urethrography for assessing urethral strictures. Eur Radiol 14:137–144

Barthelmes L, Chezhian C, Thomas KJ (2002) Progression to wet gangrene in penile necrosis and calciphylaxis. Int Urol Nephrol 34:231–235

Berrocal T, Gaya F, Arjonilla A (2005) Vesicoureteral reflux: can the urethra be adequately assessed by using contrast-enhanced voiding US of the bladder? Radiology 234:235–241

Berrocal T, Gaya F, Arjonilla A, Lonergan GJ (2001) Vesicoureteral reflux: diagnosis and grading with echo-enhanced cystosonography versus voiding cystourethrography. Radiology 221:359–365

Bertolotto M, Neumaier CE (1999) Penile sonography. Eur Radiol 9 [Suppl 3]:S407–412

Bertolotto M, Serafini G, Dogliotti L et al (2005) Primary and secondary malignancies of the penis: ultrasound features. Abdom Imaging 30:108–112

Bruce M, Averkiou M, Tiemann K et al (2004) Vascular flow and perfusion imaging with ultrasound contrast agents. Ultrasound Med Biol 30:735–743

Carbone M, Rossi E, Iurassich S et al (1999) [Assessment of microvascularization around the plaques in Peyronie's disease with Doppler color ultrasonography, power Doppler and ultrasonography contrast media]. Radiol Med (Torino) 97:66–69

Cassano E, Rizzo S, Bozzini A et al (2006) Contrast enhanced ultrasound of breast cancer. Cancer Imaging 6:4-6

Cosgrove D (2004) Future prospects for SonoVue and CPS. Eur Radiol 14 [Suppl 8]:P116-124

Cosgrove D (2006) Ultrasound contrast agents: an overview. Eur J Radiol 60:324-330

Greis C (2004) Technology overview: SonoVue (Bracco, Milan). Eur Radiol 14 [Suppl 8]:P11-15

Krix M, Weber MA, Krakowski-Roosen H et al (2005) Assessment of skeletal muscle perfusion using contrast-enhanced ultrasonography. J Ultrasound Med 24:431-441

Lencioni R, Pinto F, Di Giulio M et al (1998) [Contrast media in ultrasonography. Assessment of impotence]. Radiol Med (Torino) 95:75-80

Mate A, Bargiela A, Mosteiro S et al (2003) Contrast ultrasound of the urethra in children. Eur Radiol 13:1534-1537

Mentzel HJ, Vogt S, Patzer L et al (1999) Contrast-enhanced sonography of vesicoureterorenal reflux in children: preliminary results. AJR Am J Roentgenol 173:737-740

Pavlica P, Barozzi L, Menchi I (2003) Imaging of male urethra. Eur Radiol 13:1583-1596

Piscaglia F, Bolondi L (2006) The safety of Sonovue in abdominal applications: retrospective analysis of 23,188 investigations. Ultrasound Med Biol 32:1369-1375

Rubaltelli L, Khadivi Y, Tregnaghi A et al (2004) Evaluation of lymph node perfusion using continuous mode harmonic ultrasonography with a second-generation contrast agent. J Ultrasound Med 23:829-836

Sarteschi L, Morelli G, Menchini-Fabris G (2003) Induratio penis plastica. In: Sarteschi M, Menchini-Fabris G (eds) Ecografia andrologica. Athena, Modena, pp 195-201

Weber MA, Krix M, Jappe U et al (2006) Pathologic skeletal muscle perfusion in patients with myositis: detection with quantitative contrast-enhanced US-initial results. Radiology 238:640-649

Subject Index

3D, see three-dimensional

A

Adaptive Filtering 7
Alcoholism 18
Amputation 92
Anatomy, cavernous arteries 12
– fascia 11
– vascularization of the penile tip 29
– Buck's fascia 11
– bulbourethral arteries 12
– cavernosal-spongiosal communications 32
– cavernous veins 13
– Colles' fascia 11
– color Doppler ultrasonography 28
– – urethral arteries 29
– – cavernous arteries, 28
– – dorsal arteries 29
– – helicine arterioles 31
– – veins 33
– – arterial communications 31
– corpora cavernosa 12
– dartos 11
– dorsal arteries 12
– duplex Doppler interrogation, arterial communications 34
– – cavernosal-spongiosal communications 36
– – cavernous arteries 33
– – dorsal arteries 34
– – helicine arteries 34
– emissary veins 13
– grey-scale ultrasonography 26
– helicine arteries 13
– lymphatics 14
– muscles 12
– nerves 14
– skin 11
– subtunical venular plexus 13
– tunica albuginea 11
– urethra 164
– vasculature 12
– veins 13
Arterial insufficiency, arterial communications 50, 51
– color Doppler ultrasonography 46
– spectral Doppler 48
Audiovisual Sexual Stimulation 42

B

Balanitis, see inflammation
Balanoposthitis, see inflammation
Blunt penile trauma 91
– trauma, ultrasonography 98
Broadband Doppler Technology 5
– Transducers 1, 42

C

Calciphylaxis 180
Capacitive micromachined ultrasonic transducers 2
Cavernositis, see inflammation
Cellulitis, see inflammation
CEUS, anatomy 184
– contrast agents 184
– erectile dysfunction 187
– examination 184
– fibrosis 190
– malformations 187
– penile ischemia 189
– Peyronie's disease 187
– trauma 187
– tumors 188
– urethra 191
Circumcision 139
CMUT see Capacitive micromachined ultrasonic transducers 2
Coded transmission 2
Color Doppler ultrasonography, Timing 45
– Environment 42
Compound, see compounding
Compounding, frequency 6
– spatial 5
Contrast enhanced ultrasonography, see CEUS
Coronary artery disease, penile ultrasonography 22
Cysts 175
– dermoid 177
– epidermoid 175
– median raphe 175
– sebaceous 177

D

Diabetes, 18
Dynamic aperture 4

E

EHGS 41
Erectile dysfunction, arterial insufficiency 17
– – arteriography 51
– – assessment 39
– – cavernosal-spongiosal communications 50
– – cavernosography 51
– – CEUS 187

Erectile dysfunction (*Continued*)
- classification 16
- color Doppler ultrasonography 22, 46
- CT
- definition 21
- diagnosis 21
- epidemiology 16
- grey-scale ultrasonography 45
- helicine arteries 47
- medications 18
- pathophysiology 17
- spectral Doppler 48
- vasculogenic 17
- venogenic 17
- venoocclusive see - venogenic
- ultrasonographic technique 44
Erection, physiology 15
Evaluation Hardness Grading Scale 41
Extended Field of View 7

F

Fibrosis, 72, 84, 91, 153
- cavernosography 160
- cavernosometry 160
- CEUS 190
- circumscribed, 155
- differential diagnosis 159
- diffuse 154
- distal 155
- Doppler ultrasonography, 158
- MRI 160
- proximal 155
- ultrasonography 155
Fibrous hamartoma 178
Focusing 4
Fracture 91

I

Idiopatic dorsal vein thrombosis 178
IIEF 39
Image equalization algorithms
Impotence, see erectile dysfunction
Induratio penis plastic, see Peyronie's disease
Inflammation, abscesses 148
- balanitis 147
- balanoposthitis 147
- cavernositis 148
- cellulitis 147
- CT 149
- Mondor phlebitis 148
- MRI 149
- ultrasonography, abscesses 149
- - balanitis 148
- - cavernositis 149
- - cellulitis 149
- - Mondor phlebitis 149
Innervation 14
International Index of Erectile Function 39
Intracavernosal injection 25, 43, 61, 116, 155

- Complications 52, 155
- priapism 52, 71, 72, 85
IPP, see Peyronie's disease

K

Kelami syndrome, see urethra

L

Lengthening procedures 58, 129, 134

M

Magnetic resonance imaging, see MRI
Metastatic priapism, ultrasonography 86
Microbubbles, see CEUS
Multiple-Frequency imaging 4

N

Non-penetrating trauma, see blunt trauma

O

Onchocerchiasis 181

P

Papaverine, 43
Parasitic infections 180
PDE5 see Phosphodiesterase-5
Penetrating trauma, ultrasonography 95
Penile amputation see amputation
Penile amputation, see amputation
- fibrosis, see fibrosis
- fracture see fracture
- hematoma, see hematoma
- inflammation, see inflammation
- surgery, see surgery
- trauma, see trauma
- tumors, see tumor
- urethra, see urethra
Peyronie's disease, cavernosography 68
- cavernosometry 68
- CEUS 187
- clinical evaluation 56
- differential diagnosis 67
- Doppler ultrasonography 22,66
- epidemiology 55
- ESWL
- etiology 56
- extracorporeal shockwave lithotripsy
- grey scale ultrasonography 62
- grey scale ultrasonography plaque extent 64
- - involvement of the penile septum 64
- - involvement of the penile vessels 65

– – plaque calcifications 64
– – plaque echogenicity 63
– – tunica albuginea 62
– medical treatment 57
– – colchicines 57
– – interferon 57
– – pentoxifylline 57
– – potassium para-aminobenzoate 57
– – POTOBA 57
– – verapamil 57
– – vitamin E 57
– MRI 68
– natural history 55
– surgical treatment 58
– – grafting procedures 58
– – prosthesis implantation 58
– – straightening procedures 58
– TC 68
– ultrasonography, evaluation technique 61
– X-ray 68
PGE1 see Prostaglandin E1
Phenoxybenzamine 43
Phentolamine 43
Phosphodiesterase-5 inhibitors 22
Priapism, angiography 86
– anoxic see - low-flow
– complications 76
– diagnosis 74
– etiology 72
– high-flow 73
– – Doppler ultrasonography 80
– – grey-scale ultrasonography 80
– incidence 71
– ischemic see - low-flow
– low-flow 72
– – Doppler ultrasonography 85
– – grey-scale ultrasonography 84
– metastatic, ultrasonography 86
– MRI 87
– nitric oxide (NO) 72,73
– pathophysiology 72
– post-traumatic see - high-flow
– prognosis 76
– recurrent 74
– shunting procedures 75
– stuttering 74
– surgery 75
– treatment 74
– ultrasonography 79
Prostaglandin E1 43

R

retrograde urethrography, see urethra

S

Sclerosis lymphangitis 177
Segmental thrombosis 179
Sexual Health Inventory for Men 41
SHIM 41

Shortening procedures 58, 129, 134
Smoking 18
Sparganosis 181
Surgery, cavernosometry 142
– CT
– deformity 129
– erectile dysfunction 126
– lengthening procedures 58, 129, 134
– MRI
– penile cancer 110, 125
– Peyronie's disease 58, 129
– phalloplasty 127, 141
– prosthesis implantation 58, 126, 136
– retrograde urethrography 142
– revascularization 126, 137
– sex reassignment 127, 128, 141
– shortening procedures 58, 129, 134
– ultrasonography, augmentation procedures 140
– – circumcision 139
– – lengthening procedures 134
– – penile prosthesis 136
– – phalloplasty 141
– – postoperative complications 133
– – revascularization 137
– – sex reassignment 141
– – shortening procedures 134
– – shunting procedures 75, 140
– – straightening procedures 134
– – urethra 141
– venous ligation 126

T

Three-Dimensional (3D) Imaging 8
– Rendering 8
Transdermal drug delivery 44
Transurethral drug delivery 44
Trauma, CEUS 187
– CT 104
– management 91
– MRI 104
– ultrasonography 95
– – cavernosal hematoma 98
– – Extra-albugineal hematoma 98
– – Hematoma 98
– – intracavernosal hemorrhage 99
– – isolated septal hematoma 102
– – penile fracture 100
– – posttraumatic erectile dysfunction 22,103
– – rupture of the suspensory ligament 99
– – uretra trauma 102
– vascular injury 99
– X-ray 104
Tumor, CEUS 188
– clinical presentation 108
– CT 120
– epidemiology 107
– incidence 107
– MRI 121
– pathology 107
– prognosis 112
– staging 109

Tumor (*Continued*)
treatment 110
– ultrasonography, epithelioid sarcoma 118
– – hemangioma 118
– – Kaposi's sarcoma 118
– – lymphoma 119
– – metastases 120
– – neurilemmoma 118
Tumors, ultrasonography 115
– – , staging 116

U

Ultrasonography, technique 25
Ultrasound, see ultrasonography
Uretha, cysts 171
Urethra, anatomy 163
– CEUS 191
– CT 172
– diverticula 169
– fistulae 171
– Kelami syndrome 182
– malformations 166
– manipulation syndrome 182
– MRI 172
– retrograde urethrography 163
– sonourethrography 165
– stenosis 167
– stones 170
– syringocele 170
– trauma 171
– tumors 171
– ultrasonography, anatomy 164
– – cysts 171
– – diverticula 170
– – fistulae 171
– – malformations 166
– – stenosis 169
– – stones 170
– – syringocele 170
– – technique 164
– – trauma 171
– – tumors 172
– voiding cystourethrography 163
Uretral injury 91
US, see ultrasonography

V

Vasoactive drug delivery 43
Venogenic dysfunction, color Doppler ultrasonography 47
– spectral Doppler 51
Venous Leak see erectile dysfunction, venogenic
voiding cystourethrography, see urethra

W

Wideband Imaging 4

X

XRES 7

List of Contributors

Ciro Acampora, MD
Azienda Ospedaliera A. Cardarelli
Via Cardarelli 9
Napoli, 80131
Italy

Libero Barozzi, MD
Department of Radiology
University Hospital S. Orsola-Malpighi
Via Massarenti 9
Bologna, 40138
Italy

Anthony J. Bella, MD FRCS(C)
Assistant Professor, Division of Urology
Department of Surgery and Associate Scientist
(Neuroscience)
Ottawa Health Research Institute
University of Ottawa,
The Ottawa Hospital – Civic Campus
B3 - Division of Urology
1053 Carling Avenue
Ottawa, K1Y 4E9
Canada

Emanuele Belgrano, MD
Professor and Chairman
Department of Urology
University of Trieste
Ospedale di Cattinara
Strada di Fiume 447
Trieste, 34124
Italy

Manuel Belgrano, MD
Department Radiology
University of Trieste
Ospedale di Cattinara
Strada di Fiume 447
Trieste, 34124
Italy

Sara Benvenuto, MD
Department of Urology
University of Trieste
Ospedale di Cattinara
Strada di Fiume 447
Trieste, 34124
Italy

Michele Bertolotto, MD
Department of Radiology
University of Trieste
Ospedale di Cattinara
Strada di Fiume 447
Trieste, 34124
Italy

William O. Brant, MD
PO Box 40,000
Vail
CO 81658
USA

Stefano Bucci, MD
Department of Urology
University of Trieste
Ospedale di Cattinara
Strada di Fiume 447
Trieste, 34124
Italy

Matteo Coss, MD
Department of Radiology
University of Trieste
Ospedale di Cattinara
Strada di Fiume 447
Trieste, 34124
Italy

Maria A. Cova, MD
Professor and Chairman
Department of Radiology
University of Trieste
Ospedale di Cattinara
Strada di Fiume 447
Trieste, 34124
Italy

Massimo De Matteis, MD
Department of Radiology
University Hospital S. Orsola-Malpighi
Via Massarenti 9
Bologna, 40138
Italy

List of Contributors

Lorenzo E. Derchi, MD
Professor and Chairman
Department of Radiology
DICMI University of Genova
Ospedale S. Martino
Largo Rosanna Benzi 8
Genova, 16132
Italy

Víctor Destéfano, MD
Instituto Nacional de Enfermedades Neoplasicas
"Dr. Eduardo Caceres Graziani"
Av. Angamos 2520
Lima 34 (Surquillo)
Peru

Micheline Djouguela Fute, MD
Dept Radiology
University of Trieste
Ospedale di Cattinara
Strada di Fiume 447
Trieste, 34124
Italy

Nicoletta Gandolfo, MD
U.O. Radiologia
Ospedale S. Corona
Via XXV Aprile
Pietra Ligure, 17027
Italy

Francesca Lacelli, MD
U.O. Radiologia
Ospedale S. Corona
Via XXV Aprile
Pietra Ligure, 17027
Italy

Giovanni Liguori, MD
Department of Urology
University of Trieste
Ospedale di Cattinara
Strada di Fiume 447
Trieste, 34124
Italy

Andrea Lissiani, MD
Department of Urology
University of Trieste
Ospedale di Cattinara
Strada di Fiume 447
Trieste, 34124
Italy

Tom F. Lue, MD
Professor and Vice Chair
Emil Tanagho Endowed Chair in Clinical Urology
Deparment of Urology
University of California
400 Parnassus Ave, A633
San Francisco
CA 94143-0738
USA

Paola Martingano, MD
Department of Radiology
University of Trieste
Ospedale di Cattinara
Strada di Fiume 447
Trieste, 34124
Italy

Fabio Pozzi Mucelli, MD
Department of Radiology
University of Trieste
Ospedale di Cattinara
Strada di Fiume 447
Trieste, 34124
Italy

Carlo E. Neumaier, MD
Department of Diagnostic Imaging
National Cancer Institute
Largo Rosanna Benzi 10
Genova, 16132
Italy

Giuseppe Ocello, MD
Department of Urology
University of Trieste
Ospedale di Cattinara
Strada di Fiume 447
Trieste, 34124
Italy

Pietro Pavlica, MD
Department of Radiology
University Hospital S. Orsola-Malpighi
Via Massarenti 9
Bologna, 40138
Italy

Nadia Perrone, MD
U.O. Radiologia
Ospedale S. Corona
Via XXV Aprile
Pietra Ligure, 17027
Italy

Riccardo Pizzolato, MD
Department of Radiology
University of Trieste
Ospedale di Cattinara
Strada di Fiume 447
Trieste, 34124
Italy

Mariela Pow-Sang, MD
Instituto Nacional de Enfermedades Neoplasicas
"Dr. Eduardo Caceres Graziani"
Av. Angamos 2520
Lima 34 (Surquillo)
Peru

CARMELO PRIVITERA, MD
Servizio di Radiologia Ospedale Vittorio Emanuele
Azienda Ospedaliera
Universitaria V. Emanuele, Ferrarotto, S.Bambino
Via Plebiscito 628
Catania, 95100
Italy

DANIELA SANABOR, MD
Department of Radiology
University of Trieste
Ospedale di Cattinara
Strada di Fiume 447
Trieste, 34124
Italy

GIANFRANCO SAVOCA, MD
Department of Urology
Ospedale Fondazione San Raffaele Giglio
Contrada Pietrapollastra
Cefalù, 90015
Italy

LUCA SCOFIENZA, MD
U.O. Radiologia
Ospedale S. Corona
Via XXV Aprile
Pietra Ligure, 17027
Italy

GIOVANNI SERAFINI, MD
U.O. Radiologia
Ospedale S. Corona
Via XXV Aprile
Pietra Ligure, 17027
Italy

ANDREA SPADACCI, MD
Department of Radiology
University of Trieste
Ospedale di Cattinara
Strada di Fiume 447
Trieste, 34124
Italy

CARLO TROMBETTA, MD
Associate Professor, Department of Urology
University of Trieste
Ospedale di Cattinara
Strada di Fiume 449
Trieste, 34149
Italy

MAJA UKMAR, MD
Department of Radiology
University of Trieste
Ospedale di Cattinara
Strada di Fiume 447
Trieste, 34124
Italy

MASSIMO VALENTINO, MD
Department of Radiology
University Hospital S. Orsola-Malpighi
Via Massarenti 9
Bologna, 40138
Italy

ROBERTA ZAPPETTI, MD
Department of Radiology
University of Trieste
Ospedale di Cattinara
Strada di Fiume 447
Trieste, 34124
Italy

MEDICAL RADIOLOGY Diagnostic Imaging and Radiation Oncology
Titles in the series already published

DIAGNOSTIC IMAGING

Innovations in Diagnostic Imaging
Edited by J. H. Anderson

Radiology of the Upper Urinary Tract
Edited by E. K. Lang

The Thymus - Diagnostic Imaging, Functions, and Pathologic Anatomy
Edited by E. Walter, E. Willich, and W. R. Webb

Interventional Neuroradiology
Edited by A. Valavanis

Radiology of the Pancreas
Edited by A. L. Baert, co-edited by G. Delorme

Radiology of the Lower Urinary Tract
Edited by E. K. Lang

Magnetic Resonance Angiography
Edited by I. P. Arlart, G. M. Bongartz, and G. Marchal

Contrast-Enhanced MRI of the Breast
S. Heywang-Köbrunner and R. Beck

Spiral CT of the Chest
Edited by M. Rémy-Jardin and J. Rémy

Radiological Diagnosis of Breast Diseases
Edited by M. Friedrich and E.A. Sickles

Radiology of the Trauma
Edited by M. Heller and A. Fink

Biliary Tract Radiology
Edited by P. Rossi, co-edited by M. Brezi

Radiological Imaging of Sports Injuries
Edited by C. Masciocchi

Modern Imaging of the Alimentary Tube
Edited by A. R. Margulis

Diagnosis and Therapy of Spinal Tumors
Edited by P. R. Algra, J. Valk, and J. J. Heimans

Interventional Magnetic Resonance Imaging
Edited by J. F. Debatin and G. Adam

Abdominal and Pelvic MRI
Edited by A. Heuck and M. Reiser

Orthopedic Imaging
Techniques and Applications
Edited by A. M. Davies and H. Pettersson

Radiology of the Female Pelvic Organs
Edited by E. K.Lang

Magnetic Resonance of the Heart and Great Vessels
Clinical Applications
Edited by J. Bogaert, A.J. Duerinckx, and F. E. Rademakers

Modern Head and Neck Imaging
Edited by S. K. Mukherji and J. A. Castelijns

Radiological Imaging of Endocrine Diseases
Edited by J. N. Bruneton
in collaboration with B. Padovani and M.-Y. Mourou

Trends in Contrast Media
Edited by H. S. Thomsen, R. N. Muller, and R. F. Mattrey

Functional MRI
Edited by C. T. W. Moonen and P. A. Bandettini

Radiology of the Pancreas
2nd Revised Edition
Edited by A. L. Baert. Co-edited by G. Delorme and L. Van Hoe

Emergency Pediatric Radiology
Edited by H. Carty

Spiral CT of the Abdomen
Edited by F. Terrier, M. Grossholz, and C. D. Becker

Liver Malignancies
Diagnostic and Interventional Radiology
Edited by C. Bartolozzi and R. Lencioni

Medical Imaging of the Spleen
Edited by A. M. De Schepper and F. Vanhoenacker

Radiology of Peripheral Vascular Diseases
Edited by E. Zeitler

Diagnostic Nuclear Medicine
Edited by C. Schiepers

Radiology of Blunt Trauma of the Chest
P. Schnyder and M. Wintermark

Portal Hypertension
Diagnostic Imaging-Guided Therapy
Edited by P. Rossi
Co-edited by P. Ricci and L. Broglia

Recent Advances in Diagnostic Neuroradiology
Edited by Ph. Demaerel

Virtual Endoscopy and Related 3D Techniques
Edited by P. Rogalla, J. Terwissscha Van Scheltinga, and B. Hamm

Multislice CT
Edited by M. F. Reiser, M. Takahashi, M. Modic, and R. Bruening

Pediatric Uroradiology
Edited by R. Fotter

Transfontanellar Doppler Imaging in Neonates
A. Couture and C. Veyrac

Radiology of AIDS
A Practical Approach
Edited by J.W.A.J. Reeders and P.C. Goodman

CT of the Peritoneum
Armando Rossi and Giorgio Rossi

Magnetic Resonance Angiography
2nd Revised Edition
Edited by I. P. Arlart, G. M. Bongratz, and G. Marchal

Pediatric Chest Imaging
Edited by Javier Lucaya and Janet L. Strife

Applications of Sonography in Head and Neck Pathology
Edited by J. N. Bruneton
in collaboration with C. Raffaelli and O. Dassonville

Imaging of the Larynx
Edited by R. Hermans

3D Image Processing
Techniques and Clinical Applications
Edited by D. Caramella and C. Bartolozzi

Imaging of Orbital and Visual Pathway Pathology
Edited by W. S. Müller-Forell

Pediatric ENT Radiology
Edited by S. J. King and A. E. Boothroyd

Radiological Imaging of the Small Intestine
Edited by N. C. Gourtsoyiannis

Imaging of the Knee
Techniques and Applications
Edited by A. M. Davies and V. N. Cassar-Pullicino

Perinatal Imaging
From Ultrasound to MR Imaging
Edited by Fred E. Avni

Radiological Imaging of the Neonatal Chest
Edited by V. Donoghue

Diagnostic and Interventional Radiology in Liver Transplantation
Edited by E. Bücheler, V. Nicolas, C. E. Broelsch, X. Rogiers, and G. Krupski

Radiology of Osteoporosis
Edited by S. Grampp

Imaging Pelvic Floor Disorders
Edited by C. I. Bartram and J. O. L. DeLancey
Associate Editors: S. Halligan, F. M. Kelvin, and J. Stoker

Imaging of the Pancreas
Cystic and Rare Tumors
Edited by C. Procacci and A. J. Megibow

High Resolution Sonography of the Peripheral Nervous System
Edited by S. Peer and G. Bodner

Imaging of the Foot and Ankle
Techniques and Applications
Edited by A. M. Davies,
R. W. Whitehouse, and J. P. R. Jenkins

Radiology Imaging of the Ureter
Edited by F. Joffre, Ph. Otal,
and M. Soulie

Imaging of the Shoulder
Techniques and Applications
Edited by A. M. Davies and J. Hodler

Radiology of the Petrous Bone
Edited by M. Lemmerling and
S. S. Kollias

Interventional Radiology in Cancer
Edited by A. Adam, R. F. Dondelinger,
and P. R. Mueller

**Duplex and Color Doppler Imaging
of the Venous System**
Edited by G. H. Mostbeck

Multidetector-Row CT of the Thorax
Edited by U. J. Schoepf

Functional Imaging of the Chest
Edited by H.-U. Kauczor

**Radiology of the Pharynx
and the Esophagus**
Edited by O. Ekberg

**Radiological Imaging
in Hematological Malignancies**
Edited by A. Guermazi

**Imaging and Intervention in
Abdominal Trauma**
Edited by R. F. Dondelinger

Multislice CT
2nd Revised Edition
Edited by M. F. Reiser, M. Takahashi,
M. Modic, and C. R. Becker

**Intracranial Vascular Malformations
and Aneurysms**
From Diagnostic Work-Up
to Endovascular Therapy
Edited by M. Forsting

Radiology and Imaging of the Colon
Edited by A. H. Chapman

Coronary Radiology
Edited by M. Oudkerk

**Dynamic Contrast-Enhanced Magnetic
Resonance Imaging in Oncology**
Edited by A. Jackson, D. L. Buckley,
and G. J. M. Parker

**Imaging in Treatment Planning
for Sinonasal Diseases**
Edited by R. Maroldi and P. Nicolai

Clinical Cardiac MRI
With Interactive CD-ROM
Edited by J. Bogaert, S. Dymarkowski,
and A. M. Taylor

Focal Liver Lesions
Detection, Characterization, Ablation
Edited by R. Lencioni, D. Cioni,
and C. Bartolozzi

Multidetector-Row CT Angiography
Edited by C. Catalano and
R. Passariello

Paediatric Musculoskeletal Diseases
With an Emphasis on Ultrasound
Edited by D. Wilson

Contrast Media in Ultrasonography
Basic Principles and Clinical Applications
Edited by Emilio Quaia

**MR Imaging in White Matter Diseases of
the Brain and Spinal Cord**
Edited by M. Filippi, N. De Stefano,
V. Dousset, and J. C. McGowan

Diagnostic Nuclear Medicine
2nd Revised Edition
Edited by C. Schiepers

Imaging of the Kidney Cancer
Edited by A. Guermazi

**Magnetic Resonance Imaging in
Ischemic Stroke**
Edited by R. von Kummer and T. Back

Imaging of the Hip & Bony Pelvis
Techniques and Applications
Edited by A. M. Davies, K. J. Johnson,
and R. W. Whitehouse

**Imaging of Occupational and
Environmental Disorders of the Chest**
Edited by P. A. Gevenois and
P. De Vuyst

Contrast Media
Safety Issues and ESUR Guidelines
Edited by H. S. Thomsen

Virtual Colonoscopy
A Practical Guide
Edited by P. Lefere and S. Gryspeerdt

Vascular Embolotherapy
A Comprehensive Approach
Volume 1: *General Principles, Chest,
Abdomen, and Great Vessels*
Edited by J. Golzarian. Co-edited by
S. Sun and M. J. Sharafuddin

Vascular Embolotherapy
A Comprehensive Approach
Volume 2: *Oncology, Trauma, Gene
Therapy, Vascular Malformations,
and Neck*
Edited by J. Golzarian. Co-edited by
S. Sun and M. J. Sharafuddin

Head and Neck Cancer Imaging
Edited by R. Hermans

Vascular Interventional Radiology
Current Evidence in
Endovascular Surgery
Edited by M. G. Cowling

Ultrasound of the Gastrointestinal Tract
Edited by G. Maconi and
G. Bianchi Porro

Imaging of Orthopedic Sports Injuries
Edited by F. M. Vanhoenacker,
M. Maas, J. L. M. A. Gielen

**Parallel Imaging in
Clinical MR Applications**
Edited by S. O. Schoenberg, O. Dietrich,
and M. F. Reiser

MRI and CT of the Female Pelvis
Edited by B. Hamm and R. Forstner

Ultrasound of the Musculoskeletal System
S. Bianchi and C. Martinoli

Spinal Imaging
Diagnostic Imaging of the Spine and
Spinal Cord
Edited by J. W. M. Van Goethem,
L. van den Hauwe, and P. M. Parizel

**Radiation Dose from Adult and Pediatric
Multidetector Computed Tomography**
Edited by D. Tack and P. A. Gevenois

Computed Tomography of the Lung
A Pattern Approach
J. A. Verschakelen and W. De Wever

Clinical Functional MRI
Presurgical Functional Neuroimaging
Edited bei C. Stippich

Imaging in Transplantation
Edited by A. A. Bankier

**Radiological Imaging of the Digestive
System in Infants and Children**
Edited by A. S. Devos and
J. G. Blickman

Pediatric Chest Imaging
Chest Imaging in Infants and Children
2nd Revised Edition
Edited by J. Lucaya and J. L. Strife

**Radiological Imaging
of the Neonatal Chest**
2nd Revised Edition
Edited by V. Donoghue

Radiology of the Stomach and Duodenum
Edited by A. H. Freeman and E. Sala

Imaging in Pediatric Skeletal Trauma
Techniques and Applications
Edited by K. J. Johnson and E. Bache

**Percutaneous Tumor Ablation in
Medical Radiology**
Edited by T. J. Vogl, T. K. Helmberger,
M. G. Mack, and M. F. Reiser

**Screening and Preventive Diagnosis with
Radiological Imaging**
Edited by M. F. Reiser, G. van Kaick,
C. Fink, and S. O. Schoenberg

Color Doppler US of the Penis
Edited by M. Bertolotto

Image Processing in Radiology
Current Applications
Edited by E. Neri, D. Caramella,
and C. Bartolozzi

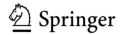

MEDICAL RADIOLOGY Diagnostic Imaging and Radiation Oncology
Titles in the series already published

RADIATION ONCOLOGY

Lung Cancer
Edited by C.W. Scarantino

Innovations in Radiation Oncology
Edited by H. R. Withers
and L. J. Peters

**Radiation Therapy
of Head and Neck Cancer**
Edited by G. E. Laramore

**Gastrointestinal Cancer –
Radiation Therapy**
Edited by R.R. Dobelbower, Jr.

**Radiation Exposure
and Occupational Risks**
Edited by E. Scherer, C. Streffer,
and K.-R. Trott

**Radiation Therapy of Benign Diseases
A Clinical Guide**
S. E. Order and S. S. Donaldson

**Interventional Radiation
Therapy Techniques – Brachytherapy**
Edited by R. Sauer

Radiopathology of Organs and Tissues
Edited by E. Scherer, C. Streffer,
and K.-R. Trott

**Concomitant Continuous Infusion
Chemotherapy and Radiation**
Edited by M. Rotman
and C. J. Rosenthal

**Intraoperative Radiotherapy –
Clinical Experiences and Results**
Edited by F. A. Calvo, M. Santos,
and L.W. Brady

**Radiotherapy of Intraocular
and Orbital Tumors**
Edited by W. E. Alberti and
R. H. Sagerman

**Interstitial and Intracavitary
Thermoradiotherapy**
Edited by M. H. Seegenschmiedt
and R. Sauer

**Non-Disseminated Breast Cancer
Controversial Issues in Management**
Edited by G. H. Fletcher and S.H. Levitt

**Current Topics in
Clinical Radiobiology of Tumors**
Edited by H.-P. Beck-Bornholdt

**Practical Approaches to
Cancer Invasion and Metastases
A Compendium of Radiation
Oncologists' Responses to 40 Histories**
Edited by A. R. Kagan with the
Assistance of R. J. Steckel

Radiation Therapy in Pediatric Oncology
Edited by J. R. Cassady

Radiation Therapy Physics
Edited by A. R. Smith

Late Sequelae in Oncology
Edited by J. Dunst and R. Sauer

Mediastinal Tumors. Update 1995
Edited by D. E. Wood and
C. R. Thomas, Jr.

**Thermoradiotherapy
and Thermochemotherapy**
Volume 1:
Biology, Physiology, and Physics
Volume 2:
Clinical Applications
Edited by M.H. Seegenschmiedt,
P. Fessenden, and C.C. Vernon

**Carcinoma of the Prostate
Innovations in Management**
Edited by Z. Petrovich, L. Baert,
and L.W. Brady

**Radiation Oncology
of Gynecological Cancers**
Edited by H.W. Vahrson

**Carcinoma of the Bladder
Innovations in Management**
Edited by Z. Petrovich, L. Baert,
and L.W. Brady

**Blood Perfusion and
Microenvironment of Human Tumors
Implications for
Clinical Radiooncology**
Edited by M. Molls and P. Vaupel

**Radiation Therapy of Benign Diseases
A Clinical Guide
2nd Revised Edition**
S. E. Order and S. S. Donaldson

**Carcinoma of the Kidney and Testis,
and Rare Urologic Malignancies
Innovations in Management**
Edited by Z. Petrovich, L. Baert,
and L.W. Brady

**Progress and Perspectives in the
Treatment of Lung Cancer**
Edited by P. Van Houtte,
J. Klastersky, and P. Rocmans

**Combined Modality Therapy of
Central Nervous System Tumors**
Edited by Z. Petrovich, L. W. Brady,
M. L. Apuzzo, and M. Bamberg

**Age-Related Macular Degeneration
Current Treatment Concepts**
Edited by W. A. Alberti, G. Richard,
and R. H. Sagerman

**Radiotherapy of Intraocular
and Orbital Tumors
2nd Revised Edition**
Edited by R. H. Sagerman,
and W. E. Alberti

**Modification of Radiation Response
Cytokines, Growth Factors,
and Other Biolgical Targets**
Edited by C. Nieder, L. Milas,
and K. K. Ang

Radiation Oncology for Cure and Palliation
R. G. Parker, N. A. Janjan,
and M. T. Selch

**Clinical Target Volumes in Conformal and
Intensity Modulated Radiation Therapy
A Clinical Guide to Cancer Treatment**
Edited by V. Grégoire, P. Scalliet,
and K. K. Ang

**Advances in Radiation Oncology
in Lung Cancer**
Edited by Branislav Jeremić

New Technologies in Radiation Oncology
Edited by W. Schlegel, T. Bortfeld,
and A.-L. Grosu

**Technical Basis of Radiation Therapy
4th Revised Edition**
Edited by S. H. Levitt, J. A. Purdy,
C. A. Perez, and S. Vijayakumar

**CURED I · LENT
Late Effects of Cancer Treatment
on Normal Tissues**
Edited by P. Rubin, L. S. Constine,
L. B. Marks, and P. Okunieff

**Clinical Practice of Radiation Therapy for
Benign Diseases
Contemporary Concepts and Clinical
Results**
Edited by M. H. Seegenschmiedt,
H.-B. Makoski, K.-R. Trott, and
L. W. Brady

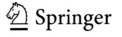